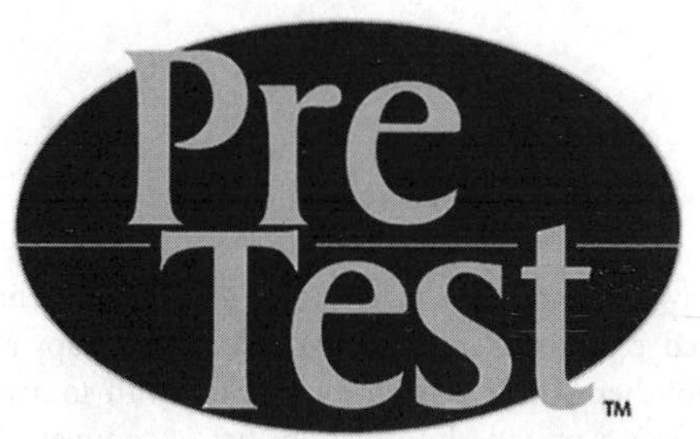

Microbiology

PreTest™ Self-Assessment and Review

Notice

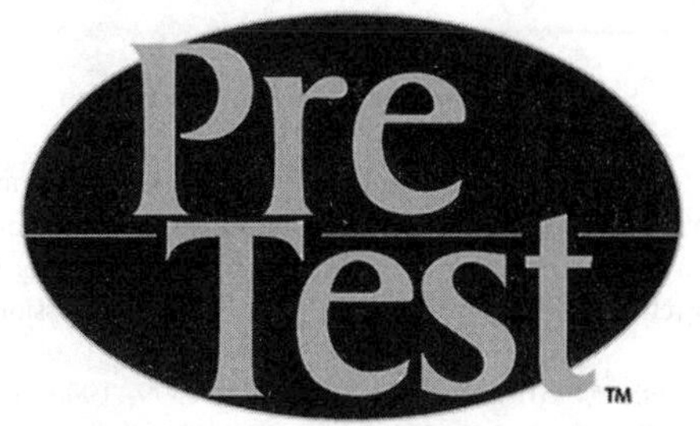

Microbiology

PreTest™ Self-Assessment and Review

14th Edition

Matthew B. Grisham, PhD
Professor and Chair
Department of Immunology and Molecular Microbiology
Texas Tech University Health Sciences Center
Lubbock, Texas

With contributions by:

Robert K. Bright, PhD
W. LaJean Chaffin, PhD
Jane A. Colmer-Hamood, BS, PhD
Abdul N. Hamood, MS, PhD
Afzal A. Siddiqui, MPhil, PhD
David C. Straus, PhD

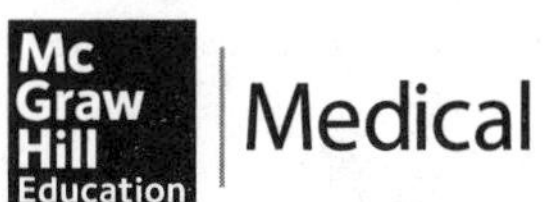

New York Chicago San Francisco Athens London Madrid
Mexico City Milan New Delhi Singapore Sydney Toronto

Microbiology: PreTest™ Self-Assessment and Review, 14th Edition

1 2 3 4 5 6 7 8 9 0 DOC/DOC 18 17 16 15 14 13

ISBN 978-0-07-179104-5
MHID 0-07-179104-3

This book was set in Berkeley by Thomson Digital.
The editors were Catherine A. Johnson and Cindy Yoo.
The production supervisor was Richard Ruzycka.
Project management was provided by Garima Sharma, Thomson Digital.
The cover designer was Maria Scharf.
RR Donnelley was printer and binder.

This book is printed on acid-free paper.

Library of Congress Cataloging-in-Publication Data

Microbiology (Grisham)
Microbiology : PreTest self-assessment and review / [edited by] Matthew B. Grisham.—14th edition.
p. ; cm.
Preceded by Microbiology / [edited by] James D. Kettering. 13th ed. c2010.
Includes bibliographical references and index.
ISBN 978-0-07-179104-5 (paperback : alk. paper)—ISBN 0-07-179104-3 (paperback : alk. paper)
I. Grisham, Matthew B., editor. II. Title.
[DNLM: 1. Microbiological Phenomena—Examination Questions. QW 18.2]
QR46
616.9'041—dc23

2013030615

McGraw-Hill Education LLC books are available at special quantity discounts to use as premiums and sales promotions, or for use in corporate training programs. To contact a representative, please visit the Contact Us pages at www.mhprofessional.com.

Student Reviewers

Constance Mennella
University of Medicine and Dentistry of New Jersey
School of Medicine
Class of 2010

Leland Stillman
University of Virginia
School of Medicine
Class of 2014

Contents

Parasitology

Immunology

Contributors

Robert K. Bright, PhD
Associate Professor
Department of Immunology and Molecular Microbiology
School of Medicne
Texas Tech University Health Sciences Center
Lubbock, Texas
Immunology
Relevant High Yield Facts and Revisions

W. LaJean Chaffin, PhD
Professor
Department of Immunology and Molecular Microbiology
School of Medicine
Texas Tech University Health Sciences Center
Lubbock, Texas
Mycology
Relevant High Yield Facts and Revisions

Jane A. Colmer-Hamood, BS, PhD
Associate Professor
Department of Immunology and Molecular Microbiology
Texas Tech University Health Sciences Center
Lubbock, Texas
Physiology and Molecular Microbiology
Virology
Relevant High Yield Facts and Revisions

Abdul N. Hamood, MS, PhD
Professor
Department of Immunology and Molecular Microbiology
School of Medicine
Texas Tech University Health Sciences Center
Lubbock, Texas
Physiology and Molecular Microbiology
Bacteriology
Relevant High Yield Facts and Revisions

Afzal A. Siddiqui, MPhil, PhD
Grover E. Murray Professor
Departments of Immunology and Molecular Microbiology; Internal Medicine; Pathology
Clinical Professor, Pharmacy Practice
Director, Center for Tropical Medicine and Infectious Diseases
Texas Tech University Health Sciences Center
Lubbock, Texas
Parasitology
Relevant High Yield Facts and Revisions

David C. Straus, PhD
Professor
Department of Immunology and Molecular Microbiology
Texas Tech University Health Sciences Center
Lubbock, Texas
Bacteriology
Rickettsiae, Chlamydiae, and Mycoplasma
Relevant High Yield Facts and Revisions

Introduction

Microbiology: PreTest™ Self-Assessment and Review, 14th Edition, allows medical students to comprehensively and conveniently assess and review their knowledge of microbiology and immunology. The 500 questions provided here have been written with the goal to parallel the topics, format, and degree of difficulty of the questions found in the United States Medical Licensing Examination (USMLE) Step 1.

The High-Yield Facts in the beginning of the book are provided to facilitate a rapid review of microbiology. It is anticipated that the reader will use these High-Yield Facts as a quick overview prior to proceeding through the questions.

Each question in the book is followed by four or more answer options to choose from. In each case, select the best response to the question. Each answer is accompanied by a specific page reference to a text that provides background to the answer and a short discussion of issues raised by the question and answer. A bibliography listing all the sources can be found following the last chapter.

To simulate the time constraints imposed by the licensing exam, an effective way to use this book is to allow yourself one minute to answer each question in a given chapter. After you finish going through the questions in the section, spend as much time as you need verifying your answers and carefully reading the explanations provided. Special attention should be given to the explanations for the questions you answered incorrectly; however, you should read every explanation even if you've answered correctly. The explanations are designed to reinforce and supplement the information tested by the questions. For those seeking further information about the material covered, consult the references listed in the bibliography or other standard medical texts.

Acknowledgments

The authors wish to thank Ms. Alicia Gauna and Ms. Jennifer Bright for their help in the preparation of the manuscript. The authors would also like to acknowledge the use of the Public Health Image Library offered by the Centers for Disease Control and Prevention.

High-Yield Facts

PHYSIOLOGY AND MOLECULAR BIOLOGY

- Koch postulates: (1) specific organism must be in diseased animal; (2) organism must be isolated in pure culture; (3) organism should produce exact disease in healthy, susceptible animal; and (4) organism must be re-isolated from infected animal.
- Gram stain: (1) fixation; (2) crystal violet; (3) iodine treatment; (4) decolorization (alcohol/acetone); and (5) counterstain (safranin). Gram-positive when the color is purple; gram-negative when the color turns red.
- Gram stain poor for: *Chlamydia* (intracellular location), *Mycoplasma* (no cell wall), *Rickettsia* (small size), *Treponema* (too thin, spirochete, use darkfield microscope), *Mycobacterium* (use acid-fast stain), and *Legionella* (use silver stain).
- Bacterial shapes: bacilli (rod), cocci (spherical), and spirilla (spiral).
- Bacterial aggregates: diplococci (eg, *Neisseriae*), streptococci (chains), tetrads (fours), staphylococci (clusters), and sarcinae (cubes).
- Flagella: monotrichous—single polar flagellum; lophotrichous—cluster of flagella at pole; amphitrichous—flagella at both poles; and peritrichous—flagella encircling the cell.
- Type VII pili = F (sex) pili; important in bacterial conjugation.
- Conjugation—DNA transferred from one bacterium to another; transduction—viral transfer of DNA from one cell to another; and transformation—cellular uptake of purified DNA or naked DNA from the environment.
- Peptidoglycan (murein or mucopeptide) layer: unique to prokaryotes (glycan polymers of sugar *N*-acetylglucosamine [NAG] and *N*-acetylmuramic acid [NAM] cross-linked by a short peptide). Cross-linking enzymes are transpeptidases (targets for β-lactam antibiotics).
- Bacterial structures: peptidoglycan (support); cell wall/membrane (antigenic); outer membrane (lipopolysaccharide [LPS]/endotoxin); plasma membrane (oxidative/transport enzymes); ribosome (protein synthesis); periplasmic space (hydrolytic enzymes and β-lactamases); capsule (antiphagocytic polysaccharide except *Bacillus anthracis*, which is D-glutamate); pilus/fimbria (adherence, conjugation); flagellum

(motility); spore (heat, chemical, dehydration resistance, consists of dipicolinic acid); plasmid (genes for toxins, enzymes, antibiotic resistance); glycocalyx (adherence, made of polysaccharide); and inclusion bodies (no membrane; store glycogen, polyphosphate, poly-β-hydroxybutyric acid).

- Gram-positive: teichoic acid unique.
- Gram-negative: LPS/endotoxin unique.
- LPS/endotoxin: lipid A covalently linked to polysaccharide core outer membrane and then unique "O antigen" polysaccharide repeat; LPS/endotoxin causes an acute-phase protein response in vivo (release of TNF-α, IL-1, and IL-6), causing fever, and the like.
- Lysozyme: breaks down glycan backbone bonds of peptidoglycan. Spheroplast: partial cell wall lysozyme digestion.
- Protoplast: complete cell wall lysozyme digestion, causing a spherical shape of bacteria.
- Exponential or geometric growth: cell number = $a(2^n)$, where a is number of starting cells and n equals number of generations.
- Bacterial growth curves (four phases): (1) lag (no cellular division, cell size increases); (2) exponential (regular doubling time, essential nutrients decrease, toxins increase); (3) stationary (cell division rate = cell death rate) stage at which spores are formed; and (4) death (cell energy stores deplete, exponential death due to low population equilibrium).
- Bacteriostatic: agent **inhibits** multiplication; growth resumes upon removal of agent.
- Bactericidal: agent **kills** bacteria; irreversible.
- Sterile: free from all forms of life.
- Disinfectant: chemical kills bacteria but is toxic to tissue.
- Septic: pathogenic organism is present in living tissue.
- Aseptic: pathogenic organism is not present in living tissue. (virology—no bacterial agents are present.)
- Passive transport: no energy required, movement down the concentration gradient, no carrier molecule (protein molecule that attaches to metabolic molecule needed inside the bacterium) that can cross the cell wall and cell membrane. The food goes in and the waste goes out.
- Active transport: requires energy, movement against the concentration gradient.
- Bacterial pathogenesis: (1) antiphagocytic (cell wall proteins—protein A in *Staphylococcus aureus* and protein M in *Streptococcus pyogenes*,

capsules, pili/fimbriae *Neisseria gonorrhoeae*); (2) adherence factors (pili/fimbriae, lipoteichoic acid, glycocalyx, adhesion); (3) enzymes (coagulase, collagenase, fibrinolysin, hyaluronidase, lecithinase, mucinase); and (4) toxins (exotoxins, endotoxins/LPS).

- Exotoxins: polypeptide, highly fatal even in low doses, toxoids as vaccines, mostly heat labile, secreted, both gram-negative and gram-positive.
- Endotoxins: LPS, low toxicity, no toxoids, no vaccines, heat stable, released on lysis, only gram-negative.
- Free radicals of oxygen (superoxides) kill anaerobic bacteria exposed to air. Superoxide dismutase is a potent bacterial antioxidant. The peroxidases in bacteria are protective.
- Obligate anaerobes: lack catalase and/or superoxide dismutase and are susceptible to oxidative damage, foul smelling, produce gas in tissue (eg, *Actinomyces*, *Bacteroides*, and *Clostridium*).
- Superoxide dismutase catalyzes: $2O_2^- + 2H^+ \rightarrow H_2O_2 + O_2$
- Catalase catalyzes: $2H_2O_2 \rightarrow 2H_2O + O_2$
- Myeloperoxidase catalyzes: $Cl^- + H_2O_2 \rightarrow ClO^- + H_2O$
- Sites of action of antimicrobial agents include cell wall synthesis, cell-membrane integrity, DNA replication, protein synthesis, DNA-dependent RNA polymerase, and folic acid metabolism.

VIROLOGY

- *Virology terminology*: virion, capsid, capsomere, nucleocapsid, and genome.
- Viral genomes:
  - *DNA viruses*:
    - Herpesviruses, hepadnaviruses, poxviruses, adenoviruses, papillomaviruses, polyomaviruses, and parvoviruses.
    - All DNA viruses are double-stranded (ds), except parvoviruses (ss).
    - All DNA viruses have linear DNA, except papillomaviruses and polyomaviruses (ds, circular) and hepadnaviruses (incomplete ds, circular).
  - *RNA viruses*:
    - (+)ssRNA (same as mRNA) viruses: picornaviruses, caliciviruses, flaviviruses, togaviruses, hepeviruses, astroviruses, and coronaviruses.
    - Retroviruses contain two strands of (+)ssRNA that is NOT mRNA (diploid).

- (–)ssRNA viruses: orthomyxoviruses, paramyxoviruses, rhabdoviruses, bunyaviruses, arenaviruses, filoviruses, hepatitis D virus; require viral RNA polymerase within the virions.
- dsRNA viruses: reoviruses; require viral RNA polymerase within the virions.
- Segmented RNA viruses: orthomyxoviruses, reoviruses, bunyaviruses, and arenaviruses.
- *Viral replication*:
  - Obligate intracellular parasites, use viral attachment proteins to attach to host cell receptors.
  - Growth cycle: attachment, entry, uncoating, macromolecular synthesis, assembly, and release.
  - Viral disease patterns: acute, chronic, persistent (virions produced), and latent (no virions produced).
  - DNA viruses replicate in the host nucleus EXCEPT poxviruses.
  - RNA viruses replicate in the host cytoplasm EXCEPT influenza viruses.
  - Viruses that use reverse transcriptase (RT) have cytoplasmic and nuclear replication phases:
    - Retroviruses: vRNA–RT→ vDNA in cytoplasm; vDNA integrates into host chromosome; host RNA polymerase (RNAP) produces vRNA in nucleus.
    - Hepadnaviruses: vDNA to nucleus; host RNAP produces vRNA genome template; vRNA–RT→ vDNA in cytoplasm.

Hepatitis Viruses

- Hepatitis A virus (HAV): Picornavirus; (+)ssRNA; fecal–oral transmission, no chronic carriers; killed virus vaccine.
- Hepatitis B virus (HBV): Hepadnavirus; partially complete circular dsDNA; parental, sexual, vertical (intrapartum, postpartum) transmission; acute and chronic disease; hepatocellular carcinoma; and recombinant HBsAg vaccine.
- Hepatitis C virus (HCV): Flavivirus; (+)ssRNA; parental or sexual transmission; acute and chronic disease; and hepatocellular carcinoma.
- Hepatitis D virus (HDV): Delta virus; (–)ssRNA; defective virus, requires HBV coinfection; acute and chronic infections.
- Hepatitis E virus (HEV): Hepevirus; (+)ssRNA; fecal–oral transmission; no chronic carriers; high mortality in pregnant women.

DNA Viruses

- Parvovirus B19: ssDNA; causes fifth disease/erythema infectiosum (slapped cheek appearance).
- Papillomavirus (HPV): circular dsDNA; causes common warts, HVP types 1, 4; condyloma accuminatum, HPV 6, 11; cervical and other genital carcinomas, HPV 16, 18; recombinant vaccines for HPV 6/11/16/18 and HPV 16/18.
- Polyomaviruses: circular dsDNA; BK virus, hemorrhagic cystitis; JC virus, progressive multifocal leukoencepalopathy; disease occurs only in immunocompromised.
- Adenoviruses: dsDNA; pharyngoconjunctivitis in children, ARDS in young adults (especially military), and gastroenteritis (serotypes 40/41).
- Herpesviruses: dsDNA; latent infections occur with all; reactivation infections occur with immunocompromisation.
- Herpes simplex virus type 1: primarily oral; latent in neurons, especially trigeminal ganglia; cold sores, keratitis, sporadic encephalitis (temporal lobe); and acyclovir.
  - HSV 2: primarily genital; latent in neurons, especially sacral ganglia; herpes genitalis; neonatal disease; sexually transmitted; and acyclovir.
  - Varicella-zoster virus (VZV): latent in neurons; primary infection, chickenpox, lesions occur in crops; reactivation infection, shingles, lesions occur in dermatomal distribution; acyclovir, valacyclovir; and live attenuated virus vaccine.
  - Cytomegalovirus (CMV): ubiquitous; direct contact, sexual, vertical transmission; causes retinitis and pneumonitis in immunocompromised; neonates suffer from CMV inclusion disease; ganciclovir, and foscarnet.
  - Epstein–Barr virus (EBV): infects B lymphocytes; infectious mononucleosis, positive for heterophile antibodies (monospot test); specific EBV antigens also used to diagnose infection—early antigen (EA), viral capsid antigen (VCA), Epstein–Barr nuclear antigen (EBNA).
  - HHV6: roseola infantum.
  - HHV8: Kaposi sarcoma in AIDS.
- Poxviruses: largest, most complex viruses, and dsDNA.
  - Variola virus: smallpox, extinct since 1977; potential bioterrorism agent.

- Vaccinia virus: vaccine strain against smallpox; can cause infection especially in immunocompromised.
- Molluscipoxvirus: molluscum contagiosum; pearly nodular lesions.

Positive ssRNA Viruses

- Picornaviruses (+ssRNA): polioviruses, coxsackieviruses A and B, echoviruses, enteroviruses, HAV, and rhinoviruses.
  - All enteroviruses multiply in upper respiratory and gastrointestinal tracts; mild upper respiratory infections (URI), rashes, aseptic meningitis (lymphocytic pleocytosis, normal glucose, and normal/slightly elevated protein).
  - Poliovirus: paralytic poliomyelitis; eradicated in the United States; two vaccines, Salk inactivated and Sabin live attenuated vaccines; US now uses killed vaccine only.
  - Coxsackievirus A: herpangina, hand-foot-and-mouth disease.
  - Coxsackievirus B: myocarditis.
  - Rhinoviruses: multiply only in URT; common cold.
- Flaviviruses: all arthropod-borne EXCEPT HCV.
  - Encephalitis (meningitis): West Nile virus, St. Louis encephalitis virus.
  - Fever with rash, hemorrhagic fever: dengue viruses, yellow fever viruses.
- Togaviruses: all arthropod-borne EXCEPT rubella virus
  - Encephalitis: alphaviruses—Eastern equine encephalitis virus, Western equine encephalitis virus, and Venezuelan equine encephalitis virus.
  - Rubella virus: rubella or German measles; causes severe birth defects; live attenuated vaccine.
- Coronaviruses: most strains cause common cold; also severe acute respiratory syndrome (SARS).
- Retroviruses:
  - HIV-1: diploid genome, *gag, env, pol* genes; major proteins, p24 (diagnosis), gp120 and gp 41 attachment, reverse transcriptase (RT), integrase (IN), protease (PR); RT, IN, PR targets for antiretroviral therapy; acute retroviral syndrome, AIDS (CD4 T-cell count <200/μL), and/or AIDS-defining opportunistic infections (*Cryptosporidium, Pneumocystis, Mycobacterium avium-intracellular*, many others), cancers (Kaposi sarcoma, others), dementia, or wasting.
  - HTLV-1: acute T-cell leukemia/lymphoma; tropical spastic paraparesis.

Negative ssRNA Viruses

- Require virion-associated RNA-dependent RNA polymerase.
- Paramyxoviruses:
  - Measles virus: measles (rubeola or hard measles)—cough, coryza, conjunctivitis, photophobia, Koplik spots; maculopapular rash; pneumonia, encephalitis; SSPE; and live attenuated vaccine.
  - Mumps virus: mumps (swelling of salivary, parotid glands); aseptic meningitis, orchitis; and live attenuated vaccine.
  - Respiratory syncytial virus: bronchiolitis and pneumonia in infants; ribavirin, palivizumab.
  - Parainfluenza viruses: croup.
- Rhabdovirus: (rabies virus): bullet-shaped appearance; causes rabies; skunks, raccoons, foxes, coyotes/dogs, and bats are main reservoirs in the United States; animal bite transmission through saliva; control animal vectors; Negri body—eosinophilic intracytoplasmic inclusion body in infected cells (brain, nuchal skin, and cornea).
- Orthomyxoviruses: Influenza viruses A and B; segmented genomes; genetic drift, minor antigen changes IA, IB; genetic shift, major antigen change to new hemagglutinin (H) and/or neuraminidase (N), IA only; oseltamivir, zanamivir for treatment; previously amantidine, rimantidine but most circulating strains resistant.
- Bunyaviruses: La Crosse virus, California encephalitis virus; hantaviruses.
- Arenaviruses: lymphocytic choriomeningitis virus; viruses that cause hemorrhagic fever (Lassa virus, Tacaribe virus).

dsRNA Viruses: Double-Shelled Capsids

- Rotaviruses: cause infantile diarrhea, live attenuated vaccine.
- Coltivirus: Colorado tick fever.

BACTERIOLOGY

- Gram-positive cocci: staphylococci catalase +, streptococci catalase –.
- *Staphylococcus aureus*: Mannitol-salt agar (selective and differential), yellow colonies, **coagulase** +, mannitol +, catalase +; some are methicillin resistant (MRSA), some have vancomycin resistance emerging (VISA); protein A binds IgG Fc inhibiting phagocytosis, causes rapid-onset food poisoning (preformed enterotoxin), toxic shock syndrome, scalded skin

syndrome, osteomyelitis, acute bacterial endocarditis (IV drug users), abscesses, and recurrent infection in chronic granulomatous disease (CGD).

- *Staphylococcus saprophyticus*: second leading cause of urinary tract infection (UTI) in young sexually active females.
- Streptococci: β-hemolytic divided into groups (13 groups: A-O) based on cell wall carbohydrate antigens. Group A divided into >50 types based on M proteins (virulence, specific immunity), catalase negative.
- *Streptococcus pyogenes* (group A): hyaluronic acid capsule, carbohydrate antigen, M protein, bacitracin sensitive, cellulitis, rheumatic fever, glomerulonephritis, necrotizing fasciitis, erysipelas, and scarlet fever.
- Viridans: include *S. mitis*, and so on. Normal oral flora, α-hemolytic, subacute bacterial endocarditis after dental/oral surgery.
- *Enterococcus* (used to be called *Streptococcus) faecalis* (group D): normal intestinal flora, subacute bacterial endocarditis after pelvic/abdominal surgery, UTIs, growth in 6.5% NaCl.
- *Streptococcus agalactiae* (group B): sometimes normal vaginal flora; in dairy products (cattle pathogen); neonatal sepsis; (CAMP) test +.
- Peptostreptococci: normal oral/vaginal flora, endocarditis, and lung abscess.
- *Streptococcus pneumoniae*: pneumonia, meningitis, otitis media (children), optochin sensitive, bile soluble, use Quellung reaction (capsule Ags, host Abs), and pneumococcal polyvalent vaccine.
- Dick test: test susceptibility to scarlet fever.
- Schultz-Charlton test: determine if rash is due to erythrogenic toxin of scarlet fever.
- Gram-negative cocci (*Neisseria*): oxidase +, diplococci, polysaccharide capsule, endotoxin, associated with C5, C6, V7, C8 complement deficiency; pathogenic forms: Thayer-Martin agar –, chocolate agar +, nutrient agar –, 37°C growth +, room temperature –; nonpathogenic forms: Thayer-Martin agar –, chocolate agar +, nutrient agar +, 37°C growth +, and room temperature +.
- *Neisseria meningitidis*: capsule, endotoxin, toxemia, petechiae, hemorrhage, disseminated intravascular coagulation (DIC), and Waterhouse–Friderichsen syndrome.
- Bacterial meningitis: in <40-year-old = *S. pneumoniae*; >40-year-old = *S. pneumoniae*; 2 to 6 months + neonates = Group B streptococci, *Escherichia coli*; and neonates to 5-year-old children = *N. meningitidis*.
- *Neisseria gonorrhoeae:* pili, endotoxin, IgA protease, pharyngitis, proctitis, pelvic inflammatory disease (PID), urethritis, and cervicitis.

- Gram-positive bacilli: aerobic (*Bacillus*); anaerobic (*Clostridium*), killed by autoclave. All are spore formers.
- *Bacillus anthracis*: polypeptide capsule, exotoxin, and anthrax (Woolsorters disease).
- *Bacillus cereus:* food poisoning (food reheated once), enterotoxin.
- *Clostridium*: no cytochrome enzymes, no catalase, and no superoxide dismutase.
- *Clostridium tetani*: noninvasive, neurotoxins (prevents release of neural inhibitory transmitters such as γ-aminobutyric acid [GABA] and glycine), lockjaw, spastic paralysis; give toxoid/antitoxin.
- *Clostridium botulinum*: noninvasive, exotoxins (prevents acetylcholine release), flaccid paralysis, and antitoxin (honey ingestion in infancy).
- *Clostridium perfringens*: invasive, enterotoxin, food poisoning, myonecrosis, collagenase, lecithinase, and gas gangrene.
- *Clostridium difficile*: Pseudomembranous colitis can occur after broad-spectrum antibiotic usage.
- *Corynebacterium diphtheriae*: Gram-positive rod, metachromatic granules, exotoxin (inhibits EF-2 and protein synthesis).
- *Listeria monocytogenes*: Gram-positive rod in cerebrospinal fluid (CSF), compromised host, neonate, diarrhea after eating raw cheeses, and tumbling motility.
- *Salmonella*: motile Gram-negative rod, enteric fever, food poisoning; *Salmonella typhi* = human pathogen; other species = animal pathogens; motile; and nonlactose fermenter.
- *Shigella*: nonmotile Gram-negative rod, more virulent than *Salmonella*, bloody diarrhea, shigellosis is human disease, oral–anal route (fingers, flies, food, and feces), toxin inhibits protein synthesis.
- *Escherichia coli*: Gram-negative rod, most common UTI, sepsis (serious); enterohemorrhagic *E. coli* (EHEC) (colitis, hemolytic uremic syndrome—verotoxin, hamburger, beef); enteroinvasive *E. coli* (EIEC) (fever, bloody stool, and diarrhea); enterotoxigenic *E. coli* (ETEC) (traveler diarrhea); enteropathogenic *E. coli* (EPEC) (infant fever and diarrhea, nonbloody stool).

E	E	E	E
Hamburger	Invasive	Traveler diarrhea	Pediatric
E	E	E	E
C	C	C	C

- *Pseudomonas aeruginosa*: Gram-negative rod, antibiotic resistance, blue–green pigments; causes UTI, wounds, burns, greenish-yellow sputum.

- *Klebsiella*: Gram-negative, large capsule; causes UTI, pneumonia, especially in alcoholics (currant jelly sputum).
- *Haemophilus influenzae*: Gram-negative rod; causes meningitis, otitis, sinusitis, and epiglottitis.
- *Proteus*: Gram-negative rod, result in swarming growth; produce urease (urea → NH_3); also produced by *Helicobacter pylori* and *Ureaplasma urealyticum*; causes UTI, wounds, renal stones, and large staghorn calculi.
- *Gardnerella vaginalis*: Gram-negative, "clue cells"; vaginitis with discharge (fishy smell, conduct Whiff test).
- *Bordetella pertussis*: Gram-negative, capsule form, pili, killed vaccine, causes whooping cough.
- *Yersinia pestis*: Gram-negative, "safety pin" (bipolar staining), causes plague (bubonic/pneumonic), spread by rat flea.
- *Francisella tularensis*: Gram-negative, spread by skinning rabbits (jackrabbits), causes tularemia.
- *Pasteurella multocida*: Gram-negative, spread by cat/dog bites; causes cellulitis, "shipping fever."
- *Brucella*: Gram-negative, detected by dye sensitivity test; causes undulant fever.
- *Mycobacterium tuberculosis*: acid-fast, causes tuberculosis, detected by acid-fast stain, Lowenstein–Jensen medium, purified protein derivative (PPD) testing.
- *Mycobacterium leprae*: acid fast, causes leprosy, cannot be cultured.
- *Haemophilus ducreyi*: Gram negative, causes painful lesion, chancroid (syphilis: painless chancre).
- *Treponema pallidum*: Gram negative, detected by Venereal Disease Research Laboratories (VDRL) tests, fluorescent treponemal antibody absorption (FTA-ABS), and IgM antibody; use penicillin G for treatment; has three stages (1—initial chancre, 2—whole body rash, 3—chronic inflammation causing tissue destruction) spirochetes, dark-field microscopy.
- *Borrelia:* Gram negative, aniline dyes (Wright/Giemsa), *Ixodes* tick, relapsing fever, Lyme disease, acute necrotizing ulcerative gingivitis, spirochete.
- *Legionella pneumophila*: Legionnaires disease, fulminating pneumonia, Gram-negative rod, airborne through contaminated water (air-conditioner cooling system).
- Exotoxin: heat labile.

- Endotoxin (LPS): heat stable.
- Diphtheria/*Pseudomonas* exotoxin: act via ADP-ribosylation of EF-2, thus protein synthesis inhibited.
- *Escherichia coli*, *Vibrio cholerae*, *B. cereus* heat-labile enterotoxin: ADP ribosylation of G_s protein turns G_s protein on, thus activating adenylate cyclase, leading to ↑cAMP and diarrhea.
- *Bordetella pertussis*: Gram negative, heat-labile enterotoxin: ADP-ribosylation of G_i protein turns off G_I protein, thereby activating adenylate cyclase, leading to ↑cAMP and nasal discharge.
- *Vibrio*: oxidase positive; one flagellum; curved, "comma-shaped" Gram-negative rod; halophilic (except *V cholerae*). All are Gram negative.
- *Vibrio parahaemolyticus*: spread by contaminated seafood, causes diarrhea.
- *Vibrio vulnificus*: spread by contaminated marine animals (oyster ingestion), causes diarrhea, skin lesions (handling).
- Resistant nosocomial infections: vancomycin-resistant enterococci (VRE), treat with quinupristin–dalfopristin; methicillin-resistant *S. aureus* (MRSA), treat with vancomycin; and vancomycin-indeterminate *S. aureus* (VISA), consider new treatment options such as linezolid or quinupristin/dalfopristin.
- *Mycobacterium tuberculosis* causes initial primary pulmonary infection that may enter chronic latent granulomatosis stage or result in reactivation of disease characterized by hemoptysis, loss of weight, and fever.
- Penicillin-resistant pneumococci (*S. pneumoniae*) Gram positive, may account for up to 40% of isolates of *S. pneumoniae*. Third- or fourth-generation cephalosporins may be used as alternative treatment as well as vancomycin and rifampin.
- *Campylobacter* (GE) and *Helicobacter* (PUD) are both helical-shaped bacteria. *Campylobacter* causes a food-borne GI illness, most commonly from undercooked meat. Both bacteria are susceptible to antibiotics such as tetracycline. *Helicobacter* may be treated with Pepto-Bismol, metronidazole, and amoxicillin. All are gram negative.

Media-Selective Examples

- Bile esculin agar—used to identify Enterococcus from non-Group D cocci.
- Bordet-Gengou agar—used for isolating *B. pertussis*.
- Chocolate agar—used to identify fastidious organisms (*Neisseria* and *Haemophilus*).

- Thayer-Martin agar—used to identify *Neisseria.*
- Mueller-Hinton agar—used for susceptibility testing.
- EMB agar and MacConkey agar—used to identify enterobacteriaceae (enterics).
- Fletcher medium—used to identify *Listeria.*
- Loeffler medium—used to identify *C. diphtheriae.*
- Lowenstein–Jensen medium—used to identify mycobacteria.
- Middlebrook 7H10—used to identify mycobacteria.
- Mannitol salt agar—used to identify staphylococci, specific for *S. aureus.*
- Selenite broth—used to identify enrichment for *Salmonella/Shigella.*

RICKETTSIAE, CHLAMYDIAE, AND MYCOPLASMAS

Rickettsiae

- *Rickettsia*, *Coxiella*, *Orientia*, *Anaplasma*, and *Ehrlichia*—main genera. All are obligate intracellular parasites due to limited adenosine triphosphate (ATP) production. Insect vectors include ticks, mites, and body lice.
- Rocky Mountain spotted fever—*caused by Rickettsia rickettsii*, spread by ticks, invades capillaries, causing vasculitis. Rash commonly progresses from extremities to trunk. Diagnosis is usually serologic, using cross-reacting antibodies to *Proteus vulgaris* OX strains.
- Treat with tetracyclines, doxycycline.
- *Coxiella burnetii*—reservoir is livestock; inhalation transmission. Causes Q fever, an atypical pneumonia.
- *Ehrlichia*—infects monocytes, granulocytes; tick transmission.
- *Anaplasma*: *A. phagocytophilum* causes human granulocytic ehrlichiosis.
- *Orientia tsutsugamushi*: causes scrub typhus.

Chlamydiae

- Obligate intracellular parasites that require host ATP. Possess a modified Gram-negative cell wall, a true bacterium.
- Unusual life cycle—infectious elementary bodies bind to receptors and enter cells, forming an intracellular reticulate body. Dividing reticulate bodies form new elementary bodies. Reticulate bodies form inclusion bodies in the host cell.
- *Chlamydia trachomatis* is sensitive to sulfa drugs, and stains with iodine (glycogen staining). Serotypes A, B, and C cause trachoma, a chronic follicular keratoconjunctivitis, often resulting in blindness (leading cause worldwide).

- Serotypes D to K cause reproductive tract infections, pneumonia, and inclusion conjunctivitis. Chlamydial genital infections are widespread and common. Neonatal infections often result in inclusion conjunctivitis. Treat with erythromycins or tetracyclines.
- Serotypes L1, L2, and L3 cause lymphogranuloma venereum.
- Identify genital infections with molecular probes, fluorescent antibody (FA) staining for tissues, grow in McCoy cell cultures.
- *Chlamydophila psittaci* uses birds as primary hosts. Humans develop an atypical pneumonia from inhaling the organism. Diagnosis is usually serology, not iodine staining.
- *Chlamydophila pneumoniae* (TWAR) causes human bronchitis, pneumonia, and sinusitis. Treat with azithromycin.

Mycoplasma

- Bacteria with no cell wall.
  - Grown on laboratory media; do not Gram stain accurately.
  - *Mycoplasma pneumoniae*—causes sore throat through atypical pneumonia (walking pneumonia); treat with tetracyclines or erythromycins.
  - *Ureaplasma urealyticum*—urethritis, prostatitis; forms tiny colonies, require urea for growth.

MYCOLOGY

- Fungi (molds [moulds] and yeasts) are eukaryotic—cell membranes have ergosterol (not cholesterol) and the difference is a drug target.
- Fungal structures—hyphae (molds) or yeast cells.
- Dimorphism—ability to grow in two forms, for example change from hyphal to yeast forms (or spherules of *Coccidioides* spp.).
- Hyphae amass into a mycelium; septate hyphae have cross-walls; nonseptate hyphae have no or rare cross-walls.
- Yeasts—oval cells that replicate by budding or by fission (*P. marneffii*).
- Spores and conidia—reproductive structures; blastoconidia—yeast buds; conidia—produced by hyphae (some species produce both macro- and microforms); endospores—produced in spherule by *Coccidioides* spp.; arthroconidia—modified hyphal cells released by fragmentation. Sporangiospores produced within sporangium, for example *Mucor* spp.
- Laboratory test—Sabouraud agar is standard fungal medium.
- Identification—macroscopic (colony) and microscopic morphology, biochemical tests, immunologic tests, or DNA probes.

Antifungal Drugs

- Drugs that target ergosterol–ergosterol biosynthesis: inhibition of squalene epoxidase (tolnaftate, allylamines); inhibition of P450 14-α-demethylase (imidazoles and triazoles); bind to ergosterol disturbing membrane structure (polyenes).
- Antimetabolite: flucytosine inhibition of RNA and DNA synthesis.
- Echinocandins: inhibition biosynthesis cell wall glucan.
- Drug resistance mechanisms—uptake and metabolism (flucytosine); mutation subunit β-1,3-glucan synthase (echinocandins); mutation and/or overexpression of target and/or efflux pumps (azoles). Alteration or decrease ergosterol content (polyenes).

Superficial Skin, Cutaneous Dermatophyte, and Subcutaneous Infections

- *Malassezia* spp.—etiology of pityriasis (tinea) versicolor, a superficial infection with hyper- or hypopigmentation of skin; microscopic analysis skin scraping shows "spaghetti and meatballs" appearance.
- Dermatophytes—three genera: *Trichophyton* spp. affects skin, hair, and nails; *Microsporum* spp. affects hair and skin; *Epidermophyton* affects nail and skin.
- Tineas cause by dermatophytes—ringworm (*T. capitis*—scalp infection involving hair; *T. corporis*—infection glabrous skin; *T. cruris* infection groin-aka jock itch; *T. pedis* aka athlete's foot; *T. unguim*-nail infection aka onychomycosis caused by dermatophytes); hyaline hyphae and arthroconidia in tissue.
- *Sporothrix schenckii*—thermally dimorphic fungus found on plants and in soil (mold form); subcutaneous inoculation of puncture wound, for example from a thorn, or occasionally scratch from infected cat; develop subcutaneous infection at location with spread along draining lymphatic (rose gardener's disease); yeast form in tissue.

Systemic Infections Due to Dimorphic Fungi

- *Histoplasma capsulatum*—mold in the environment with tuberculate macroconidia and small nondistinction microconidia; small, oval budding yeast in cells of the reticuloendothelial system (RES).
- Eastern half United States—Ohio and Mississippi river valleys, especially important—birds and bat caves.

- Primary disease—asymptomatic to pneumonia.
- Disseminated disease—especially in immunosuppressed and AIDS patients. May be acute or subacute with mucocutaneous lesions common in subacute.
- Laboratory tests—history plus blood smears and culture, antigen detection.
- *Coccidioides* spp.—found in a sandy environment, especially deserts (in southwestern USA, lower part of California, Arizona, New Mexico, and Texas); drying hyphae fragment into arthroconidia; inhaled arthroconidia develop into spherules containing endospores.
- Primary disease—valley fever—asymptomatic to self-limited pneumonia.
- Disseminated form more often in men than in women, risk greater immunocompromised individuals and pregnant women, risk appears increased among those of African American or Filipino ancestry; affects skin, bone, joints, and meninges.
- Laboratory—culture is hazardous and a proper technique is necessary if done; sputum, urine, and bronchial washes may show spherules. Detection of antibodies in serum.
- *Blastomyces dermatitidis*—environment mold, hyphae with conidia on stalks; tissue—large yeast cell with broad-based bud.
- Same geographical area as *Histoplasma*, conidia are inhaled.
- Primary disease—asymptomatic to pneumonia.
- Disseminated disease—skin most common manifestation and may be presenting complaint.
- Laboratory—culture and examination tissue for large yeast cells, broad-based buds.

Opportunistic Mycoses

- *Aspergillus fumigatus*—hyphae with branches at acute angles and small conidia; ubiquitous in environment.
- Noninvasive fungus balls (aspergilloma) in lung cavities; colonization in ears and nasal cavity.
- Opportunistic (eg, immunosuppressed patient) invasive disease may be localized in lungs or disseminate to generalized disease and may be life threatening.
- *Candida albicans*—normal flora of cutaneous and mucocutaneous surface usually in yeast form. Hyphae and pseudohyphae are generally

additionally present in infection. *C. albicans* most frequent isolate in most studies; other *Candida* spp. include *C. glabrata* and *C. tropicalis*.

- Cutaneous or mucocutaneous infection associated morbidity. For example, thrush in neonates, AIDS; denture stomatitis; and vaginitis.
- Systemic—candidemia; may hematogenously disseminate any organ, including kidney, brain, eye, and skin. Life threatening. Risk factors include immunosuppression and catheters.
- *Cryptococcus neoformans*—yeast with large capsule.
- Environment—soil with bird (especially pigeons) droppings.
- Primary disease—primary pulmonary (often asymptomatic).
- Disseminated infections frequently manifest in USA as meningitis; underlying risk includes prolonged treatment corticosteroids, malignancy, and AIDS.
- Laboratory test—India ink mount body fluids, tissue stains highlight capsule; culture; latex agglutination—CSF (capsular antigen).
- *Cryptococcus gattii*—geographically limited, less frequently isolated and associated vegetation (not guano); may be more likely to infect immunocompetent individuals and most cases may have primary pulmonary symptoms.
- *Mucor*, *Rhizopus*, and *Absidia*—nonseptate hyphae.
- Environment—common organisms.
- Opportunist infections—rhinocerebral infections; acidosis, eg, diabetics.
- Laboratory test—broad, nonseptate hyphae with 90° angles on branching but often too few to see; culture.
- *Pneumocystis jiroveci*—exposure common—seldom causes disease except in immunocompromised, especially AIDS patients and debilitated infants; causes interstitial pneumonia (old name: *P. carinii*, isolated from rats, while *P. jiroveci* from humans).
- Laboratory tests—organisms not culturable and rely stains (eg, H&E, silver, Giemsa) to detect asci (cysts), spores, etc.
- Treatment—TMP-SMX, pentamidine (not antifungals; organism lacks ergosterol).

PARASITOLOGY

- Protozoa are single-celled animals. Trophozoites are motile (ingested RBC are often seen inside), while cysts (four nuclei and chromatid body are characteristic) are involved in transmission.

- Amoebas.
- *Entamoeba histolytica*—disease of the large intestine; amebic dysentery—trophozoites feed on red blood cells (RBCs), causing flask-shaped ulcers. Also liver and lung abscesses possible.
- *Naegleria*—free-living amoeba in hot water sources; causes primary amebic meningoencephalitis (PAM); rapid onset of symptoms, with death possible in days.
- *Acanthamoeba*—free-living amoebas; cause granulomatous amoebic encephalitis (GAE); found in tap water, freshwater, seawater, and other such sources.
- Flagellates.
- *Giardia lamblia*—worldwide distribution, animal reservoirs; cysts in water sources. Trophozoites attach to intestine, causing watery diarrhea and malabsorption (beaver fever). Cramping, light-colored, fatty stools; also acquired from day-care centers or while camping.
- *Trichomonas vaginalis*—trophozoite with undulating membrane and polar flagella; presents with yellow discharge that has a fishy odor; males usually asymptomatic; sexually transmitted. No cyst stage.
- *Trypanosoma brucei*—flagellates transmitted by tsetse fly; cause African sleeping sickness. Winterbottom sign (swelling of the posterior cervical lymph node is characteristic of disease).
- *Trypanosoma cruzi*—Chagas disease transmitted by kissing bug; prevalent mostly in South and Central America; causes cardiomegaly, megacolon. Romana sign or chagoma (swelling around the eye caused by the entry of *T. cruzi*).
- Leishmania—sandfly vectors; cause visceral, cutaneous, and mucocutaneous lesions.
- *Cryptosporidium parvum*—found in US waters; causes a self-limited diarrhea. Symptoms severe in immunocompromised patients, especially those with CD4 counts <200/µL.
- Plasmodium species cause malaria. *Anopheles* mosquito vectors; complicated life cycles; *P. vivax* (Schuffner dots, enlarged RBC), *P. ovale* (crenated RBC), *P. malariae* (daisy head schizont), *P. falciparum* (signet ring, normal-size RBC, sausage-shaped gametocyte), and an emerging species *P. knowlesi* (similar to *P. malariae* morphologically).
- *Toxoplasma gondii*—reservoir is cats. Humans ingest cysts from cat feces or undercooked meats; especially dangerous to human fetus as it affects congenital development.

SUMMARY POINTS TO REMEMBER ABOUT PROTOZOAN PARASITES

Transmission

- Ingestion (eg, *Giardia*, *Entamoeba*).
- Direct penetration via insect bite (eg, Malaria, *Trypanosoma*).
- Transplacental penetration (eg, *Toxoplasma*).

Diagnosis

- Many infections may be diagnosed by microscopic examination of the feces (eg, *Giardia*, *Entamoeba*), blood (eg, Malaria, *Trypanosoma)* or bone marrow (*Leishmania*).
- Serologic tests are available but cross-reactivity with other parasites may be a problem.

Clinical Manifestations

- Can be nonspecific and clinically unremarkable and nonspecific (eg, diarrhea and abdominal discomfort [intestinal parasites]) to very species-specific (eg, Chagas disease).

Prevention and Treatment

- Avoidance with the source of infective stage.
- Personal hygiene.
- Vector control.
- Important drugs to remember (metronidazole for intestinal protozoa; quinine derivatives; atovaquone–proguanil; artemisinin derivatives.
- No vaccine for any protozoan parasite. Some vaccines for malaria have shown promise in clinical trials.
- Flukes.
- *Fasciolopsis buski*—affects intestines; cysts on water plants ingested; causes diarrhea.
- *Clonorchis sinensis*—affects liver; transmitted from raw or undercooked fish; biliary tree localization and liver location.
- *Fasciola hepatica*—sheep liver fluke; humans can become infected by ingestion of metacercariae on aquatic plants.
- *Schistosoma*—also called blood flukes; portal hypertension and hepatosplenomegaly (*S. mansoni*, *S. japonicum*). Cystitis and urethritis (*S. haematobium*) with hematuria, which can progress to bladder cancer.
- Cestodes—segmented flatworms with complicated life cycles.

- *Taenia solium* (pork) and *T. saginata* (beef)—larval forms (cysticercosis) found in undercooked meat. Adult tapeworms develop in the intestine. *T. solium* eggs when ingested by human can develop into cysticercosis.
- *Diphyllobothrium latum*—fish tapeworm; fish in freshwater lakes, undercooked fish ingested; depletes host of vitamin B12.
- *Echinococcus granulosus*—dog tapeworm. Humans are intermediate hosts and ingest eggs from sheep or dog feces, hydatid cysts of liver, *anaphylaxis* if burst.
- Nematodes—roundworms.
- *Ascaris lumbricoides*—may cause intestinal blockage.
- *Enterobius vermicularis* (pinworm)—eggs in bedclothes, detected in scotch tape test, etc; retroinfection common; widespread in the United States.
- *Necator americanus*—New World hookworm.
- *Ancylostoma duodenale*—Old World hookworm; eggs found in soil; penetrate bare feet.
- *Strongyloides stercoralis* (threadworm)—found in tropics, southeast United States; is similar to hookworms; no eggs, only larval forms. Hyperinfection can develop in patients on steroid therapy with high mortality.
- *Trichuris trichiura* (whipworm)—found in tropics; spreads when eggs are ingested, or due to poor sanitation; causes mucoid or bloody diarrhea, anal prolapse.
- *Trichinella spiralis* (pork roundworm)—larvae ingested in pork or wild game meat. Larvae may calcify in muscle of intermediate host.
- Tissue nematodes—filarial worms. None are significant in the United States.
- *Onchocerca volvulus*—also called river blindness. Blackfly is the vector of disease. The preferred treatment is ivermectin.
- *Loa loa*—day-biting fly is the vector.
- *Wuchereria bancrofti*—mosquito vectors; may cause elephantiasis by blocking lymphatics.

SUMMARY POINTS TO REMEMBER ABOUT WORMS

Transmission—Oral

- Human feces. Feco-oral transmission is important in several worms. Soiling by infected human feces is responsible for infestation by *Ascaris*, *Enterobius*, *Trichuris*, and cysticercus larvae (larval *T. solium*).

- Animal feces. Humans become infected with the eggs of *Echinococcus granulosus* (hydatid cysts) by eating products that have been contaminated by animal excreta.
- Infected meat. Eating raw or insufficiently cooked meat, which contains larvae, leads to infection by adult *Taenia*.
- Infected fish. Eating raw or insufficiently cooked fish may lead to infection with trematodes such as *Clonorchis*.
- Infected crabs and crayfish. Eating larval-infested, raw, or insufficiently cooked crabs may lead to paragonimiasis (lung fluke).
- Contaminated plants. Infection with the giant intestinal fluke (Fasciolopsiasis) occurs via the consumption of several kinds of raw plants, for example water nut and water chestnut, on which larvae are encysted.
- Contaminated water. Drinking water containing cyclops (small crustaceans) infected with *Dracunculus*, leads to guinea worm infection (almost eradicated only 1000 infected people).

Transmission—Skin Penetration

- Larvae of *Strongyloides* and hookworm enter through the skin from the soil. *Schistosome* cercariae penetrate the skin when humans come into contact with infested water.

Clinical Manifestations

- Can be nonspecific and clinically unremarkable and nonspecific (eg, diarrhea, abdominal discomfort, nausea, and anorexia [intestinal nematodes]) to very species-specific (eg, cysticercosis and hydatid cyst disease).

Prevention and Treatment

- Avoidance with the source of infective stage. Inspection of meat. Storage and proper cooking of meat.
- Anthelmintic treatment—praziquantel, albendazole, mebendazole, and ivermectin are the basic drugs.

IMMUNOLOGY

- Two types of immune response: (1) adaptive or acquired (specific, slow primary response, rapid secondary response), and (2) innate (native or natural, rapid).

- Innate immunity: limited specificity, no immunological memory, first line of defense (epithelial), biochemical defenses (stomach ↓pH, GI proteolytic enzymes, and bile), phagocytes (polymorphonuclear neutrophils [PMNs] and monocytes, macrophages), natural killer (NK) cells, soluble mediators (complement, acute-phase proteins such as C-reactive protein, cytokines such as ILs, IFNs, CSFs), inflammation (C5a: chemotaxis, C3b: opsonization, neutrophils).
- Adaptive immunity: specific, antigen-driven, discriminates self from non-self, possesses memory, divided into (1) humoral immunity (B cells, plasma cells) and (2) cell-mediated immunity (T helper cells, T cytotoxic cells—CTLs).
- Antibodies (B lymphocytes/plasma cells): main functions are (1) *neutralize* toxins/viruses, (2) *opsonize* bacteria, and (3) *complement activation.*
- Antibodies (five isotypes): IgG, IgA, IgM, IgD, and IgE (based on Fc heavy-chain differences), two light chains (kappa and lambda) and two heavy chains held together by disulfide bonds, the hinge region is polyproline, paratope binds antigen and is composed of heavy and light chains. Pepsin yields $F(ab)_2$ and papain yields two Fab fragments and one Fc fragment.
- Antibody concentrations (serum): IgG > IgA > IgM > IgD > IgE.
- IgG: crosses the placenta (Rh incompatibility, hemolytic disease of newborn), 80% of serum antibody, binds (activates) complement, four subclasses (IgG1, IgG2, IgG3, and IgG4), main antibody in secondary (recall or memory) response.
- IgA: secretory antibody, serum (monomer), secretions (dimers), two subclasses, dimer (J chain), does not bind complement.
- IgM: pentamer, binds complement, first to appear after infection, elevated in congenital/perinatal infections.
- IgD: susceptible to proteolytic degradation, found with surface IgM on mature B lymphocytes.
- IgE: cytotropic/reaginic antibody, allergy antibody, type I hypersensitivity (mast cells/basophils protective in worm infections), lowest concentration in serum.
- Bence Jones proteins: multiple myeloma—large amounts of κ/λ light chains in urine excretion.
- Natural killer cells: marker is CD16 (IgG Fc receptor).
- B cells: antibody producers contributing to allergy (IgE), autoimmunity, host defense (opsonize, neutralize, complement activate).

- B-cell markers: Fc receptor, C3 receptor, CD21 (receptor for EB virus), and CD10 (common acute lymphoblastic leukemia antigen [CALLA]).
- T cells: host defense (fungi, viruses, *M. tuberculosis*), allergy (type IV—delayed hypersensitivity), antibody regulation, graft/tumor rejection.
- T-cell markers: CD2, TCRαβ-CD3, CD28, CD4 (also receptor for HIV) or CD8, CD44 (migration).
- Complement deficiencies: (1) C1 esterase inhibitor: angioedema; (2) decay-accelerating factor (DAF): paroxysmal nocturnal hemoglobinuria; (3) C3 deficiency: severe, recurrent infections (sinus and respiratory)—pneumonococci; (4) C5 to C9 deficiency: disseminated gonococcemia.
- Major histocompatibility complex (MHC) Class I: exists on all nucleated cells—MHC I + peptide = ligand for CD8 T cells.
- MHC Class II: exists on antigen-presenting cells (macrophages/dendritic cells), important to organ rejection—MHC II + peptide = ligand for CD4 T cells.
- Cytokines: IFN-α, β (antiviral), TNF (inflammation, fever, acute-phase reactants, cachexia), IL-1 (fever/pyrogen, acute-phase proteins), IL-2 (T-cell stimulator), IL-3 (bone marrow stimulator), IL-4 (IgE production), IL-5 (proeosinophil, antihelminths), IL-6 (acute-phase proteins, B-cell differentiation), IL-8 (inflammation, chemotaxis), IL-12 and IFN-γ NK cell stimulator, T_H1 stimulator, active cytotoxic lymphocyte stimulator, promotes cell-mediated immunity.
- Acute-phase cytokines: IL-1, IL-6, and TNF-α.
- Mitogens: B lymphocytes (LPS), T lymphocytes (phytohemagglutinin [PHA] and Con A), both B and T cells (pokeweed mitogen [PWM]).
- Enzyme-linked immunosorbent assay (ELISA)-sensitive presumptive diagnosis of HIV infection, western blot specific, definitive diagnosis of HIV infection → both detecting anti-HIV antibodies in patient sera; detection of HIV RNA by nucleic acid amplification of viral load is best predictor of "progression to AIDS."
- Immunodeficiencies: (1) primary—rare and *cause* disease; and (2) secondary—common and the *result* of disease.
- Primary immunodeficiencies: Bruton agammaglobulinemia—no B cells, low antibodies, small tonsils, only males; DiGeorge syndrome (congenital thymic aplasia)—third and fourth pharyngeal pouches development failure, no thymus, no T cells, no parathyroid (hypocalcemia), and recurrent viral, fungal, protozoal infections; severe combined immunodeficiency disease (SCID)—no T or B cells, defective IL-2 receptor, deficiency

adenosine enzyme, recurrent infections (viral, bacterial, fungal, and protozoal); Wiskott Aldrich syndrome—B- and T-cell deficiency, low IgM, high IgA, normal IgE; ataxia telangiectasia—defective DNA repair; Chèdiak–Higashi disease—autosomal-recessive defect in phagocytosis; CGD—NADPH oxidase deficiency, increased opportunistic pathogens, phagocytic deficiency; chronic mucocutaneous candidiasis—*C. albicans* T-cell dysfunction.

- Immunodeficiency characterized by unusual and recurrent infections.
- B-cell (antibody) deficiency—bacterial infections.
- T-cell deficiency—viral, fungal, and protozoal infections.
- Phagocytic cells deficiency—pyogenic infections (bacterial), skin infections, and systemic bacterial opportunistic infections.
- Complement deficiencies—pyogenic infections (bacterial).
- Hypersensitivity: (1) type I (anaphylaxis, immediate-type hypersensitivity, IgE); (2) type II (cytotoxic hypersensitivity); (3) type III (immune complex hypersensitivity); and (4) type IV (cell-mediated, delayed-type hypersensitivity).
- Type I: mast cell/basophil, IgE, vasoactive amines, asthma, anaphylaxis, local wheal, and flare.
- Type II: IgM, IgG bind antigen and lyse cell, autoimmune hemolytic anemia, Goodpasture syndrome, and erythroblastosis fetalis.
- Type III: immune complex, serum sickness, Arthus reaction → antibody–antigen complexes.
- Type IV: lymphokines released from activated T lymphocytes, TB skin test, contact dermatitis, transplant rejection, and lupus (SLE).
- Autoantibodies: systemic lupus erythematosus (antinuclear antibodies, anti-dsDNA, anti-Smith); drug-induced lupus (antihistone); rheumatoid arthritis (anti-IgG); celiac disease (antigliadin), Goodpasture syndrome (antibasement membrane); Hashimoto thyroiditis (antimicrosomal); scleroderma Calcinosis Raynaud Esophagus Sclerosis Teleangiectasiae (CREST) (anticentromere); and scleroderma diffuse (anti-scl-70).
- Active immunity: induced after exposure to foreign antigens, memory established, slow primary response, and rapid secondary (recall or memory) response.
- Vaccines: (1) capsular polysaccharide vaccines (*Streptococcus, N. meningitidis, H. influenzae*); (2) toxoid vaccines (*C. diphtheriae, C. tetani, B. pertussis*); (3) purified protein vaccines (*B. pertussis, Borrelia burgdorferi, B. anthracis*); (4) live, attenuated bacterial vaccines (*M. bovis* for

tuberculosis/BCG, *F. tularensis*); (5) killed bacterial vaccines (*V. cholerae*, *Y. pestis*, *R. rickettsiae*/typhus, *C. burnetii*/Q fever); (6) killed, live, attenuated, and polysaccharide vaccines (*S. typhi*).

- Adjuvants (human vaccines): aluminum hydroxide, lipid, or oil-in-water emulsion.
- Passive humoral immunity: administration of preformed antibody in immune globulin preparations, no memory established, rapid onset (eg, tetanus antitoxin, botulinum antitoxin, diphtheria antitoxin), antitoxin = immune globulins.
- Passive cellular immunity: administration of specific lymphocytes (NK cells, T cells), short lived, may not result in memory, adaptive cell therapy (ACT).

Physiology and Molecular Microbiology

Questions

1. A 28-year-old female with folliculitis is not responsive to a 10-day treatment course with penicillin. An enzyme produced by the etiologic agent is most likely responsible for this treatment failure. At which site on the molecule shown does this enzyme act to destroy penicillin?

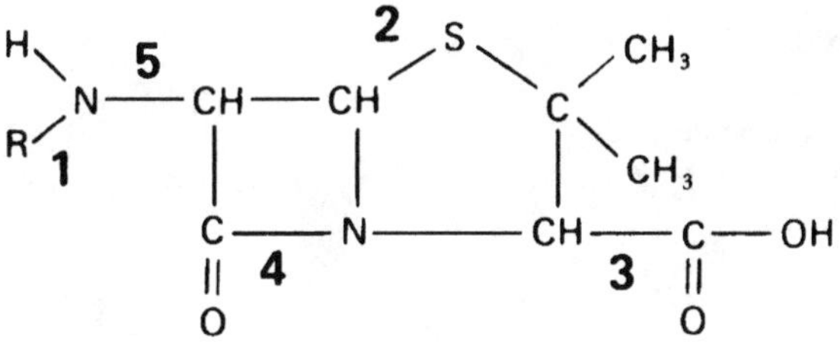

```
                        2   S               CH3
H       5                 /   \           /
  \                      /     \         /
   N ——— CH ——— CH              C
  /       |      |               \
R    1    |      |            |   CH3
          |      |            |
          C ——— N ——————— CH ——— C ——— OH
          ||  4                3   ||
          O                        O
```

a. 1
b. 2
c. 3
d. 4
e. 5

2. A 35-year-old male was treated with an aminoglycoside for an infection with a gram-negative rod. Which of the following bacterial processes is involved in transport of this antibiotic into the cell?

a. Facilitated diffusion
b. Fermentation
c. Group translocation
d. Oxidative phosphorylation
e. Transpeptidation

3. A 36-year-old male developed a painful purulent urethral discharge following a 2-week vacation to Thailand. A Gram stain reveals gram-negative diplococci. Iron, which it obtains through surface receptors, is essential for the expression of the microorganism's virulence factors. From which of the following molecules does it obtain iron?

a. Ferric oxide
b. Lactoferrin
c. Lipopolysaccharide (LPS)
d. Pyocyanin
e. Siderophores

4. A female medical student is admitted to the emergency department with symptoms of severe urinary tract infection (UTI). The *Escherichia coli* strain isolated from urine produced extended-spectrum β-lactamase. In which anatomic area of the cell would this enzyme be located?

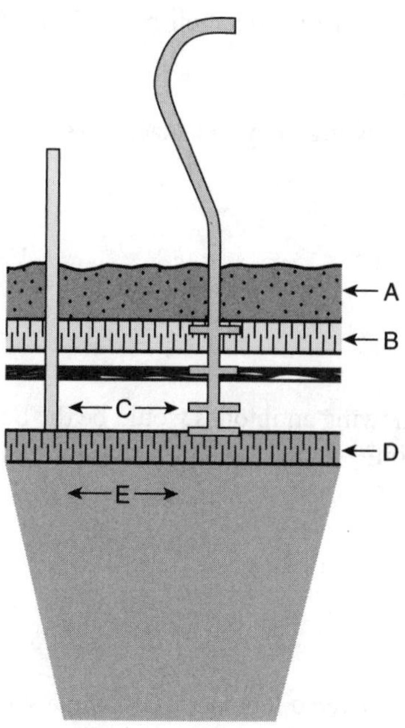

Structure of gram-negative bacterium.

a. A
b. B
c. C
d. D
e. E

Questions 5 and 6

A 52-year-old male develops abscesses following surgery to repair an abdominal gunshot wound. Gram stain of the foul-smelling exudate from his abscess reveals numerous polymorphonuclear leukocytes (PMNs or neutrophils) and several gram-negative rods that did not grow on blood plates in the presence of O_2. Metabolism of O_2 results in toxic reactive oxygen species.

5. Which of the following enzymes inactivates superoxide free radicals (O_2^-)?

a. ATPase
b. Catalase
c. Permease
d. Peroxidase
e. Superoxide dismutase

6. Which of the following antibiotics would be the best choice for treating this patient's infection?

a. Ampicillin
b. Chloramphenicol
c. Ciprofloxacin
d. Gentamicin
e. Metronidazole

7. A teenaged boy suffered a foot laceration while swimming in a polluted water area in a river. He did not seek medical treatment, and the wound developed a foul-smelling exudate. One of the bacteria isolated from the abscess exudate was missing superoxide dismutase, catalase, and a peroxidase. Which of the following statements best describes this microorganism?

a. It is a capnophile
b. It is a facultative anaerobe
c. It is a microaerophile
d. It is an anaerobe
e. It is an obligate aerobe

Questions 8 and 9

A 20-year-old pregnant female patient presents to the emergency room with a 4-day history of fever, chills, and myalgia. Two days prior to this, she had noted painful genital lesions that had begun as vesicles. Pelvic examination revealed extensive vesicular and ulcerative lesions on the left labia minora and majora with marked edema, and inguinal lymphadenopathy.

8. Which of the microorganisms causing genital ulcers can be demonstrated by dark field microscopy?

a. *Chlamydia trachomatis* LGV serovars
b. *Haemophilus ducreyi*
c. Herpes simplex virus type 2
d. *Klebsiella granulomatis*
e. *Treponema pallidum*

9. Which of the following tests would prove that the patient is infectious for herpes simplex virus (HSV) type 2?

a. Culture
b. Detection of HSV2-specific IgM
c. Direct immunofluorescent assay
d. Nucleic acid amplification testing
e. Tzanck smear

10. Gram-negative diplococci were demonstrated in a Gram stain of urethral drainage from an 18-year-old male who presented with symptoms of urethritis. Continuous passage of this strain on laboratory medium resulted in the reversion of a fimbriated to a nonfimbriated strain. Which of the following is the most likely implication of this phenomenon?

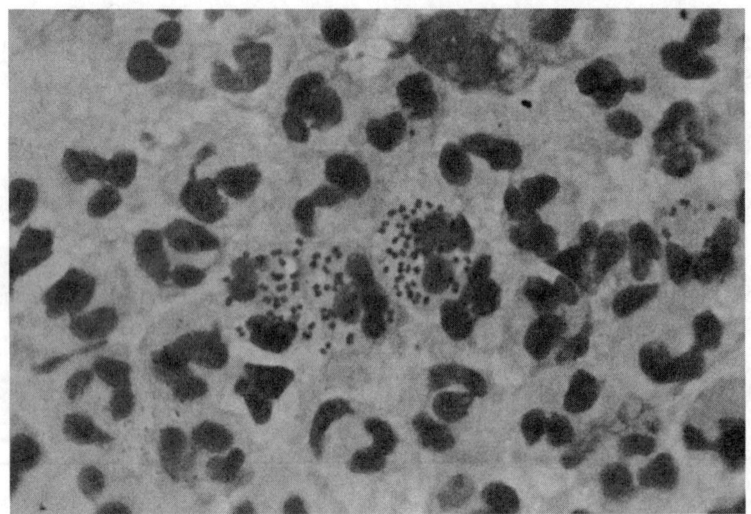

Gram-stained photomicrograph showing intracellular gram-negative diplococci and numerous PMNs. *(Courtesy of Bill Schwartz; Public Health Image Library, Centers for Disease Control and Prevention, 1971.)*

a. A negative capsule strain
b. Death of the organism
c. Inability to colonize the mucosal epithelium
d. Loss of serologic specificity
e. Reversion to a gram-positive stain

11. Twenty-eight hours after eating undercooked chicken, a 50-year-old farmer presents to the emergency room with abdominal pain, cramping, bloody diarrhea, and nausea. An isolate from the stool is biochemically identified as *Salmonella enterica*; however, the isolate cannot be serotyped. Which of the following has this organism lost?

a. Capsule
b. Flagella
c. Mannose receptor
d. Pili
e. O-specific polysaccharide

12. A 2-year-old infant is diagnosed with meningitis. A lumbar puncture reveals numerous neutrophils and gram-positive cocci in pairs that appear encapsulated. She is admitted to the hospital and started on intravenous (IV) β-lactams. Which of the following targets would most likely play a role in the development of resistance to this antibiotic in the most likely etiologic agent of this child's meningitis?

a. Bactoprenol
b. DNA gyrase
c. Penicillin-binding protein
d. Reverse transcriptase
e. RNA polymerase

13. A cattle farmer develops necrotic lesions on his arms and face following a traumatic encounter with a bull. Selective inhibition of synthesis of dipicolinic acid by the etiologic agent of the infection would most likely inhibit the formation of the infective structure. Which of the following would be inhibited?

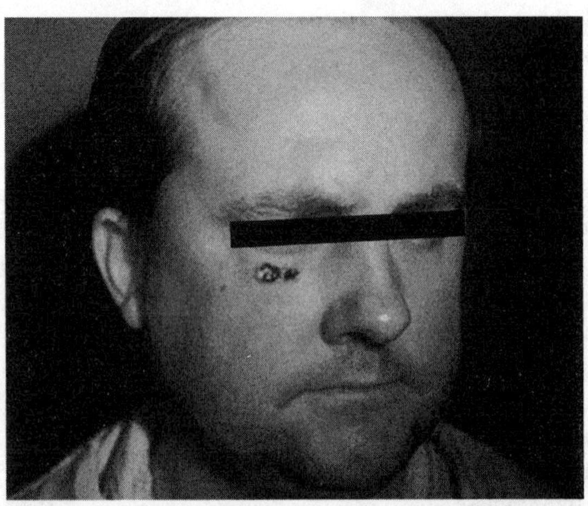

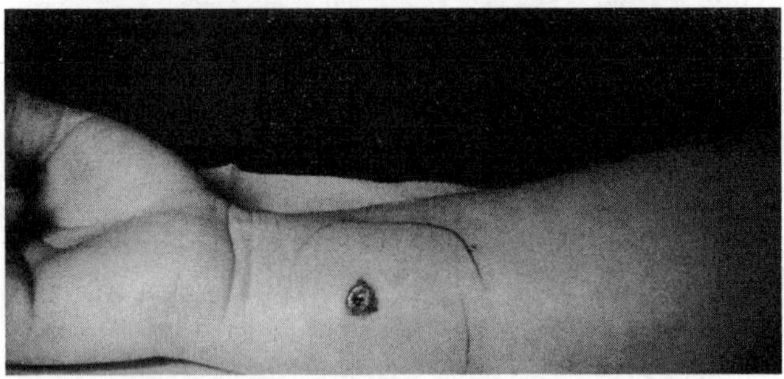

(Courtesy of Public Health Image Library, Centers for Disease Control and Prevention.)

a. Bacterial spore formation
b. Bacterial vegetative cells
c. Fungal arthrospores
d. Fungal microconidia
e. Mycobacterial vegetative cells

Questions 14 and 15

A 30-year-old male presents to the emergency room with high fever and malaise, which he reports that it began 4 days ago and got progressively worse each day. He appears underweight and very ill. Physical examination reveals needle marks in both antecubital fossae. Upon listening for heart sounds, you hear a distinctive systolic heart murmur. You order blood cultures and make a presumptive diagnosis of acute bacterial endocarditis. Following is the growth curve of the organism growing in a nutrient medium at 35°C with both O_2 and added CO_2 present.

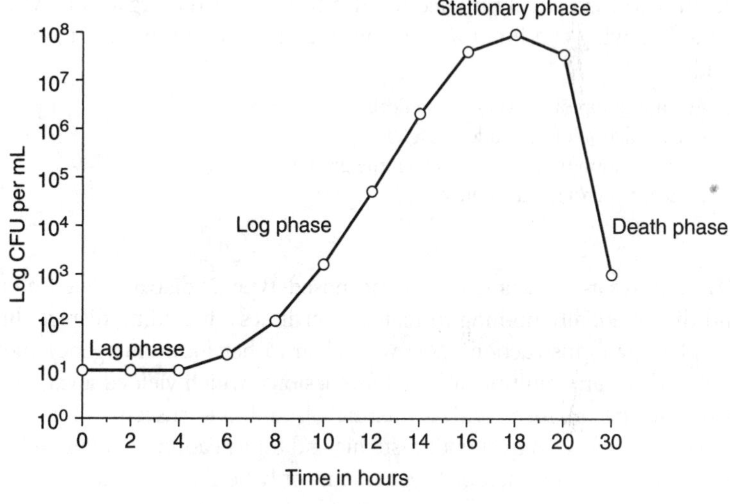

Growth curve–*Escherichia coli*

14. In which of the following growth phases would the organism most likely be resistant to β-lactam antibiotics?

a. Lag phase
b. Log phase
c. Stationary phase
d. Death phase

15. On which of the following growth phases would treatment with gentamicin have a maximal effect?

a. Lag phase
b. Log phase
c. Stationary phase
d. Death phase

16. An outbreak of diarrhea is thought to be related to a group of vendors who were selling hot dogs at the county fair. Stool cultures are positive for *Shigella* in almost all individuals who ate the hot dogs. Growth of the isolated colonies in nutrient liquid medium without the transfer to fresh medium will eventually induce the death phase of the organism. Which of the following is a limiting factor in microbial growth under laboratory conditions?

a. Accumulation of oxygen-free radicals
b. Accumulation of peroxide
c. Accumulation of toxic products in the growth medium
d. Loss of superoxide dismutase
e. Oxygen

17. A 62-year-old woman with diagnosed type 2 diabetes lived alone and did essentially nothing to manage her illness, including disregarding her physician's instructions. She was taken to her local emergency room (ER) with severe, multiple infected foot lesions, which yielded a variety of opportunistic microbes with a mixture of antibiotic susceptibilities. The physician decided to treat with systemic and topical antimicrobials. Which of the following antimicrobial agents must only be used topically?

a. Bacitracin
b. Gentamicin
c. Itraconazole
d. Penicillin
e. Vancomycin

18. A 42-year-old alcoholic man presents with fever, chills, cough, and chest x-ray suggestive of pneumonia. The Gram-stained smear of sputum shows many PMNs and gram-positive cocci in pairs and chains. Which of the following is the correct order of the procedural steps when performing the Gram stain?

a. Fixation, crystal violet, alcohol/acetone decolorization, safranin
b. Fixation, crystal violet, iodine treatment, alcohol/acetone decolorization, safranin
c. Fixation, crystal violet, iodine treatment, safranin
d. Fixation, crystal violet, safranin
e. Fixation, safranin, iodine treatment, alcohol/acetone decolorization, crystal violet

19. A 78-year-old man presents to the local emergency department with a severe headache and stiff neck. The cerebrospinal fluid (CSF) specimen is cloudy. Analysis reveals 400 white blood cells per cubic millimeter (95% PMNs), a protein concentration of 75 mg/dL, and a glucose concentration of 20 mg/dL. While in the ER, a resident does a Gram stain of the CSF but mistakenly forgets the iodine treatment step. If the meningitis is caused by *Streptococcus pneumoniae*, how will the bacteria seen on the resident's slide appear?

a. All the cells will be blue
b. All the cells will be decolorized
c. All the cells will be purple
d. All the cells will be red
e. All the cells will lyse; thus, no Gram stain results will be obtained
f. Half of the cells will be red and the other half will be blue

20. A 28-year-old female just returned from a 1-week cruise with stops along the coast of Mexico. Forty-eight hours after her return she is reported to have headache, fever, abdominal cramps, and constipation. Over the next 5 days, her fever increases with continued complaints of myalgias, malaise, and anorexia. A blood culture is positive for *S. enterica* ser. Typhi. Her condition improves with a treatment course of a ciprofloxacin. Which of the following is the function of porins that would prevent the effective use of this antimicrobial?

a. Hydrolysis of hydrophilic antimicrobials
b. Metabolism of phosphorylated intermediates
c. Serologic stabilization of the O antigen
d. Inactivation of hydrophobic antimicrobials
e. Transfer of molecules through the outer membrane

21. A 21-year-old man was bitten by a tick while hiking in Michigan. Four months later, he presented to his doctor complaining of swelling and pain in his left knee. A screening test for Lyme disease was equivocal. An IgG western blot was performed using the patient's serum against proteins of *Borrelia burgdorferi* and *Borrelia turicatae* is shown below. Which of the following is an accurate interpretation of the test?

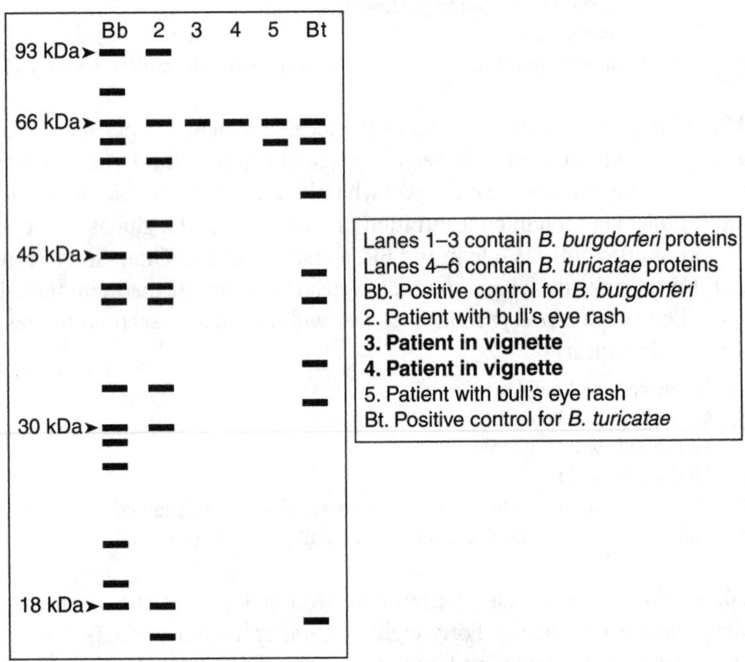

Western blot for *Borrelia burgdorferi*-specific IgG antibodies. Five of 10 specific bands for *B. burgdorferi* must be present for test to be considered positive. (18, 21 [OspC], 28, 30, 39 [BmpA], 41 [Fla], 45, 58 [not GroEL], 66, and 93 kDa.)

a. The patient has early Lyme disease
b. The patient has early disseminated Lyme disease
c. The patient late disseminated Lyme disease
d. The pattern most likely represents nonspecific reactivity
e. The screening test should be repeated

Questions 22 and 23

Over 30 individuals, attendees of a home improvement conference and their family members, are hospitalized with bloody diarrhea. Several children of the attendees develop fever, abdominal pain, and severe hematological abnormalities. An investigation establishes that all of these individuals developed symptoms following consumption of hamburgers from the same fast-food restaurant chain. Although other individuals ate the same hamburgers, they did not report any symptoms.

22. Which of the following tests is the best to detect the most likely etiologic agent of this outbreak?

a. Gram stain of stool specimens
b. Immunoassay for Shiga toxin-producing *Escherichia coli*
c. Polymerase chain reaction (PCR) for *Campylobacter*
d. Serologic testing for *Salmonella enterica* antibodies
e. Stool culture

23. The clinical laboratory is trying to develop a molecular assay to detect the suspected agent. Nucleotide primers are available for the virulence gene. Which of the following molecular methods is best and the most rapid for detecting this gene in the stool sample?

a. DNA sequencing
b. Dot blot hybridization
c. PCR
d. Real-time PCR
e. Southern blot hybridization

24. An outbreak of a diarrhea is suspected to be related to hamburgers that were served at a fast food restaurant. Stool cultures from the patrons and the food handlers were positive for *Salmonella*. To assess if the outbreak was caused by a specific *Salmonella* strain, investigators obtained chromosomal DNA from the isolated strains, purified the DNA samples, and digested the samples with *Xba*I, a restriction enzyme that produces large DNA fragments. The results are shown in the below figure. What molecular technique was used to produce these results?

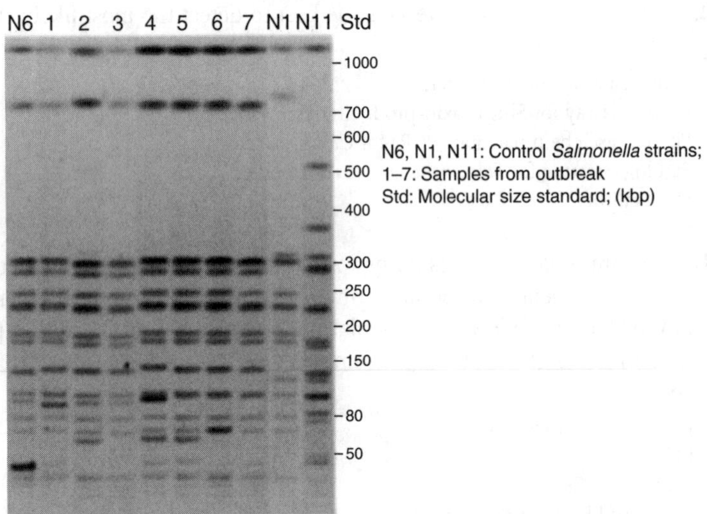

(Modified from Egorova S, Timinouni M, Demartin M, et al. Ceftriaxone-resistant Salmonella enterica *serotype Newport, France. Emerg Infect Dis 2008. http://wwwnc.cdc.gov/eid/article/14/6/07-1168.htm; accessed* 01-09-2013.*)*

a. Cloning
b. PCR
c. Pulsed-field gel electrophoresis
d. Sodium dodecyl sulfate polyacrylamide gel electrophoresis
e. Southern blot hybridization

25. Some of the *E. coli* bacteria that were originally isolated from a contaminated salad were tetracycline resistant while the others were susceptible. However, when tetracycline-resistant and -susceptible strains were grown together, all of them became tetracycline resistant. This efficient transfer of resistance depends on which of the following?

a. Cell lysis and the release of DNA from donor bacteria
b. Competent cells
c. Conjugative plasmids
d. Recombinase enzymes
e. Transposons

26. A high school-aged young woman presented to her family physician with what appeared to be an acute uncomplicated UTI. She was treated with a β-lactam antimicrobial, but her symptoms persisted. *E. coli* was isolated from the infection, but many of the organisms appeared Gram-stain variable and rounded. The rounded forms were identified as spheroplasts. Which of the following statements about the *E. coli* cells shown in the microphotograph below is most characteristic of the organism observed in this infection?

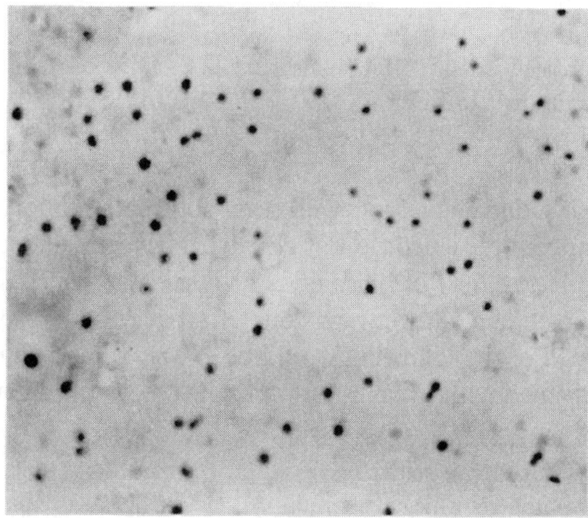

a. They are commonly referred to as endospores
b. They are osmotically stable
c. They resulted from treatment with the β-lactam
d. They have formed cell walls

27. A 3-year-old girl from a family that does not believe in immunization presents to the emergency room with a sore throat, fever, malaise, and difficulty breathing. A gray membrane covering the pharynx is observed on physical examination. *Corynebacterium diphtheriae* is confirmed as the etiologic agent of this infection. Which of the following is required to prove that *C. diphtheriae* is the etiologic agent of this child's infection?

a. Demonstration of cysteinase production
b. Isolation of *C. diphtheriae* from throat culture
c. Metachromatic granules seen on methylene blue stain
d. Pleomorphic gram-positive bacilli seen on Gram stain
e. Toxigenicity demonstrated by the Elek test

28. A 3-year-old girl from a day care center is brought to the local public health clinic because of a severe, intractable cough. During the previous 10 days, she had a persistent cold that had worsened. The cough developed the previous day and was so severe that vomiting frequently followed it. The child appears exhausted from the coughing episodes. A blood cell count shows a marked leukocytosis with a predominance of lymphocytes. Which of the following is most appropriate for diagnosis of this child's illness?

a. Culture alone
b. Culture plus PCR
c. Direct fluorescence assay (DFA) alone
d. DFA plus culture
e. PCR alone

29. A 55-year-old male presents with severe bilateral pulmonary infiltrate, elevated temperature, leucocytosis, elevated enzymes, and elevated creatine kinase. He and six of his friends had recently visited their favorite restaurant, which had a large water fountain that was misty on the day of his visit. Which of the following would be expected on a Gram stain that was counterstained with safranin for 3 minutes (prolonged counterstain)?

a. Strongly staining gram-positive bacilli
b. Weakly staining gram-positive bacilli
c. Strongly staining gram-negative bacilli
d. Weakly staining gram-negative bacilli
e. Strongly staining gram-negative cocci
f. Weakly staining gram-negative cocci

Questions 30 to 33

The following five growth curves are lettered (A to E) corresponding to an expected growth curve if certain antibiotics were added to an exponentially growing culture of *E. coli*. The arrow indicates when antibiotics were added to the growing culture.

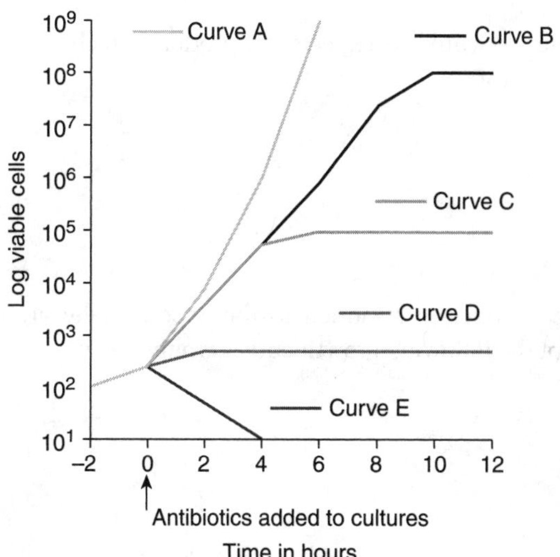

Growth curves in the presence or absence of antibiotics.

30. Penicillin treatment would be expected to produce which one of the following growth curves?

a. A
b. B
c. C
d. D
e. E

31. Chloramphenicol would be expected to produce which one of the following growth curves?

a. A
b. B
c. C
d. D
e. E

32. Sulfonamide would be expected to produce which one of the following growth curves?

a. A
b. B
c. C
d. D
e. E

33. If no antibiotics were added to the exponentially growing culture, which one of the following growth curves would result?

a. A
b. B
c. C
d. D
e. E

34. Several strains of *S. pneumoniae* are isolated from various patients. Some demonstrate high virulence while others appear to be nonvirulent. Mixing these cultures in the laboratory causes the nonvirulent strains to become pathogenic in laboratory animal experiments. Uptake by a recipient cell of soluble DNA released from a donor cell is defined as which of the following?

a. Conjugation
b. Frameshift mutation
c. Homologous recombination
d. Transduction
e. Transformation

35. A nonspore-forming, gram-positive bacillus was isolated from a throat specimen from a primary school-aged child who had not been vaccinated with the DTaP vaccine. The strain isolated carried a bacteriophage on which the gene for toxin was encoded. How did this strain become toxigenic?

a. Conjugation
b. Frameshift mutation
c. Homologous recombination
d. Transduction
e. Transformation

36. An increase in antibiotic resistance has been observed in *Staphylococcus aureus*, *Pseudomonas aeruginosa*, and *E. coli* strains isolated from patients in medical centers. Direct transfer of a plasmid between two bacteria is defined as which of the following?

a. Conjugation
b. Frameshift mutation
c. Homologous recombination
d. Transduction
e. Transformation

37. *E. coli* has a doubling time of 30 minutes in human urine at room temperature. A patient had 1000 bacteria per mL of urine when a urine specimen was collected. How many bacteria would be present if the specimen sat at room temperature for 4 hours before being plated for culture in the laboratory?

a. 4000
b. 16,000
c. 64,000
d. 256,000
e. 512,000

38. A 24-year-old female presented with pain during urination. Gram stain of the uncentrifuged urine revealed the presence of gram-negative rods. What virulence factor is essential for the survival of these uropathogenic bacteria in the urinary tract?

a. Pili
b. LPS (endotoxin)
c. Heat labile toxin
d. Flagella
e. Capsule

39. A 30-year-old hospitalized patient with an intravenous (IV) catheter developed fever and systemic infection. The source of the infection was bacteria that contaminated the catheter during its insertion. The IV catheter had to be removed because the bacteria grew within the catheter forming a biofilm. Biofilm development depends on the ability of the bacteria to produce which of the following?

a. Endotoxin
b. Periplasm
c. Polysaccharides
d. Porins
e. Teichoic acid

40. A 55-year-old British teacher presents with weight loss, weakness, muscle atrophy, and declining cognitive function. Her history reveals that her favorite meal is soup made with cow brain, which she has eaten almost every week since she was 10 years old. Which of the following best describes the most likely etiologic agent of her symptoms?

a. Abnormally folded protein
b. Capsid containing DNA
c. Enveloped capsid containing RNA
d. Multicellular cyst-forming organism
e. Unicellular organism with one chromosome

41. Over 200 isoniazid-resistant strains of *Mycobacterium tuberculosis* isolated from different patients in the northwestern region of Russia are screened by a PCR-restriction fragment length polymorphism assay. This analysis reveals a 93.6% prevalence of a specific G to C mutation in the *katG* in strains from patients with both newly and previously diagnosed cases of tuberculosis. Which of the following best describes the type of mutation that resulted in isoniazid resistance in these strains?

a. Deletion
b. Inversion
c. Missense
d. Nonsense
e. Transversion replacement

42. Seven closely related isolates of *Candida albicans* exhibited progressive decreases in susceptibility to posaconazole. Sequencing of the gene involved in azole resistance in these strains revealed predicted proteins with single amino acid changes. Which of the following best describes the type of mutation that has resulted in decreased susceptibility to posaconazole in these strains?

a. Deletion
b. Inversion
c. Missense
d. Nonsense
e. Transversion replacement

43. A 25-year-old man presents to the emergency room with several red, swollen, tender bite wounds on both arms that he stated occurred yesterday when he rescued his dog from a dogfight involving three other dogs, whose owner(s) is unknown. His right wrist and left elbow are also swollen and there is axillary lymphadenopathy on the left side. Gram stain of purulent material from the worst wound shows small gram-negative pleomorphic coccobacilli. The patient reports his last tetanus vaccination was 2 years ago. In addition to antibiotics, which of the following should be included in this patient's treatment?

a. Hepatitis B virus prophylaxis
b. IV immunoglobulins (nonspecific)
c. Rabies prophylaxis
d. Tetanus prophylaxis
e. Varicella-zoster prophylaxis

44. A patient presents to the emergency room with vomiting, diarrhea, high fever, and delirium. Upon physical examination, you notice large buboes, which are painful on palpation, and purpura and ecchymoses suggestive of disseminated intravascular coagulation. Gram stain on aspirate of a bubo reveals gram-negative rods with bipolar staining. Which of the following antibiotics is the drug of choice for empiric therapy?

a. Ceftazidime
b. Chloramphenicol
c. Penicillin
d. Streptomycin
e. Vancomycin

45. A 3-year-old girl who has missed several scheduled immunizations presents to the emergency room with a high fever. She is irritable and has a stiff neck. Fluid from a spinal tap reveals 20,000 white blood cells per milliliter with 85% polymorphonuclear cells. Which of the following is the drug of choice for empiric therapy against organisms of childhood meningitis?

a. Ceftriaxone
b. Erythromycin
c. Gentamicin
d. Penicillin
e. Vancomycin

46. During the course of his hospital stay, a severely burned 60-year-old male develops a rapidly disseminating bacterial infection. Small gram-negative rods that are oxidase positive are cultured from green pus taken from the burn tissue. Which combination of antibiotics is the best choice for empiric therapy against this etiologic agent?

a. Ceftazidime plus vancomycin
b. Erythromycin plus imipenem
c. Penicillin plus gentamicin
d. Piperacillin/tazobactam plus cephalothin
e. Ticarcillin/clavulanate plus tobramycin

47. Laboratory results of a clinical specimen from a patient with hospital-acquired pneumonia reveal the presence of methicillin-resistant *Staphylococcus aureus* (MRSA). Which of the following drugs is the best empiric treatment?

a. Ceftazidime
b. Dicloxacillin
c. Penicillin
d. Tobramycin
e. Vancomycin

48. A young, essentially healthy woman was concerned about her loss of job time due to recurrent UTIs. Her physician prescribed an antibiotic, which would control microbial nucleotide synthesis by inhibiting dihydrofolic acid reductase in bacteria up to 50,000 times more than in mammalian cells. Which of the following agents work by this mechanism?

a. Ampicillin
b. Amphotericin
c. Chloramphenicol
d. Levofloxacin
e. Trimethoprim

49. A 52-year-old woman presents with fever of 103°F, headache, right flank pain, nausea and vomiting, and urinary frequency with hematuria and dysuria. Renal ultrasound demonstrates a right urinary stone with right hydronephrosis. Which of the following antibiotics is the most appropriate treatment option?

a. Ampicillin
b. Amphotericin
c. Chloramphenicol
d. Penicillin
e. Trimethoprim/sulfamethoxazole

50. A 75-year-old African American male with neurogenic bladder presents to the emergency room with hypertension, fever up to 104.6°F, and nausea and vomiting. The urine from his foley catheter gives a positive culture for an antibiotic-resistant strain of *Enterococcus faecalis*. He had previously been given an antibiotic that binds to D-alanine-D-alanine. To which of the following antibiotics is this isolate most likely resistant?

a. Ampicillin
b. Amphotericin
c. Chloramphenicol
d. Levofloxacin
e. Vancomycin

51. A patient with leukemia has a chest CT finding that suggests aspergillosis. Which of the following antimicrobials affects ergosterol synthesis and would most likely be used in this patient's treatment?

a. Amphotericin B
b. Caspofungin
c. Griseofulvin
d. Micafungin
e. Voriconazole

52. A 6-year-old girl is diagnosed with meningitis. A lumbar puncture reveals numerous neutrophils and gram-negative diplococci. She is admitted to the hospital for antibiotic treatment, which is complicated by the fact that she is known to be allergic to β-lactams. What is the mechanism of action of the alternative drug of choice to treat this infant's meningitis?

a. Blocks tRNA binding to the A site
b. Causes misreading of mRNA
c. Inhibits formation of the peptide bond
d. Prevents translocation
e. Results in premature termination

53. A clinical laboratory performs real-time PCR for detection of MRSA in the area where specimens are plated. The supervisor discovers that the last 50 specimens tested were positive. However, companion cultures were positive for only 15 of the specimens. What is the most likely reason for this discrepancy?

a. Real-time PCR is more sensitive than culture
b. Real-time PCR is more specific than culture
c. The PCR instrument needs to be calibrated
d. The PCR workstation has been contaminated with MRSA DNA

54. Guests at a party consumed beef broth that was boiled earlier in the day but left at room temperature for several hours. The individuals presented with symptoms of food poisoning, including watery diarrhea and abdominal cramps, 8 to 10 hours later. The symptoms lasted 24 hours. The agent that caused the symptoms is most likely which of the following?

a. Spore-forming gram-positive bacilli
b. Gram-positive cocci
c. Gram-negative bacilli
d. An opportunistic fungus
e. An enteric virus

55. A 25-year-old male presented with severe urethritis. Over the past 2 days, he had developed fever and chills. Gram stain of the urethral discharge revealed the presence of gram-negative diplococci. The fever and chills are most likely due to the release of excessive amounts of which bacterial component?

a. Capsule
b. Exotoxin
c. Lipooligosaccharide (LOS)
d. Opacity protein
e. Pili

56. A 2-year-old had been treated three times with ampicillin for acute otitis media. Fluid aspirated from his middle ear during placement of tympanostomy tubes grows *Moraxella catarrhalis*, which is resistant to ampicillin. Which enzyme is responsible for this resistance?

a. Acetyltransferase
b. β-Lactamase
c. Catalase
d. DNase
e. Phosphotransferase

57. A patient admitted to surgical intensive care for dehiscence of her surgical incision was screened for MRSA by PCR for the *mecA* gene. Nasal, rectal, and wound swabs were submitted for testing. The nasal and wound samples were positive for MRSA by PCR; however, the wound culture grew *Staphylococcus epidermidis* but no MRSA. What is the most likely reason for the discrepancy in the results of testing on the wound samples?

a. The culture was performed improperly
b. The PCR was contaminated
c. The *S. epidermidis* isolate carries the *mecA* gene
d. The wrong primers were used in the PCR

58. *Neisseria meningitidis*, group B, is identified as the cause of a local meningitis outbreak in a military training camp. Which of the following protects this organism from complement-mediated phagocytosis by neutrophils?

a. Opacity proteins
b. Polysaccharide capsule
c. Pili
d. Lipooligosaccharide
e. Catalase

59. A child attending classes in a preschool is noted by his teacher to have several skin lesions on his arms. The lesions are pustular in appearance and some have broken down and are covered with a yellow crust. Which of the following protects the most likely etiologic agent of this child's infection from phagocytosis and provides serologic specificity?

a. Erythrogenic toxin
b. Hyaluronic acid
c. Lipoteichoic acid
d. M protein
e. Streptolysin O

60. A pharmacologic compound intended for injection was contaminated with gram-negative bacilli during production. The product was filtered before packaging. Quality control cultures were sterile so the product was shipped for use. However, numerous persons who received the product developed fever and several developed hypotension. Which of the following was most likely responsible for the reaction observed in these patients?

a. Bacterial polysaccharides
b. Hyaluronic acid
c. Lipopolysaccharide
d. Protein toxin
e. Teichoic acid

61. A 64-year old female with a history of COPD visited her physician because of recent poor health symptoms, including cough, fever and night sweats, weakness, and 20-pound weight loss. Chest x-ray demonstrated a nodular infiltrate in the upper lobe. Laboratory staining of sputum revealed acid-fast organisms. Which characteristic of the most likely organism is responsible for this staining result?

a. Ergosterol
b. Glycolipids
c. Hyaluronic acid
d. Peptidoglycan
e. Teichoic acid

62. In 2001, a number of governmental offices received mailed envelopes that contained an unknown white powder. Several employees were contaminated and developed cutaneous and/or inhalational anthrax. Which of the following is responsible for the antiphagocytic properties of this organism?

a. D-glutamic acid capsule
b. Hyaluronic acid
c. Lethal factor
d. M protein
e. Protective antigen

63. Twelve elderly residents living in an assisted care facility suffered from sinusitis, otitis media, and mild pneumonias during midwinter. Despite the fact that they had all received the 13-valent pneumococcal conjugate vaccine recently licensed for adults, *S. pneumoniae* was isolated from 10 of the patients. Which of the following is the best explanation for the pneumococcal infections?

a. Elderly patients do not mount good immune responses to vaccines
b. Some patients will not respond to the vaccine
c. The capsular type responsible was not present in the vaccine
d. The vaccine was defective

Physiology and Molecular Microbiology

Answers

1. The answer is d. (*Katzung, Ch 43. Murray, Ch 17. Ryan, Ch 23.*) The structural integrity of the β-lactam ring in penicillins is essential for their antimicrobial activity. Many resistant strains of staphylococci produce a β-lactamase (penicillinase) that cleaves the β-lactam ring of penicillin at the carbon-nitrogen bond (4 in diagram). Other organisms, including coliform bacteria and *Pseudomonas*, produce cephalosporinases, metallo-β-lactamases, and carbapenamases that cleave the β-lactam rings of cephalosporins and/or carbapenems, as well as penicillins, at the same site. Penicillin amidase inactivates penicillin by disrupting the bond between the radical and nitrogen in the free amino group (1 in diagram). Bonds 2, 3, and 5 are not commonly broken by bacterial enzymes.

2. The answer is d. (*Katzung, Ch 45. Murray, Ch 13. Ryan, Ch 21, 23.*) Aminoglycosides passively diffuse across the outer membrane of gram-negative bacteria through porins. The passage of aminoglycosides into the cytoplasm is an active process dependent on oxidative phosphorylation (d). Facilitated diffusion (a) involves specific protein carriers. Group translocation (c) occurs in the absence of oxygen. Fermentation (b) is a mechanism for production of energy. Transpeptidation (e) is a reaction involving the transfer of one or more amino acids from one peptide chain to another, or in the addition of amino acids to the growing peptide chain during translation.

3. The answer is b. (*Murray, Ch 12, 26. Ryan, Ch 21, 30.*) Unlike *E. coli*, *Salmonella*, *Pseudomonas*, and other gram-negative bacilli, *Neisseria gonorrhoeae* does not produce siderophores (e). Instead the pathogenic *Neisseria* obtain iron through surface receptors that interact with lactoferrin (b) and transferrin, host molecules that sequester iron. Ferric oxide (a) is produced by some environmental bacteria. LPS (c) does not play a role in the iron uptake or metabolism of the bacteria. Pyocyanin (d) is a blue redox pigment produced by *P. aeruginosa* that can generate reactive oxygen intermediates and affect the electron transport chain and vesicular transport of eukaryotic cells.

4. The answer is c. (*Murray, Ch 12. Ryan, Ch 21.*) The periplasm is the space between the outer membrane and the cytoplasmic membrane of gram-negative bacteria. The periplasmic space (c) in *E. coli* has been shown to contain enzymes involved in transport, degradation, and synthesis, including β-lactamase. The other structures are labeled in the diagram above (capsule—A; outer membrane—B; cytoplasmic membrane—D; cytoplasm). The chromosome and other structures found within or on the cell surface, such as the flagellum and pilus present in the diagram, were not indicated among the choices.

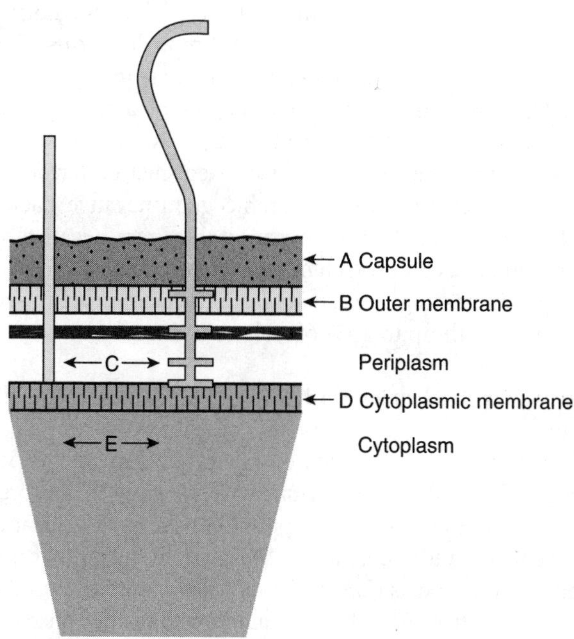

5. The answer is e. (*Murray, Ch 13. Ryan, Ch 21.*) Toxic oxygen radicals, superoxide and hydrogen peroxide, are generated during aerobic metabolism. Superoxide dismutase (e) catalyzes the reaction that detoxifies superoxide ($2O_2^- + 2H^+ \rightarrow H_2O_2 + O_2$). Both catalase (b) and peroxidase (d) detoxify hydrogen peroxide, but peroxidases also act on lipid peroxides. The reaction catalyzed by catalase is $2H_2O_2 \rightarrow 2H_2O + O_2$. ATPase (a) converts ATP into ADP plus a free phosphate ion. Permeases (d) are membrane transport proteins that facilitate the passage of specific molecules across into or out of the cell.

6. The answer is e. (*Katzung, Ch 44-46. Murray, Ch 13, 38. Ryan, Ch 21, 29.*) The etiologic agent of this man's infection is an anaerobe, most likely *Bacteroides fragilis*. Ampicillin (a) is unlikely to be successful as most isolates of *B. fragilis* produce β-lactamase. Chloramphenicol (b) is rarely used in the United States because of its toxicity, although it is used for treatment of serious rickettsial infection such as Rocky Mountain spotted fever and as an alternative for treatment of bacterial meningitis in patients who have hypersensitivity to penicillins and cephalosporins. Ciprofloxacin (c), a fluoroquinolone antibiotic, has no spectrum of activity against anaerobes. Oxygen is necessary for transport of aminoglycosides like gentamicin (d) into the bacterial cell; thus, they have no spectrum of activity against anaerobes. Of the drugs listed, metronidazole (e) is the best choice for infections with anaerobic gram-negative bacilli. Additional antibiotics with activity against anaerobic gram-negative bacilli are carbapenems and β-lactam/β-lactamase inhibitor combinations. *Bacteroides* has become increasingly resistant to clindamycin, which used to be a good alternative, with up to 25% of isolates now resistant.

7. The answer is d. (*Murray, Ch 13. Ryan, Ch 21.*) Superoxide dismutase is an enzyme found in both prokaryotic and eukaryotic cells that can survive in an environment of O_2. Lack of this enzyme, as well as peroxidase and catalase, ensures that a bacterium will not grow in the presence of O_2, making it an anaerobe (d). Capnophiles (a) prefer an atmosphere with increased CO_2 and ambient O_2; *Haemophilus ducreyi* is capnophilic. Microaerophiles (c) such as *Campylobacter jejuni* prefer increased CO_2 and reduced O_2. Facultative anaerobes (b) can grow in the presence or absence of O_2. Obligate aerobes (e), such as *Mycobacterium tuberculosis*, require O_2 for growth unless they can utilize an alternative terminal electron acceptor.

8. The answer is e. (*Murray, Ch 15. Ryan, Ch 64. Workowski & Berman, sections on diagnosis.*) The microbes that cause genital ulcers are *Chlamydia trachomatis* LGV serovars 1 to 3, *Haemophilus ducreyi*, herpes simplex virus types 1 and 2, *Klebsiella granulomatis*, and *Treponema pallidum*. The various methods for diagnosis are outlined in the below table. *Treponema pallidum* (e) can be demonstrated by darkfield microscopy in primary and secondary syphilitic lesions.

Organism	Disease	Lesion	Inguinal Lymphadenopathy	Method for Diagnosis
Chlamydia trachomatis LGV	Lymphogranuloma venereum	Small ulcer or papule Painless Usually healed at presentation	Discrete swollen nodes Progressing to suppuration, draining fistulas	Special culture Serology
Haemophilus ducreyi	Chancroid	Separate shallow nonindurated ulcers Painful	Suppurative	Special culture
Herpes simplex virus	Genital herpes	Multiple clustered vesicles to coalesced ulcers Painful	Tender, discrete nodes Nonsuppurative	Viral culture Immunofluorescence PCR
Klebsiella granulomatis	Granuloma inguinale	Papular or nodular ulcerative lesion or lesions Painless	Induration of subcutaneous tissue in inguinal area	Giemsa stain of biopsy
Treponema pallidum	Syphilis	Single ulcer at primary presentation; indurated Usually painless	Rubbery nodes	Darkfield exam Immunofluorescence Serology

9. The answer is a. (*Murray, Ch 15. Ryan, Ch 64. Workowski & Berman, sections on diagnosis.*) See the table above. Culture (a) is the best method to prove *infectivity*. However, viral culture decreases in sensitivity as the lesions begin to heal, so nucleic acid amplification testing or PCR (d) is increasingly used. PCR detects viral DNA, which may be present in noninfective particles. Because herpes simplex is shed intermittently upon reactivation, negative culture or PCR does not rule out latent infection. Viral antigens, detected by direct immunofluorescent assay (c) (or enzyme immunoassay), may be present after infectious particles have been neutralized or disrupted by antivirals. Cytologic detection by Tzanck smear (e) of genital lesions or cervical Pap smear is insensitive and nonspecific and should not be relied upon. Serologic detection (b) using tests that are type-specific may be used in cases or recurrent genital symptoms or atypical symptoms with negative culture; clinical diagnosis of genital herpes without laboratory confirmation, or a partner with genital herpes. Screening of the general population should not be done.

10. The answer is c. (*Murray, Ch 12, 14, 26. Ryan, Ch 21, 22, 30.*) The vignette and figure detail a typical case of *Neisseria gonorrhoeae*. Bacteria may shift rapidly between the fimbriated (fim +) and the nonfimbriated (fim–) states. Fimbriae function as adhesions to specific surfaces and, consequently, play a major role in pathogenesis. Lack of fimbriae prevents colonization of the mucosal surface by the bacterium (c). Pili (fimbriae) are hairlike appendages that extend several millimeters from the gonococcal surface. Fim changes would have no effect on capsule presence (a) or loss of serologic specificity (d). Such changes would not cause the death of the organism (b), and *Neisseria* organisms never revert to a gram-positive staining result (e) due to the major differences found in the structures of gram-positive and gram-negative cell walls.

11. The answer is e. (*Levinson, Ch 2. Murray, Ch 12, 27. Ryan, Ch 21, 33.*) LPS, a component of the outer membrane of gram-negative microorganisms consists of three regions: lipid A, which forms the outer leaflet of the lipid bilayer outer membrane; the core polysaccharide; and the O-antigen polysaccharide (e) side chain that confers serospecificity or serotype for the Enterbacteriaceae. Strains that have lost the O antigen cannot be serotpyed. Flagella (b) confer the H antigens, which are also used in the typing of *Salmonella* strains after the O typing; strains that have lost flagella cannot be H-typed. The capsule (a) confers the K antigen; pili (d) can be conjugative or be involved in motility or adhesion (usually called fimbriae). Neither the K antigens nor the pilus- nor fimbria-related antigens are utilized in the serotyping of *Salmonella* for epidemiologic purposes. The mannose receptor (c) is found on macrophages and used by them to characterize pathogenic microbes in the host innate response.

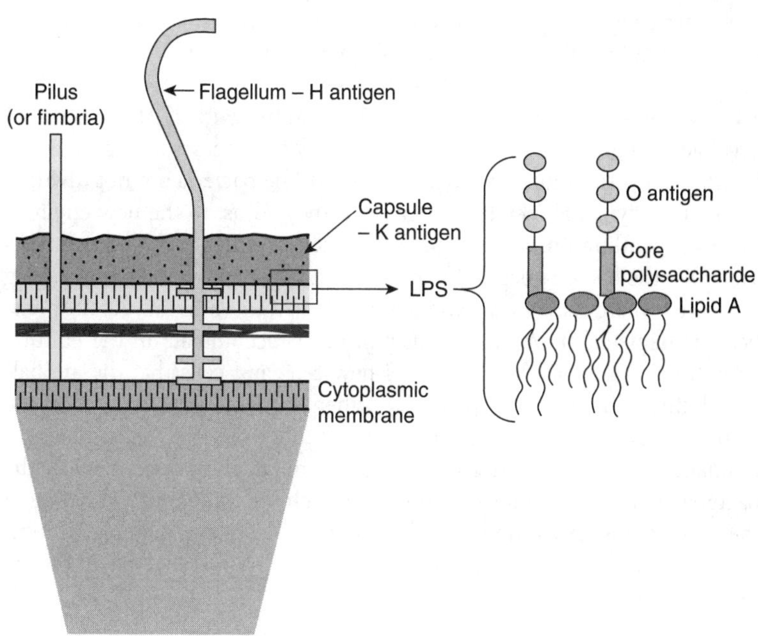

12. The answer is c. (*Levinson, Ch 10, 11. Murray, Ch 17. Ryan, Ch 23.*) Transpeptidases, or penicillin-binding proteins (PBPs) (c), are inactivated when bound to penicillin. Altered PBPs no longer bind the β-lactam antibiotic. The acquisition of a new PBP or modification of the existing one is the mechanism by which *S. pneumoniae*, the most likely etiologic of this child's meningitis, become resistant to β-lactams. Altered PBPs are also seen in *N. gonorrhoeae*, *S. aureus*, and other bacteria. Bactoprenol (a) is not known to be involved in antibiotic resistance. Fluoroquinolones target the DNA gyrase (b), while rifamycins target the bacterial RNA polymerase (e). Bacteria do not utilize reverse transcriptase (d).

13. The answer is a. (*Murray, Ch 12, 21. Ryan, Ch 21, 26.*) The vignette presents a case of cutaneous anthrax. Anthrax is acquired by cutaneous introduction, ingestion, or inhalation of endospores from contaminated animals such as cattle, sheep, and goats. Inhibition of dipicolinic acid synthesis would prevent formation of bacterial spores (a), but would not affect vegetative cells (b, e). Mycobacteria do not form spores. Dipicolinic acid is not found in fungal arthrospores (c) or microconidia (d).

14. The answer is a. (*Levinson, Ch 3, 10. Murray, 13, 17. Ryan, 21, 23.*) The bacterial growth cycle is characterized by four phases as shown in the figure for this question. In the lag phase (a), the bacteria are not dividing but exhibit dynamic metabolic activity as they adjust to the new environment. Depending on the species and the temperature, pH, and nutrients available, the bacteria begin dividing within a few hours and enter the log phase (b) where they grow exponentially for 12 to 18 hours. As nutrients become depleted and/or toxic waste products accumulate in the culture, growth slows so that the number of new cells and cells that die are balanced; this is the stationary phase (c). When nutrients are exhausted or the culture medium becomes too toxic, the number of viable cells decreases dramatically; this is the death phase (d). Similar phases occur when the bacteria are introduced into the host, although the timing may vary due to the specific host environment and the host defenses encountered. Antibiotics that affect the cell wall, such as β-lactams, are not effective in the lag phase (a).

15. The answer is b. (*Levinson, Ch 3, 10. Murray, Ch 13, 17. Ryan, Ch 21, 23.*) Aminoglycosides exert three effects on protein synthesis: (1) block initiation of translation, (2) cause incorporation of incorrect amino acids into the growing peptide chain, and (3) elicit premature termination of translation. Protein synthesis occurs throughout the growth cycle, but optimum effectiveness of aminoglycosides is seen in the log phase (b).

16. The answer is c. (*Levinson, Ch 18. Murray, Ch 18. Ryan, Ch 33.*) Differentiation of the gram-negative bacilli that cause gastroenteritis begins with aerobic (Enterobacteriaceae and *Vibrio*) versus microaerophilic (b) (*Campylobacter*) growth. Morphology on a lactose-containing selective agar such as MacConkey agar separates *Salmonella* and *Shigella*, which do not ferment lactose (a), whereas *E. coli* and *Vibrio* do. *Shigella* can be differentiated from *Salmonella* on agar containing iron; *Shigella* do not produce H_2S (c) while *Salmonella* do. *Vibrio* species are oxidase positive (d); the Enterobacteriaceae are not. Urease production (e) distinguishes *Proteus* spp. from *Salmonella*.

17. The answer is a. (*Katzung, Ch 43, 45, 48.*) Penicillin (d) is well-tolerated as is itraconazole (c). Vancomycin (e) is irritating and can result in phlebitis at the site of injection; nephrotoxicity of aminoglycosides is exacerbated by concomitant use of vancomycin, but can be controlled by careful dosage. Gentamicin (b) and other aminoglycosides are ototoxic and nephrotoxic, but these adverse effects can usually be controlled by monitoring of serum concentration and careful dosage. Bacitracin (a) is highly nephrotoxic, so much so that it cannot be administered systemically. Because bacitracin is poorly absorbed, it can be used topically, providing local antibacterial activity but no systemic toxicity.

18. The answer is b. (*Levinson, Ch 2. Murray, Ch 4. Ryan, Ch 4.*) First described in 1884 by a Danish physician, Hans Christian Gram, the Gram stain has proved to be one of the most useful diagnostic laboratory procedures in microbiology and medicine. The Gram stain procedure is characterized by the following steps: (1) *fixation* of the bacteria to the slide, (2) crystal violet (acridine dye) treatment, (3) iodine treatment, (4) *decolorization* using alcohol/acetone wash, and (4) *counterstaining* using safranin. Gram-positive bacteria have thick outer walls with no lipids, whereas gram-negative bacteria have a thin wall and an outer membrane. The difference between gram-positive and gram-negative organisms is in the cell-wall permeability to these complexes on treatment with mixtures of acetone and alcohol solvents. Thus, gram-positive bacteria retain purple iodine-dye complexes, whereas gram-negative bacteria do not retain these complexes when decolorized using an alcohol/acetone wash.

19. The answer is d. (*Levinson, Ch 2. Murray, Ch 4. Ryan, Ch 4.*) If the iodine treatment step is omitted during the Gram stain process, the purple iodine-dye complexes will not form. The crystal violet will wash away during the alcohol/acetone decolorization washing step and all cells will appear *red* (d). Gram staining of pus or fluids along with clinical findings can guide the management of an infection before culture results are available in the clinical setting.

20. The answer is e. (*Levinson, Ch 11. Ryan, Ch 21.*) Porins are protein trimers that function in outer-membrane (OM) permeability. Porins permit the transfer of molecules across the OM (e) including the passage of many antimicrobial drugs such as the fluoroquinolones. Porins participate in multidrug-resistance efflux pumps that export drugs like ciprofloxacin from the cell. Porins play no role in the metabolism required for hydrolysis of antimicrobials (a), metabolism of metabolic intermediates (b), serologic stabilization of the O antigen (c), or inactivation of hydrophobic antimicrobials (d).

21. The answer is d. (*Levinson, Ch 24. Murray, Ch 39. Ryan, Ch 37.*) The diagnosis of Lyme disease is complicated. Early Lyme disease (a) (3-30 days post-tick bite) is usually diagnosed clinically. IgM specific for *Borrelia burgdorferi* appears between 2 and 4 weeks after the lesions, peaks at 4 to 6 weeks, and disappears (returns to baseline) by 4 to 6 months. Specific IgG usually appears after 30 days and lasts as long as disease persists. Early disseminated Lyme (b) (days to weeks post-tick bite) is diagnosed by clinical suspicion, likelihood of exposure, and serology. A positive screening EIA (enzyme immunoassay) or IFA (immunofluorescence assay) for specific IgM and/or IgG, depending on timing, followed by a positive western blot is diagnostic. Late disseminated Lyme disease (c) can also be diagnosed serologically by detection of high levels of specific IgG on screening and positive IgG western blot. Patients with neuroborreliosis usually have specific IgG in the CSF. A positive western blot for Lyme disease requires the presence of at least 5 of 10 specific bands for *B. burgdorferi*: 18, 21 (OspC), 28, 30, 39 (BmpA), 41 (Fla), 45, 58 (not GroEL), 66, and 93 kDa. The pattern shown in the figure shows only one antibody-positive band, which is also present with the *B. turicatae* proteins. This indicates nonspecific reactivity (d). There is no need to repeat the screening test (e); other diagnoses for the patient's arthritis should be considered. http://www.cdc.gov/lyme/diagnosistreatment/LabTest/TwoStep/WesternBlot/

22. The answer is b. (*Levinson, Ch 9, 18. Murray, Ch 5, 27. Ryan, Ch 4, 33.*) The vignette strongly suggests that the patients were infected with a Shiga toxin-producing strain of *E. coli* (STEC). While culture on selective and differential agar can detect the presence of O157 STEC, as well as *Salmonella* and *Shigella*, stools should simultaneously be assayed for non-O157 STEC with a test that detects the Shiga toxin or the genes encoding these toxins (recommendation for identification of STEC by clinical laboratories). Culture (e) will not detect non-O157 STEC strains. Gram stain (a) would show the presence of fecal leukocytes, but cannot be used to determine the presence or absence of a particular species of gram-negative bacilli. PCR for *Campylobacter* (c) and serologic testing for *Salmonella enterica* antibodies (d) are not relevant to the case presentation. The immunoassay (EIA) for Shiga toxin-producing *E. coli* (b) is the test that will detect all strains. Because the amount of free fecal Shiga toxin in stools is often low, EIA testing of enrichment broth cultures incubated overnight is recommended rather than direct testing of stool specimens, although testing of both specimens can be done.

23. The answer is d. (*Murray, Ch 5.*) Using a DNA sequence as a template, polymerase chain reaction (PCR) (c) converts few copies of the DNA template into a million copies. Among the different applications of PCR is the diagnosis of infectious diseases. Using a heat stable DNA polymerase and short DNA segments that are complementary to the target DNA (primers), the reaction amplifies the target DNA through series of melting, annealing, and extension steps in which the complementary DNA strands are synthesized. The high sensitivity of PCR permits the detection of extremely small amount DNA within the sample. Besides its sensitivity, the assay is rapid and may detect viral DNA before the onset of the disease. The final step, which includes running the amplified product on agarose gel to visualize it, is time-consuming and not very practical for clinical settings. This disadvantage was eliminated by real-time PCR (d) in which the synthesized DNA is detected and quantified as the PCR reaction progresses in real time. The technique uses a reporter signal, a fluorescence labeled probe. The intensity of the detected fluorescence signal, which correlates with the amount of the amplified DNA target, allows detection of the PCR product earlier and eliminates the need for running the final product on agarose gel. Compared with real-time PCR, Southern blot hybridization (e) and dot blot hybridization (b) are time-consuming, require larger amount of DNA, and are not practical for clinical settings. DNA sequencing (a) analysis is an additional step that may be used to confirm the identity of the DNA amplified by PCR. It will not help in the initial diagnosis.

PCR assays to detect the *stx1* and *stx2* genes are used by many public health laboratories for diagnosis and confirmation of STEC infection. Depending on the primers used, these assays can distinguish between *stx1* and *stx2*. Most of these PCR assays are designed and validated for testing isolated colonies taken from plated media; some assays have been validated for testing on stool specimens subcultured to an enrichment broth and incubated for 18 to 24 hours. Currently, Shiga toxin PCR assays on DNA extracted from whole stool specimens are not recommended because the sensitivity is low. DNA-based Shiga toxin gene detection is not approved by FDA for diagnosis of human STEC infections by clinical laboratories.

24. The answer is c. (*Murray, Ch 5.*) Conventional agarose gel electrophoresis, in which the current runs in only one direction, is capable of separating and resolving DNA fragments no larger than 30 kbp in size. In contrast, pulsed-field gel electrophoresis (PFGE) (c) extends the size range of the resolved DNA molecules up to 5 Mbp. In PFGE, chromosomal DNA is extracted without shearing. The DNA is then digested with restriction enzymes that cut only in few places, thereby generating large DNA fragments. The fragments are separated on agarose gels by electrophoresis in which the direction of the voltage is periodically switched (pulsed). Each pulse continues for several hours allowing the separation of the large DNA fragments. PFGE is frequently used in epidemiological studies of bacterial pathogens to identify the specific strain (subtype) that caused the outbreak of food poisoning. PCR (b) and Southern blot hybridization (e) are capable of identifying a strain, such as *Listeria* or *Salmonella*, by determining specific genes within the strain but are not capable of identifying the subtype. Sodium dodecyl sulfate polyacrylamide gel electrophoresis is (d) designed to separate proteins produced by the bacteria. The subtypes are unlikely to produce different proteins. Cloning (a) is inserting a DNA fragment in a cloning vector for further analysis of the gene carried on that fragment. It will not define the bacterial subtypes.

25. The answer is c. (*Murray, Ch 13. Hartwell, Ch 14.*) Many antibiotic resistance genes in bacteria are carried on conjugative plasmids (c) also known as R factors. These plasmids are transferred from one bacterium to another, of the same or related species, by conjugation. Conjugation is a process by which the donor bacterium (male cell) is brought in direct contact with the recipient bacterium (female cell) through the conjugative pilus. In *E. coli*, the conjugative pilus is referred to as a sex pilus or F pilus. The conjugative plasmid carries genes necessary for its transfer including the pilus genes. The plasmid is transferred into the recipient cell as a strand of ssDNA, which recircularizes within the recipient cell. The complementary DNA strand is then synthesized in the recipient cell. The ssDNA in the donor cell is also replicated; thus, both the donor and the recipient now carry a copy of the plasmid. Due to the direct contact between bacteria through the pilus, conjugation is an efficient process of DNA transfer. A transposon (e) is a mobile genetic element that is capable of moving from one replicon (a chromosome or a plasmid) to another but is incapable of initiating DNA transfer. Recombinase enzymes (d) are required for the recombination process that occurs between homologous regions of DNA (as in integration of a DNA in a replicon). Competent cells (b) are part of the bacterial population that is capable of taking up DNA from a solution (naked DNA). This may occur naturally or artificially (in the laboratory). *E. coli* competent cells are only generated in the laboratory through treatment with certain chemicals. Cell lysis and release of donor DNA (a) may be part of a mechanism through which naturally competent bacteria such as *Neisseria* take up naked DNA during infection.

26. The answer is c. (*Brooks, pp 30, 161, 348. Levinson, pp 8-9, 89. Ryan, p 19.*) The organisms illustrated in the question are spheroplasts of *E. coli*. Lysozyme cleaves the β-1-4-glycosidic bond between *N*-acetylmuramic acid and *N*-acetylglucosamine. Spheroplasts are bacteria with cell walls that have been partially removed by the action of lysozyme or penicillin. Ordinarily, with disintegration of the walls, the cells undergo lysis; however, in a hypertonic medium, the cells persist and assume a spherical configuration. Endospores are formed by gram-positive bacteria in the genera *Bacillus* and *Clostridium*. It has also been shown that for *E. coli* and other gram-negative rods, exposure to minimal concentrations of antibiotics does not rupture the cell wall but promotes elongation of the cell by inhibiting the division cycle.

27. The answer is e. (*Levinson, Ch 17. Murray, Ch 14, 23. Ryan, Ch 26.*) The vignette describes a child with diphtheria. The finding of pleomorphic gram-positive bacilli on Gram stain (d) or demonstration of metachromatic granules by methylene blue stain (c) are suggestive that *C. diphtheriae* might be present. Culture for *C. diphtheriae* requires a special medium containing tellurite, such as Tinsdale agar. *C. diphtheriae* can be differentiated from other species of *Corynebacterium* by production of cysteinase (a), which causes the organism to produce colonies surrounded by a brown halo on this agar. However, isolation alone (b) is insufficient to prove that the strain caused diphtheria. Only toxigenic strains of *C. diphtheriae* cause diphtheria, so any isolate identified as *C. diphtheriae* must be tested for toxin production (e) using the Elek test. The toxin genes are carried on a lysogenic bacteriophage, and not all strains carry this phage. PCR can also be performed for the diphtheria toxin genes, but even this is not conclusive as these genes may not be expressed.

28. The answer is b. (*Levinson, Ch 19. Murray, Ch 32. Ryan, Ch 31.*) The vignette describes a child with pertussis caused by *Bordetella pertussis*. Culture of *B. pertussis* requires plating of a nasopharyngeal swab on special medium containing charcoal and blood with and without cephalexin for best result. The specimen must be collected before any antibiotics are given and the closer to onset of symptoms the better the result. However, culture alone (a) is not sufficiently sensitive. DFA is no longer recommended by the Centers for Disease Prevention and Control (CDC) due problems with both false positive and false negative tests, whether used alone (c) or with culture (d). PCR (e), which appeared at first to be more sensitive than culture, has been shown over the course of time to have about the same sensitivity as culture. Therefore, the best approach is to collect two swabs and use one for culture and one for PCR (b). Be aware there is great inconsistency in textbooks and reviews regarding the best methods for diagnosis of pertussis. The CDC is the best guide in this case.

29. The answer is d. (*Levinson, Ch 19. Murray, Ch 34. Ryan, Ch 34.*) The vignette describes a patient with legionellosis (also called Legionnaires disease). *Legionella* spp. are gram-negative bacilli that stain poorly if at all by traditional Gram stain. However, the organisms can be demonstrated by prolonged counterstaining with safranin for at least 3 minutes. Even with prolonged counterstain, the organisms still appear as weakly staining (very pale pink) gram-negative bacilli (d). The bacteria may appear coccoid, but should not be mistaken for gram-negative cocci (e, f). *Legionella* should not appear gram-positive (a, b) in a correctly performed Gram stain.

30. The answer is e. (*Katzung, Ch 43, 44, 46. Murray, Ch 13, 17. Ryan, Ch 21, 23.*) Penicillin causes lysis of growing bacterial cells. Because penicillin is bactericidal, the number of viable cells should fall immediately after introduction of the drug into the medium of an exponentially growing susceptible bacterial culture. This is represented by curve E (e).

31. The answer is d. (*Katzung, Ch 43, 44, 46. Murray, Ch 13, 17. Ryan, Ch 21, 23.*) Chloramphenicol is bacteriostatic; it causes an immediate, reversible inhibition of protein synthesis. Thus, chloramphenicol retards cell growth without causing cell death, as represented by curve D (d).

32. The answer is c. (*Katzung, Ch 43, 44, 46. Murray, Ch 13, 17. Ryan, Ch 21, 23.*) Sulfonamides are also bacteriostatic. However, sulfonamides act by competing with *para*-aminobenzoic acid in the synthesis of folate. Their effect is not apparent until intracellular stores of folate are depleted, so the inhibition is not apparent as quickly. This is represented by curve C (c).

33. The answer is b. (*Katzung, Ch 43, 44, 46. Murray, Ch 13, 17. Ryan, Ch 21, 23.*) The number of viable cells in a culture eventually will level off (reach stationary phase) even if no antibiotic is added to the environment. A key factor in this phenomenon is the limited availability of nutrients. This is represented by curve B (b). Curve A (a) is not physiologically possible for bacteria, which double their number at a constant (logarithmic) rate.

34. The answer is e. (*Levinson, Ch 4. Murray, Ch 13. Ryan, Ch 21.*) Transformation (e) is the term for uptake of exogenous or foreign DNA, which may be released from lysed cells or provided artificially in the laboratory. Conjugation (a) involves the direct passage of DNA from one bacterium (donor) to another (recipient) through a conjugative pilus (sex pilus). Transduction (d) is the transfer of DNA mediated by bacteriophages. Homologous recombination (c) may take place once DNA has entered the cell by conjugation or transformation if the closely related sequences exist on the chromosome and the exogenous DNA. A frameshift mutation (b) occurs when a small deletion or insertion (not in multiples of three) is made in a gene.

35. The answer is d. (*Levinson, Ch 4. Murray, Ch 13. Ryan, Ch 21.*) Transduction (d) is the transfer of DNA mediated by bacteriophages. In generalized transduction, the phage virus can carry any segment of the donor chromosome; in specialized transduction, the phage carries only specific genes, generally those immediately adjacent to the site of prophage insertion.

36. The answer is a. (*Levinson, Ch 4. Murray, Ch 13. Ryan, Ch 21.*) Conjugation (a) involves the direct passage of DNA from one bacterium (donor) to another (recipient) through a conjugative pilus (sex pilus). Transduction (d) is the transfer of DNA mediated by bacteriophages.

37. The answer is d. (*Levinson, Ch 3. Murray, Ch 13. Ryan, Ch 21.*) Bacteria reproduce by binary fission and thus undergo exponential (logarithmic) growth. In this question, a doubling time for *E. coli* was given at 30 minutes in urine. Therefore, after 4 hours there will be eight doubling times. Since there were 1000 bacteria per mL at the time of collection, the number of *E. coli* present after 4 hours can be calculated using the formula: $N \times 2^n$, where N equals the number at the start and n equals the number of generations. $1000 \times 2^8 = 256{,}000$. In this example, what began as a potentially insignificant number of bacteria (depending on the clinical situation) has multiplied to a significant number. If the laboratory or the clinician was unaware of the delay, the patient might have been diagnosed with a UTI when no infection was present. The figure shows the doubling of one bacterium over four doubling times.

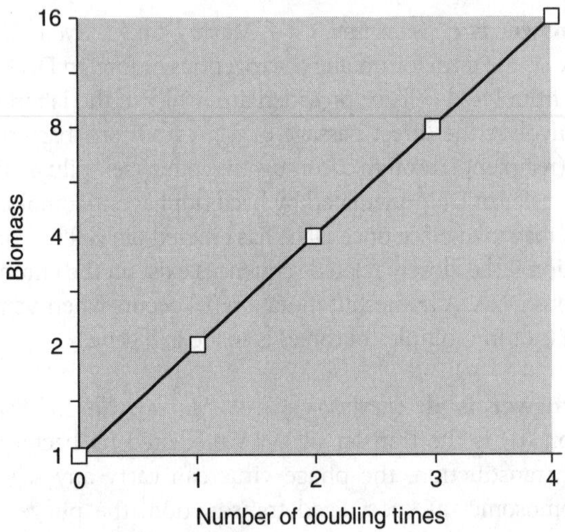

(Reproduced, with permission, from Brooks GF, et al. Jawetz's Medical Microbiology. *24th ed. New York, NY: McGraw-Hill; 2007:53.)*

38. The answer is a. (*Murray, Ch 1, 27.*) Pili (a) or fimbriae are hair-like structures that are found on the surface of many bacteria. They are composed of repeated subunits of the pilin protein. They promote bacterial adherence to each other and bacterial adherence to different host tissues. Uropathogenic *E. coli* colonize the urinary tract and resist the washing action of urine through their pili. The tip of the pilus contains a specific protein that recognizes a receptor on the host cell. The other choices are not involved in *E. coli* uropathogenesis. Capsules (e) are loose polysaccharide or protein layers that surround the gram-negative or gram-positive bacteria. Capsules are antiphagocytic, protect the bacteria from hydrophobic molecules, and promote adhere of certain bacteria such as *Streptococcus mutans* to host tissues. Flagella (d), which are anchored on the bacterial surface, are essential for bacterial motility. The heat-labile (c) and heat-stabile toxins are enterotoxins secreted by the enterotoxigenic *E. coli*. These toxins produce watery diarrhea by stimulating hypersecretion of fluids. LPS (b) composes the outer leaflet of the outer membrane in gram-negative bacteria and is an endotoxin, which stimulates innate immune responses.

39. The answer is c. (*Murray, Ch 12, 14.*) Pathogenic bacteria such as the gram-negative bacillus *Pseudomonas aeruginosa* and the gram-positive coccus *Staphylococcus aureus* colonize the surface of certain surgical appliances such as artificial heart valves and catheters. Multiple layers of the colonizing bacteria surround themselves with a polysaccharide (c) matrix, which protects them from the effect of antibiotics and host immune defenses. The remaining choices do not contribute to biofilm development. Porins (d), proteins that are located within the outer membrane of gram-negative bacteria, facilitate the transfer of hydrophilic molecules through the membrane. Teichoic acids (e) found within the cell wall of gram-positive bacteria are anionic polymers of polyglycan that provide rigidity to the cell wall. In gram-negative bacteria, the periplasmic space occupies the area between the external surface of the cytoplasmic membrane and the internal surface of the outer membrane. The periplasm (b) contains hydrolytic enzymes, virulence proteins, and components of the sugar transport systems. Endotoxin (LPS), a component of the outer membrane of gram-negative bacteria, is recognized by the host defenses and stimulates macrophages to produce cytokines.

40. The answer is a. (*Levinson, Ch 44. Murray, Ch 64. Ryan, Ch 20.*) The vignette presents a case of infectious prion disease or new-variant Creutzfeldt-Jakob disease acquired by the ingestion of the bovine spongiform encephalopathy (BSE) prion. Prions are infectious particles that are currently thought to be composed solely of protein (ie, they contain no detectable nucleic acid). Normal host prions do not cause disease, but prions synthesized from mutated genes (inherited CJD, sporadic CJD), BSE prions, and prions found in other transmissible spongiform encephalopathies are abnormally folded proteins (a). These abnormally folded proteins catalyze the refolding of normal prions into the CJD form leading to disease. Viruses have nucleic acid, either RNA or DNA, present in protein capsids (b); some viruses are enveloped (b) in lipid bilayer membranes pirated from their host. Viruses, bacteria (e), and parasites (d) can all cause CNS disease, but none are associated with the clinical picture/history of the vignette.

41. The answer is e. (*Murray, Ch 13. Ryan, Ch 21. Mokrousov, pp 1417-1424.*) Mutations result from three types of molecular changes, namely, base substitution mutation, frameshift mutation, and transposon or insertion sequences causing mutations. Inversion mutations (b) are caused by insertion sequences (ISs) or IS-like elements. Missense mutation (c) refers to base substitution resulting in a codon that causes a different amino acid to be inserted. Nonsense mutation (d) refers to base substitution generating a termination codon that prematurely stops protein synthesis. Replacement mutations (e) are transition or transversion depending on the substitution. Transition mutations are the replacement of a pyrimidine (C, T) by a pyrimidine or a purine (A, G) by a purine. Transversions (e) are the replacement of a purine by a pyrimidine or pyrimidine by a purine.

42. The answer is b. (*Murray, Ch 13. Ryan, Ch 21. Li, pp 74-80.*) The mutation described here is a missense mutation (c), or one in which base substitution resulting in a codon that causes a different amino acid to be inserted. See the answer to 41 for other responses.

43. The answer is c. (*Levinson, Ch 11. Murray, Ch 58. Ryan, Ch 17.*) The patient has bite wounds most likely infected with *Pasteurella multocida*. Since the wounds were caused by dogs whose owners were unknown, the patient should also begin rabies prophylaxis (c). There is no need for varicella-zoster prophylaxis (e) since there is no history of shingles at this time. The patient is up to date on his tetanus immunization, so tetanus prophylaxis is not needed either (d). IV immunoglobulins (nonspecific) (b) are used to treat patients with IgG deficiency. Hepatitis B virus (HBV) prophylaxis is not needed unless the bites were inflicted by a human whose HBV status was unknown and could not be determined.

44. The answer is d. (*Katzung, Ch 51. Levinson, Ch 10. Murray, Ch 17. Ryan, Ch 23.*) The patient is infected with *Yersinia pestis* and has bubonic plague. The drug of choice for plague is streptomycin (d). Gentamicin or another aminoglycoside can be substituted. Ceftazidime, chloramphenicol, penicillin, and vancomycin are not used to treat plague.

45. The answer is a. (*Katzung, Ch 51. Levinson, Ch 10. Murray, Ch 17. Ryan, Ch 23.*) The child in the question has bacterial meningitis. The most likely etiologic agents are *Haemophilus influenzae, N. meningitidis*, and *S. pneumoniae*. Ceftriaxone (a) and cefotaxime have the highest activity against these agents. Ceftazidime, another third-generation cephalosporin, has limited activity against *H. influenzae* and is not recommended unless the specific identification and susceptibility of the microorganism is known. Erythromycin, gentamicin, penicillin, and vancomycin do not cross the blood-brain barrier as well as the third-generation cephalosporins.

46. The answer is e. (*Katzung, Ch 51. Levinson, Ch 10. Murray, Ch 17. Ryan, Ch 23.*) The patient most likely has an infection with *P. aeruginosa*. The best combination for this patient is ticarcillin/clavulanate plus tobramycin (e). *P aeruginosa* is frequently resistant to multiple antibiotics, and strains acquired in hospital intensive care units and burn units can be resistant to all commonly used antimicrobials. Until the specific susceptibility for the patient's isolate is available, the best choice is an antipseudomonal penicillin (piperacillin (d) or ticarcillin) plus a β-lactamse inhibitor and an aminoglycoside. Ceftazidime (a) is consistently active against many *P. aeruginosa* strains but hospital-acquired strains may be resistant. Erythromycin (b), penicillin (c), cephalothin (d), and vancomycin (a) have no activity against *P. aeruginosa*. Fluoroquinolones make a good alternative treatment with aminoglycosides, but imipenem (b) must always be given with cilastatin.

47. The answer is e. (*Katzung, Ch 51. Levinson, Ch 10. Murray, Ch 17. Ryan, Ch 23.*) This patient has a hospital-acquired methicillin-resistant *S. aureus* (HA-MRSA) infection, for which the drug of choice is vancomycin (e). HA-MRSA are frequently resistant to multiple antibiotics, whereas community-acquired methicillin-resistant *S. aureus* (CA-MRSA) are more susceptible. For CA-MRSA, clindamycin may be a better choice. Dicloxacillin (b) and ceftazidime (a) are used to treat methicillin-susceptible *S. aureus* strains. Almost all strains of *S. aureus* in the United States produce penicillinase, so penicillin (c) should not be used. Tobramycin (d) is used mainly for serious gram-negative infections and may be effective. However, *S. aureus* strains are emerging with decreased susceptibility to vancomycin.

48. The answer is e. (*Katzung, Ch 43, 44, 46, 48. Levinson, Ch 10. Murray, Ch 17. Ryan, Ch 23.*) The mechanism of action described is that of trimethoprim (TMP) (e), a diaminopyrimidine that is a folic acid antagonist. Although TMP is commonly used in combination with sulfa drugs, its mode of action is distinct. TMP is structurally similar to the pteridine portion of dihydrofolate and prevents the conversion of folic acid to tetrahydrofolic acid by inhibition of dihydrofolate reductase. Fortunately, this enzyme in humans is relatively insensitive to TMP. Ampicillin (a), a structural analog of the natural D-Ala-D-Ala substrate for penicillin-binding protein (PBP), prevents the transpeptidase function of PBP that crosslinks the developing peptidoglycan cell well. Amphotericin (b) is an antifungal drug that binds ergosterol in the fungal membrane. Chloramphenicol (c) binds reversibly to the 50S ribosomal subunit and inhibits formation of peptide bond by inhibiting the transpeptidase function. Levofloxacin (d) blocks bacterial DNA synthesis by inhibiting bacterial topoisomerase II (DNA gyrase) and topoisomerase IV (separation of replicated chromosomal DNA).

49. The answer is e. (*Katzung, Ch 51. Levinson, Ch 18. Murray, Ch 27. Ryan, Ch 33.*) The drug of choice for complicated UTIs without sepsis is trimethoprim/sulfamethoxazole (e). Ampicillin (a) is no longer sufficiently effective against *E. coli*, *Proteus* spp., and other gram-negative bacilli associated with UTI with kidney stone formation. Chloramphenicol (c) is not used to treat UTI, and is rarely used in the United States for any infection except rickettsial infections and some cases of childhood meningitis. Penicillin (d) is not active against enteric gram-negative bacilli. Amphotericin (b) is an antifungal drug.

50. The answer is e. (*Katzung, Ch 43. Murray, Ch 20. Ryan, Ch 25.*) *Enterococcus faecalis* and other enterococci are inherently resistant to oxacillin and cephalosporins and may acquire resistance to aminoglycosides and vancomycin; yet they have remained susceptible to penicillins, especially ampicillin (a). Treatment with vancomycin (e), which binds to D-Ala-D-Ala of peptidoglycan, can select vancomycin-resistant strains (VRE) from the population of enterocci in the colon. These VRE can then cause infection. Treatment of choice for VRE UTI is ampicillin plus an aminoglycoside. Daptomycin may be substituted for either drug in case of resistance. Amphotericin (b) is an antifungal. Chloramphenicol (c) is not used to treat UTI. Levofloxacin (d) has no activity against VRE.

51. The answer is e. (*Katzung, Ch 48. Murray, Ch 69. Ryan, Ch 43.*) Voriconazole (e), an antifungal azole, is the drug of choice for treating aspergillosis in immunocompromised individuals such as the patient in the vignette who has leukemia. It is less toxic than amphotericin B (a), an alternative treatment. Antifungal azoles affect ergosterol synthesis by acting on the demethylase enzyme in the synthetic pathway. Amphotericin B binds to ergosterol and alters the permeability of the cell by forming pores in the cell membrane. The pores allow the leakage of intracellular ions and macromolecules, leading to cell death. Binding to human membrane sterols also occurs, which likely accounts for the severe toxicity of the drug. Caspofungin (b), primarily used to treat invasive candidiasis, can also be used to treat invasive aspergillosis, but it works by blocking synthesis of the glucan component of the cell wall. Nikkomycin Z (d), a drug in development, blocks chitin synthesis and has activity against *Coccidioides* and *Blastomyces* but not *Aspergillus*. Griseofulvin (c) is a topical or systemic antifungal used to treat dermatophytosis. It functions by disrupting the microtubules.

52. The answer is c. (*Katzung, Ch 51. Levinson, Ch 18. Murray, Ch 27. Ryan, Ch 33.*) The girl in the vignette most likely has *Neisseria meningitidis* meningitis. The drug of choice is ceftriaxone, which is contraindicated by the child's known β-lactam allergy due to cross-hypersensitivity. The alternative drug of choice is chloramphenicol, which inhibits formation of the peptide bond (c) through inhibition of the transpeptidase reaction. Meropenem, a second alternative, is also a β-lactam with cross-hypersensitivity. Tetracycline, which blocks tRNA binding to the A site (a), is not used to treat meningitis and should not be used in children under 10. Aminoglycosides, which cause misreading of mRNA (b) and result in premature termination (e) of translation, as well as blocking initiation of protein synthesis, are not generally used to treat meningitis except in cases caused by *Listeria*. Macrolides prevent translocation (d) and are not used to treat meningitis.

53. The answer is d. (*Murray, Ch 5, 18. Ryan, Ch 4, 24.*) In general, real-time PCR is more sensitive than culture (a), due to the ability of the assay to detect very few copies of bacterial DNA present in the specimen. Recently, many clinical laboratories have begun using real-time PCR for the *mecA* gene or the SCC*mec* cassette that carries *mecA* to detect the presence of MRSA in nasal specimens collected from patients upon admission to the hospital. Numerous studies have shown that the sensitivity of real-time PCR is slightly higher than that of optimally performed chromogenic culture for MRSA. However, even at 85% sensitivity, if the 50 positive samples were true positives, one would expect to have recovered 42 to 43 isolates in the companion cultures rather than 15. Real-time PCR was thought to be more specific than culture (b), but the appearance of increasing numbers of *mecA* gene variations has led to false-negative results due to primer mismatch and failure to amplify the gene even when present. Detecting SCC*mec* was thought to be the solution to this problem, only to come under fire because the same SCC*mec* cassette found in community-acquired MRSA is present in methicillin-resistant *S. epidermidis*, leading to misclassification of patients with MRSE. This finding has led to the development of multiplex PCR tests that detect genes specific for *S. aureus* in addition to the *mecA* gene. Unfortunately, many laboratories have implemented nucleic acid testing without having access to dedicated space for sample preparation and the PCR instrument, as described in the vignette. This frequently leads to contamination of the PCR workstation with MRSA DNA (d), which is then amplified in the reaction producing a false-positive result. Failure of the thermocycler, the PCR instrument, because it needs to be calibrated (c), is a possibility, but should have been addressed through required instrument maintenance and running of appropriate controls.

54. The answer is a. (*Murray, Ch 12, 36. Diagnosis and management of foodborne illness, pp 1-33.*) Under harsh environmental conditions, certain gram-positive bacteria convert from the vegetative state into a dormant state or spore. The spores, which are dehydrated structures, protect bacterial DNA and other contents from the effect of the intense heat, radiation, and standard disinfectants. If spores present in the food are not killed during preparation, and if the cooked food is left for several hours at room temperature, the spores will germinate allowing vegetative bacteria to produce the enterotoxin. The spore-forming gram-positive bacteria (a), *Clostridium perfringens* and *Bacillus cereus*, produce enterotoxins that cause watery diarrhea and abdominal cramps but no fever. While very similar, the vignette suggests *C. perfringens* as the etiologic agent. Onset is more rapid than with *B. cereus* diarrheal toxin, and while the types of food overlap, temperature-abused food is frequently associated with *C. perfringens*. Among the gram-positive cocci (b), *Staphylococcus aureus* produces enterotoxin, but the onset is more abrupt (1-6 hours) and fever may be present. The gram-negative bacilli (a) must first colonize the intestine and grow, even if an enterotoxin is at the root of the diarrhea. Thus, onset of symptoms occurs from 24 hours to several days after ingestion of the food. Opportunistic fungi (d) are not known to be involved in food poisoning. Enteric viruses (e) such as norovirus and rotavirus require 12 to 48 hours and 1 to 3 days, respectively, for symptoms to appear. They are more commonly associated with foods contaminated by food workers during preparation (salads, sandwiches, and fruit), or food prepared with contaminated water (salads, fruit, and ice).

55. The answer is c. (*Murray, Ch 12, 26.*) In *Neisseria*, the equivalent to LPS is lipooligosaccharide (LOS) (c), which consists of lipid A and core oligosaccharide but lacks the O antigen. By triggering an inflammatory response, LOS causes most of the symptoms during *Neisseria gonorrhoeae* infection. It activates the complement and stimulates the influx of phagocytes leading to the purulent discharge. LOS also contributes to serum resistance, which is an important feature of strains that causes systemic infection. Rapidly growing *Neisseria* releases outer membrane blebs, which contain LOS. Pili (e) mediate the initial attachment of *N. gonorrhoeae* to the surface of cervical or urethral epithelial cells. Pili are attached to the cell surface and are not released. The opacity protein (d), which provides *N. gonorrhoeae* colonies with their opaque appearance, is an outer membrane protein. It mediates binding of *N. gonorrhoeae* to epithelial cells and plays a role in cell-to-cell signaling. Similar to the pili, the opacity protein is a cell-associated factor. The capsule (a) surrounds pathogenic bacteria and provides them with antiphagocytic properties. However, *N. gonorrhoeae* is not encapsulated. Exotoxins (b), which are produced by some gram-negative and gram-positive bacteria, bind to specific receptors on the host cells and either alter the function of the host cell or destroy it. *N. gonorrhoeae* does not produce exotoxin.

56. The answer is b. (*Murray, Ch 30. Ryan, Ch 35.*) Most isolates of *Moraxella catarrhalis*, a common cause of acute otitis media, produce β-lactamase (b) making them resistant to the penicillins. They are almost all susceptible to third-generation cephalosporins, macrolides, tetracycline (contraindicated in a 2-year-old), trimethoprim/sulfamethoxazole, and ampicillin/sulbactam. Chloramphenicol acetyltransferase (a) is responsible for naturally occurring chloramphenicol resistance in bacteria. Aminoglycoside phosphotransferases (e) confer resistance to aminoglycoside antibiotics. Catalase (c) is an enzyme involved in the detoxification of the reactive oxygen species H_2O_2; DNase (d) is an enzyme that destroys DNA. Both are produced by *M. catarrhalis*, but neither is involved in antibiotic resistance.

57. The answer is c. (*Murray, Ch 5, 18. Ryan, Ch 4, 24.*) Due to variations in the *mecA* gene which confers methicillin (oxacillin) resistant, several of the real-time PCR assays used by clinical laboratories now amplify the SCC*mec* cassette that carries *mecA* in order to determine whether patients are colonized with MRSA upon admission. Any specimen testing positive is considered to harbor MRSA. However, the same SCC*mec* cassette found in community-acquired MRSA is present in methicillin-resistant *S. epidermidis* (c). Unless additional targets specific for *S. aureus* are amplified, the actual source of the amplicon could have been *S. epidermidis*, or other species of *Staphylococcus*. It is entirely possible for a person to carry MRSA in the nasal passages and be infected with a different strain of *S. aureus* that is methicillin-susceptible or with a different species of *Staphylococcus*. There is no reason to believe the PCR was contaminated (b) or that the wrong primers were used in the PCR (d). *S. epidermidis* is a common cause of surgical wound infections, gaining entry directly into the incision from the surrounding skin. There is no reason to suspect that the culture was performed improperly (a).

58 to 62. (*Levinson, Ch 7. Murray, Ch 14. Ryan, Ch 22.*) This series of questions reviews virulence factors and components of various pathogenic bacteria—*Neisseria meningitidis* (58), *Streptococcus pyogenes* (59),

Mycobacterium tuberculosis (61), and *Bacillus anthracis* (62), as well as the role of LPS as endogenous pyrogen (60). Virulence factors in general are discussed in the chapters listed above, and include capsules, pili, endotoxin (LPS, LOS), teichoic acid, catalase, and exotoxins. Bacterial (and fungal) cell wall components include peptidoglycan, teichoic acid, glycolipids or waxes, and ergosterol (fungi).

58. The answer is b. (*Levinson, Ch 16. Murray, Ch 26. Ryan, Ch 30.*) At least 13 serogroups of *N. meningitidis* have been identified by immunologic specificity of capsular antigens. Five, A, B, C, Y, and W-135, are the most important strains associated with disease. Virulence factors associated with *N. meningitidis* are the polysaccharide capsule (b), pili (c) that mediate attachment, an IgA protease, and lipooligosaccharide (d) or endotoxin that mediates the clinical manifestations. The polysaccharide capsule (b) binds serum factor H to its surface, protecting the microbe from complement-mediated phagocytosis by neutrophils unless the capsules are opsonized with antibody. This is the function of the polysaccharide *N. meningitidis* vaccine. The organism is oxidase and catalase (e) positive, but these are traits used to identify the bacterium. Opacity proteins (a) are found in *N. gonorrhoeae* where they mediate firm attachment to host cells.

59. The answer is d. (*Levinson, Ch 15. Murray, Ch 19. Ryan, Ch 25.*) *Streptococcus pyogenes*, or Group A *Streptococcus* (GAS), produces a number of virulence factors. The M protein (d) is the organism's most important antiphagocytic factor, and it conveys serologic specificity—over 100 serotypes are now known. In the early stages of growth, the bacteria have hyaluronic acid (b) capsules. This capsule (similar to human hyaluronic acid structure) is rapidly destroyed by the organism's own hyaluronidase. Also known as spreading factor, hyaluronidase plays a role in GAS cellulitis. Erythrogenic toxin (a) is a superantigen produced by some strain of GAS lysogenized by a bacteriophage carrying the toxin gene; it causes the rash of scarlet fever. A second superantigen, streptococcal pyrogenic toxin, causes streptococcal toxic shock syndrome. Streptolysin O (e) an oxygen-labile hemolysin is useful for identification of the organism and is antigenic so antistreptolysin antibodies can be used to diagnosis rheumatic fever, a sequelae of GAS infection. Lipoteichoic acid (c) is a component of the cell wall that is involved in binding of the bacterium to host fibronectin.

60. The answer is c. (*Levinson, Ch 57. Murray, Ch 7. Ryan, Ch 2.*) Lipopolysaccharide (LPS or endotoxin) (c) consists of three regions: lipid A, which forms the outer leaflet of the lipid bilayer outer membrane; the core polysaccharide; and the O-antigen polysaccharide side chain. Endotoxin is recognized by macrophages through their LPS receptors CD14 and Toll-like receptor 4. Upon this recognition, the macrophage secretes interleukin (IL)-1, IL-6, and tumor necrosis factor-α (TNF-α), which stimulate inflammatory responses including fever. This occurs whether the intact microbe is present or not. Overproduction of TNF-α can lead to hypotension. Teichoic acid (e) is also recognized by macrophages through toll-like receptors, but this substance is not present in gram-negative bacteria. Bacterial polysaccharides (a) and hyaluronic acid (b) do not elicit this type of inflammatory response. Protein toxins (d) would produce symptoms in keeping with the type of toxin and rely on the appropriate receptor being present, which may not be the case in event of systemic administration (intravenous) or injection intramuscularly.

61. The answer is b. (*Levinson, Ch 21. Murray, Ch 25. Ryan, Ch 26.*) The vignette describes *Mycobacterium tuberculosis* infection. Mycobacteria are rod-shaped, aerobic bacteria that do not form spores. While mycobacteria have peptidoglycan (d), it is highly decorated with many branched-chain polysaccharides, proteins, and lipids. The cell wall also contains mycolic acids and lipoarabinomannan, a structure functionally analogous to LPS. These glycolipids (b) make the lipid content of the cell wall approximately 60%. The acid-fast nature of mycobacteria is due to this waxy coat; only extreme conditions allow the stain to penetrate, and once inside, the stain cannot be removed by acid and alcohol. Ergosterol (a) is found in fungal cell membranes. Hyaluronic acid (b) comprises the capsule of *S. pyogenes* and is found on human cells. Mycobacteria do not contain teichoic acid (e); this is a component of gram-positive bacterial cell walls.

62. The answer is a. (*Levinson, Ch 21. Murray, Ch 21. Ryan, Ch 26.*) *Bacillus anthracis* produces an unusual capsule composed of poly-D-glutamic acid (a). The capsule prevents phagocytosis of the organisms by PMNs and is an important virulence factor. Strains that do not produce capsules are nonvirulent. Lethal factor (c) combines with protective antigen (e) to form the lethal toxin, which cleaves mitogen-activated protein kinase resulting in cell death. Protective antigen (e) also combines with edema factor to form edema toxin, a calmodulin-dependent adenylate cyclase whose action increases intracellular cAMP resulting in severe edema. Hyaluronic acid (b) composes the often short-lived capsule of *S. pyogenes*. M protein (d) of *S. pyogenes* is antiphagocytic.

63. The answer is c. (*Levinson, Ch 15. Murray, Ch 19. Ryan, Ch 25.*) There are more than 90 capsular immunotypes of *Streptococcus pneumoniae*. Immunity to *S. pneumoniae* is conveyed by antibodies against the specific capsular type. Vaccines have been formulated to contain the most commonly isolated capsular types. Originally, the *S. pneumoniae* conjugated vaccine contained seven serotypes. Unfortunately, the serotype replacement phenomenon occurred in which a nonvaccine strain began to cause disease among the vaccinated population. Over time this lead to the licensing of a 13-valent pneumococcal conjugated vaccine (PCV-13), which was recommended for children. A 23-valent nonconjugated vaccine (PV-23) was developed for children over age 2 and adults who are at risk for the disease. Recent research showed that older adults vaccinated with PCV-13 elaborated higher protective antibody titers than those immunized with PV-23. PCV-13 has now been licensed for adults 50 and older. The failure of the vaccine to protect these individuals is most likely due to the replacement phenomenon—the capsular type responsible was not present in the vaccine (c). Elderly patient do mount good immune responses to vaccines so (a) is not the likely cause. Some patients will not respond to the vaccine (b), but the effectiveness of the vaccine is higher than 17% (10/12, the number of patients who became infected). In fact, recent analyses of strains causing illness in those over 65 suggest that over 70% of the cases of invasive pneumococcal disease are covered by PCV-13. It is unlikely that the vaccine was defective (d), although this can occur.

Virology

Questions

64. A 27-year-old man presents to his primary care physician with complaints of a fever, headache, muscle aches, and swollen glands. The physician observes disseminated lymphadenopathy, pharyngitis, and a rash on the man's upper chest. The patient states that he had been to a party 2 weeks ago where he experimented with injecting drugs to get high. Needles were shared among the party-goers. A rapid latex test for human immunodeficiency virus (HIV) antibodies performed in the physician's office is negative. The doctor has a strong suspicion that this man has acute retroviral syndrome. Which of the following tests is most likely to support a diagnosis of HIV infection at this time?

a. CD4 lymphocyte count
b. HIV antibody test by enzyme-linked immunosorbent assay (EIA)
c. HIV p24 antigen
d. Reverse transcriptase polymerase chain reaction (PCR) for HIV RNA
e. Western blot for HIV antibodies

65. A 9-year-old male with a history of fever and nonspecific symptoms presents with a bright red cheeks and a macular lacy rash over his body. Which of the following viruses is the most likely cause of this disease?

a. Herpes simplex virus (HSV) type 1
b. Parvovirus B19
c. Rubella virus
d. Rubeola (measles) virus
e. Varicella-zoster virus (VZV)

66. A 24-year-old pregnant woman presents near term with lesions suspicious for primary genital herpes. Culture identifies the presence of HSV type 2. At the time of delivery, she still has active genital lesions. Which of the following should be done to avoid transmitting the virus to the baby?

a. Cesarean delivery
b. Internal fetal monitoring
c. Rupture of the membranes to speed delivery
d. Vaginal delivery

67. A 24-year-old street person, who is known to be HIV-positive, enters the community health clinic complaining of sores in his mouth. He says he has been having fevers and night sweats and thinks he has lost weight recently. Examination of his mouth reveals the lesions shown in the image. Scraping of the white patches shows budding yeast and masses of pseudohyphae. His CD4 T-cell count is 280/μL and viral load is 75,000 copies/mL. The doctor and patient agree it is time to begin antiretroviral therapy. Which of the following regimens is best for this treatment-naïve patient?

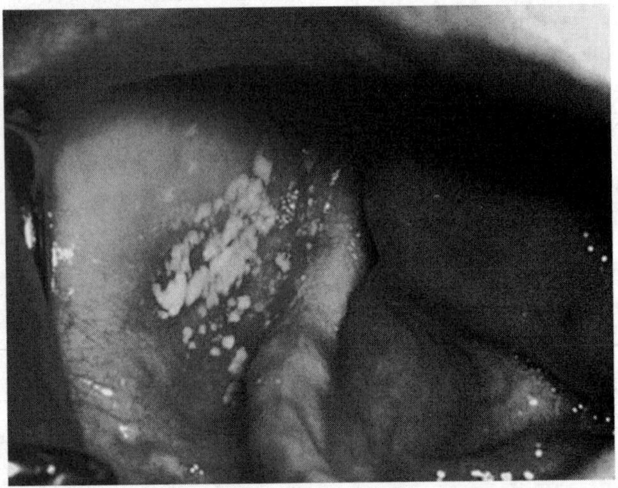

(Courtesy of CDC/Sol Silverman Jr, DDS, University of California, San Francisco 1987; ID #6066.)

a. Abacavir alone
b. Efavirenz plus tenofovir plus emtricitabine
c. Darunavir boosted with ritonavir
d. Maraviroc plus enfuvirtide plus raltegravir
e. Nevirapine alone

68. An HIV-positive patient, after treatment with tenofovir/emtricitabine plus ritonavir-boosted atazanavir, has a CD4 T-cell count of 325/μL and a viral load of less than 50 copies of HIV RNA/mL. Previously her CD4+ T-cell count was 280/μL and viral load was 100,000 copies/mL. Which of the following best describes this patient?

a. This patient is no longer in danger of opportunistic infection
b. The 5-year prognosis is excellent
c. The patient's HIV screening test is most likely negative
d. The patient is not infectious
e. The antiretroviral therapy has been effective

69. An HIV-positive patient with a viral load of 100,000 copies/mL of HIV RNA and a drop in his CD4 T-cell count from 240 to 50/μL has been diagnosed with *Pneumocystis jiroveci* pneumonia. Which of the following is the best description of the stage of this patient's HIV disease?

a. HIV infection, stage 1
b. HIV infection, stage 2
c. HIV infection, stage 3 (AIDS)
d. HIV infection, stage unknown

70. A 19-year-old college student presents to the student health clinic complaining of sore throat, fever, swollen neck lymph nodes, and malaise of several days. His complete blood count shows WBC count 22,000/μL with 10% neutrophils, 28% lymphocytes, 47% reactive lymphocytes, and 15% monocytes. His monospot test is positive. Which of the following is causing this student's infection?

a. Adenovirus
b. Cytomegalovirus
c. Echovirus
d. Epstein–Barr virus
e. Human metapneumovirus

71. During a medical checkup for a new insurance policy, a 60-year-old grandmother is found to be positive by a conventional EIA screening test for antibodies against HIV-1. She has no known risk factors for exposure to the virus. Which of the following is the most appropriate next step?

a. Immediately begin antiretroviral therapy
b. Perform the EIA screening test a second time
c. Request that a viral blood culture be done by the laboratory
d. Tell the patient that she is likely to develop AIDS
e. Test the patient for *Pneumocystis jiroveci* infection

72. A 74-year-old man who lived in Illinois developed malaise, fever, cough, and sore throat in August. Two days later, he visited his doctor because of severe headache, nausea and vomiting, and continued fever. He told his doctor that the mosquitoes had been fierce in the last 2 weeks and that he had been bitten numerous times. The doctor noted tremors in the man's hands as well as fever of 104°F, and admitted him to the hospital for tests. Examination of CSF revealed normal glucose and protein with 150 lymphocytes/μL; PCR assays for HSV and West Nile virus (WNV) on the CSF were negative. Despite supportive care, the man slipped into a coma and died. Which of the following viruses was most likely responsible for this man's illness?

a. *Coltivirus*
b. Dengue virus
c. *Erythrovirus* (parvovirus B19)
d. La Crosse virus
e. St. Louis encephalitis virus

73. A 64-year-old man complained of poor memory and difficulty with vision that was progressing rapidly and myoclonic jerks. Cerebrospinal fluid examination at a reference laboratory revealed the presence of 14-3-3 protein. Over the next 6 months his cognitive deterioration became severe and he died 2 months later. At autopsy, spongiform encephalopathy was noted. Which of the following is the most appropriate diagnosis for this man?

a. Sporadic Creutzfeldt–Jakob disease (CJD)
b. Familial CJD
c. Iatrogenic CJD
d. Variant CJD

74. In 2003, the zoonotic severe acute respiratory syndrome (SARS) coronavirus caused a pandemic in which over 8000 people were infected and the mortality rate was 10%. In 2012, a novel coronavirus was isolated from 12 persons in Saudi Arabia, Qatar, and Britain with severe respiratory illness; so far, 50% have died. Which of the following syndromes is more commonly caused by other known types of human coronaviruses?

a. Common cold
b. Herpangina
c. Meningitis
d. Pneumonia
e. Vesicular lesions

75. A 35-year-old intravenous (IV) drug abuser with known chronic hepatitis B virus (HBV) status suddenly presents with an acute hepatitis episode. He develops massive hepatic necrosis and dies. Which of the following is most likely responsible for the change in his condition?

a. A hepatitis B mutant has developed
b. He has contracted hepatitis D virus (HDV)
c. He has developed cirrhosis
d. His food contained hepatitis A virus (HAV)
e. His food contained hepatitis E virus (HEV)

76. Which of the following antiviral compounds inhibits activity of the pyrophosphate-binding site of viral DNA polymerases and is used to treat serious infections with cytomegalovirus?

a. Amantadine
b. Foscarnet
c. Ganciclovir
d. Ribavirin
e. Zidovudine

77. A clinic associated with a medical school and located in a lower income city district documents a series of cases involving echoviruses in school-age children. Most cases experienced common cold symptoms plus mild fever and maculopapular rash; some were hospitalized with acute onset of fever, headache, nuchal rigidity, and petechial rash. All experienced complete recovery within 1 week without specific antiviral therapy. Which of the following body systems is the main target of echoviruses?

a. Bloodstream
b. Central nervous system (CNS)
c. Intestinal tract
d. Lymphoid tissues
e. Upper respiratory tract

78. A newborn infant presents with vesicular skin lesions. He also had generalized symptoms suggestive of CNS and liver involvement. His mother had developed painful vesicular lesions on her genitalia several days prior to the birth of her son. She had not sought medical help until she was in heavy labor. At admission to labor and delivery, internal lesions were seen on her cervix and vaginal walls, but the birth was eminent, precluding C-section. Which of the following is the most rapid test for definitive identification of the most likely etiologic agent?

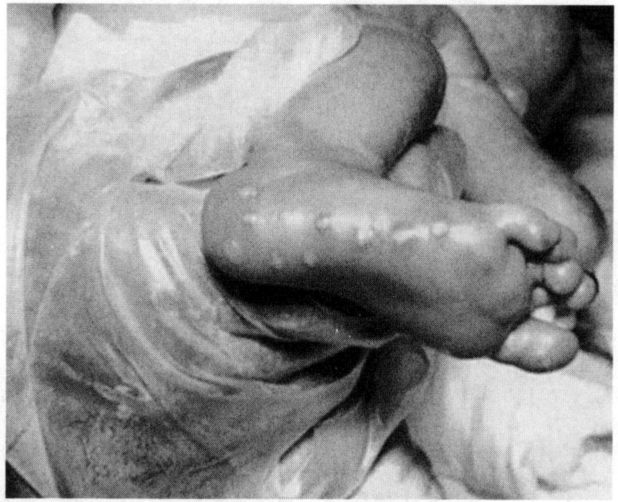

Vesicular lesions of congenital herpes. *(Courtesy of CDC.)*

a. Detection of specific HSV IgG antibodies
b. Direct immunofluorescence for HSV on cells from lesions
c. HSV PCR on cerebrospinal fluid
d. Tzanck smear
e. Viral culture of fluid from lesions

79. Several children in a day care center for preschoolers developed fever, irritability, lack of appetite, and a vesicular rash found on their hands, feet, and mouths. With which virus were these children most likely infected?

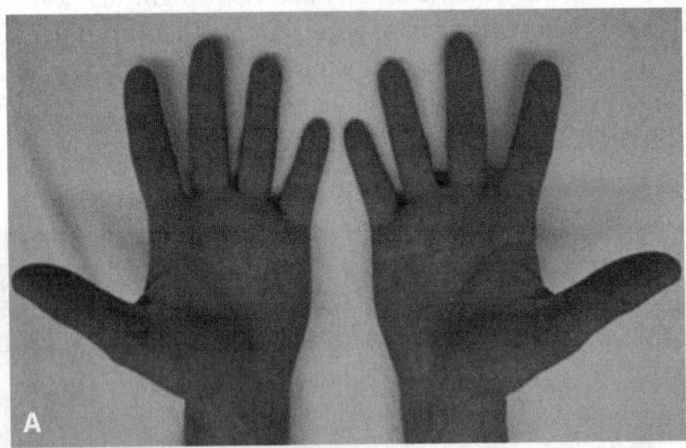

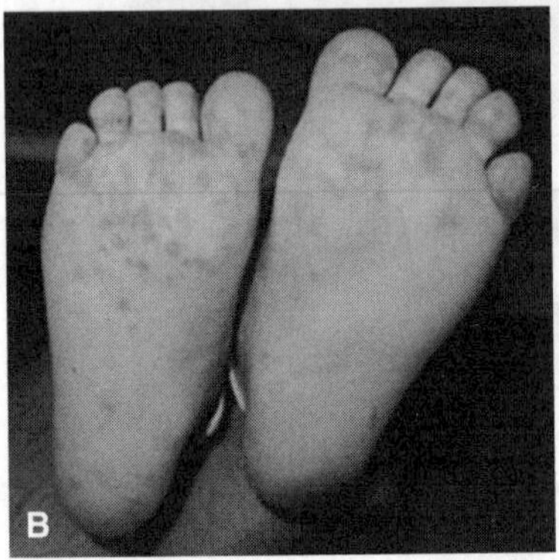

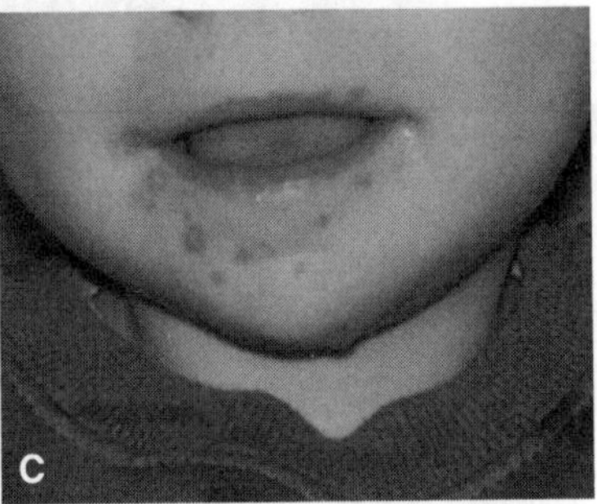

*(**A**: Courtesy of James Heilman, MD, Creative Attribution-Share Alike 3.0 Unported license; **B**: Courtesy of Ngufra, 2102-07-06, GNU Free Documentation License; **C**: Courtesy of DJ Midgley, May 2008, Creative Commons Attribution-Share Alike 3.0 Unported license.)*

a. Coronavirus
b. Coxsackievirus A
c. Orthoreovirus
d. Respiratory syncytial virus
e. Rhinovirus

80. A 15-year-old boy is taken to his pediatrician after experiencing fever, malaise, and anorexia followed by tender swelling of his parotid glands. Which of the following is the most likely complication to occur in this patient?

a. Guillain–Barré syndrome
b. Hemorrhage
c. Myocarditis
d. Oophoritis
e. Orchitis

81. An otherwise healthy 65-year-old male was in a car accident and broke several ribs on the left side. Approximately 12 days later, he developed a painful, well-circumscribed vesicular rash over the left rib cage that persists for several weeks. The rash is most likely due to which of the following?

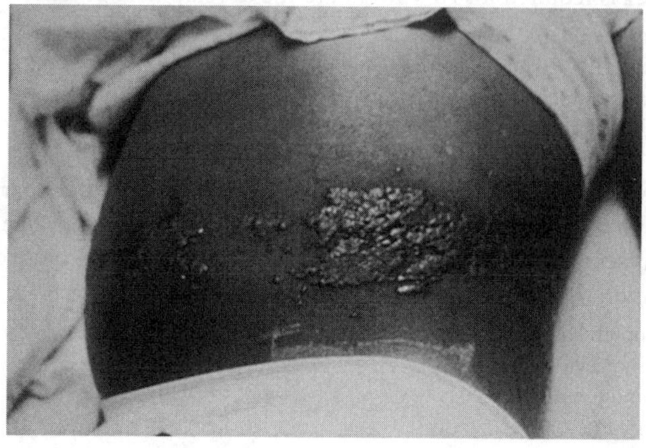

(Courtesy of CDC, 1995, ID#6886.)

a. Primary infection with HSV type 1
b. Reactivation of latent HSV type 1
c. Primary infection with Epstein–Barr virus
d. Reactivation of latent Epstein–Barr virus
e. Primary infection with VZV
f. Reactivation of latent VZV

82. A 3-year-old child who had not been immunized presents at the physician's office with symptoms of coryza, cough, conjunctivitis, and photophobia. He has a low-grade fever, and small, bluish-white ulcerations are seen on the buccal mucosa opposite the lower molars. What is the causative agent of this child's symptoms?

a. Adenovirus
b. HSV
c. Influenzavirus
d. Measles virus
e. Rubella virus

83. A sexually active woman was seen for a routine gynecologic exam that included a Pap smear. The report indicated cervical intraepithelial neoplasia. In situ hybridization showed the presence of human papillomavirus (HPV) type 16 genomes within the neoplastic cells. Which of the following processes is required for HPV to lead to the development of cancer?

a. Integration of the viral genome
b. Loss of HPV E6 and E7 genes
c. Mutation of the virus
d. Viral replication

84. Two siblings, ages 2 and 4, experience fever, rhinitis, and pharyngitis that result in laryngotracheobronchitis. Both have a harsh, bark-like cough and hoarseness. Which of the following viruses is the leading cause of their syndrome?

a. Adenovirus
b. Coxsackievirus B
c. Parainfluenza virus
d. Rhinovirus
e. Rotavirus

85. An outbreak of hepatitis occurred in an area of India with poor sanitation. Most of the patients reported fever, nausea with vomiting, and weight loss occurring over several days followed by jaundice and pruritus. Testing quickly ruled out HAV. A number of women in the area are pregnant. For which of the following are these women at risk?

a. Chronic hepatitis
b. Fetal hydrops
c. Fulminant hepatic failure
d. Guillain–Barré syndrome
e. Reye syndrome

86. An 18-year-old man was taken to an emergency medicine department because of fever and headache for 36 hours and now complaint of a stiff neck. No bacterial agents appeared to be involved and an initial diagnosis of aseptic meningitis was made. Which of the following laboratory findings in the examination of his cerebrospinal fluid led to this diagnosis?

a. Decreased protein content
b. Elevated glucose concentration
c. Eosinophilic pleocytosis
d. Lymphocytic pleocytosis
e. Neutrophilic pleocytosis

87. A street person well known to the local public health clinic appears to have acute symptoms of hepatitis and tests positive for HDV antigen. Knowing that HDV requires HBV, which of the following sets of test results shows this patient had chronic HBV infection and was superinfected with HDV?

a. HBsAg +, HBeAg +, Anti-HBcAg IgM +, Anti-HBcAg IgG –, Anti-HBsAg –
b. HBsAg +, HBeAg +, Anti-HBcAg IgM –, Anti-HBcAg IgG +, Anti-HBsAg –
c. HBsAg –, HBeAg –, Anti-HBcAg IgM –, Anti-HBcAg IgG +, Anti-HBsAg +
d. HBsAg –, HBeAg –, Anti-HBcAg IgM –, Anti-HBcAg IgG –, Anti-HBsAg +

88. A nurse develops clinical symptoms consistent with hepatitis. She recalls sticking herself with a needle approximately 5 months before, after drawing blood from a patient. Serologic tests for HBsAg, and antibodies to HBsAg and HAV are all negative; however, she is positive for HBcAg IgM antibody. Which of the following characterizes the current health state of the nurse?

a. Does not have hepatitis B
b. Has resolved hepatitis B
c. Has chronic hepatitis B
d. Is in window period of acute hepatitis B
e. Was immunized with HBsAg

89. A 65-year-old Florida fisherman forgot his insect repellent on a recent sporting trip. A week later, he developed fever, chills, headache, and flu-like symptoms. He was brought to the Emergency Department by his wife with photophobia, extreme lethargy, and severe headache. CNS examination revealed cranial nerve deficits and hemiparesis. The patient was admitted to intensive care with a grave prognosis. Which of the following is the vector that transmitted the infection from which this man is suffering?

a. Bird
b. Flea
c. Mosquito
d. Sand fly
e. Tick

90. A local school district finds a large number of student absences, with the children presenting with rhinorrhea, nasal obstruction, headache, and malaise, but no fever. A strain of rhinovirus is the most likely etiologic agent of these infections. By which method is this virus most frequently spread?

a. Fecal–oral route
b. Hand-to-hand contact
c. Respiratory droplets
d. Sexual contact
e. Vertical transmission

91. A 10-month-old infant who was born 4 weeks premature was brought to the Emergency Department with high fever, rhinorrhea, cough, and difficulty breathing. On examination, the baby had dyspnea and tachypnea; rales and wheezing were heard over both lungs. The baby was admitted to Pediatric Intensive Care where she suffered respiratory failure and was placed on mechanical ventilation. Two different types of tests for respiratory syncytial virus (*RSV* or *Pneumovirus*) were negative, as were tests for parainfluenza virus, influenza A and B viruses, and adenovirus. Which of the following viruses is the most likely etiologic agent?

a. Cytomegalovirus
b. HSV type 1
c. Human metapneumovirus
d. Parvovirus B19
e. Rhinovirus

92. A 32-year-old woman was bitten on the fingers by a feral kitten that she was trying to feed. She cleaned the wounds, and after a week, the sites healed without bacterial infection. Sixty days later, she noticed pain, itching, and numbness at the sites of the bite wounds. Alarmed, she made an appointment to see her doctor the next day. By the time of the appointment, her arm was paralyzed, and she was febrile, had a headache, and was very anxious. Her doctor sent her to the hospital for a nuchal skin biopsy, which was sent to a reference laboratory for workup. The H&E stain showed viral inclusion bodies (A, arrows) and DFA (direct fluorescent antibody test) with virus-specific antiserum was positive (B). With which virus was this woman infected?

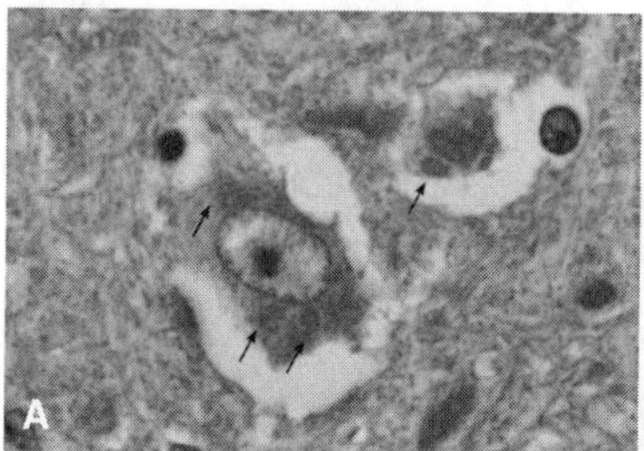

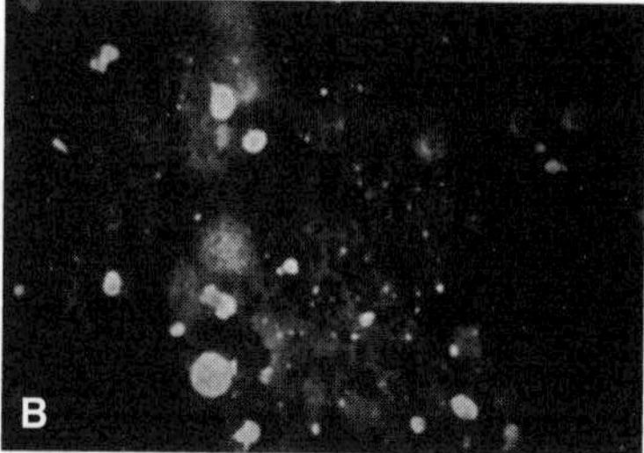

*(**A**: Courtesy of CDC/Dr Daniel P. Perl, 1971, ID#1958; **B**: Courtesy of CDC/Dr. Tierkel, ID#6455.)*

a. Cytomegalovirus
b. Eastern equine encephalitis virus (EEEV)
c. Echovirus
d. HSV type 1
e. Rabies virus

93. Kuru was a fatal disease of certain New Guinea natives and was characterized by tremors and ataxia; Creutzfeldt–Jakob disease (CJD) is characterized by both ataxia and dementia. CJD has been accidentally transferred to others by contaminated growth hormone from human pituitary glands, corneal transplants, and contaminated surgical instruments. These diseases are thought to be caused by which of the following?

a. Cell wall-deficient bacteria
b. Environmental toxins
c. Flagellates
d. Prions
e. Slow viruses

94. Recently, a recombinant vaccine bait to prevent rabies in raccoons had been used in wooded suburban communities. This bait uses a large double-stranded DNA virus that replicates in the cytoplasm as the carrier of the rabies glycoprotein gene. A woman who was immunocompromised found a bait that had broken open and picked it up to dispose of it. She subsequently developed lesions on her hands 11 days after she handled the bait. What caused these lesions?

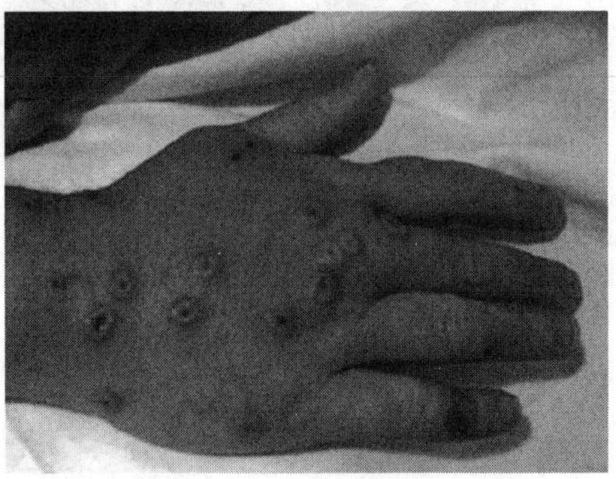

(Courtesy of CDC; MMWR 2009;58:1204-1207.)

a. Adenovirus type 5
b. Echovirus 11
c. Rabies virus
d. Vaccinia virus
e. Variola (smallpox) virus

95. A 35-year-old man developed headache, nausea, vomiting, and sore throat 8 weeks after returning from a trip abroad. He eventually refused to drink water and had episodes of profuse salivation, difficulty in breathing, and hallucinations. Two days after the patient died of cardiac arrest, it was learned that he had been bitten by a dog while on his trip. Which of the following treatments, if given immediately after the dog bite, could have helped prevent this disease?

a. Broad-spectrum antibiotics
b. High-dose acyclovir
c. IV ribavirin
d. Rabies immune globulin plus rabies vaccine
e. Tetanus immune globulin and tetanus toxoid vaccine

96. A patient who works in an industrial setting presents to his ophthalmologist with prominent subconjunctival hemorrhage, periorbital swelling, and corneal changes consistent with keratitis. The patient reported severe photophobia and the sensation that something was in his eye. Nine other workers developed similar symptoms 7 days later. The differential diagnosis should include infection with which of the following viruses?

a. Adenovirus
b. Epstein–Barr virus
c. Parvovirus
d. Respiratory syncytial virus
e. VZV

97. A hospital worker is found to be positive for hepatitis B surface antigen. Subsequent tests reveal the presence of HBeAg as well. Which of the following best describes the worker?

a. Has a biologic false-positive test for hepatitis
b. Is highly contagious
c. Is less contagious
d. Is not contagious
e. Has resolved hepatitis B

98. An extended family met for a family reunion in a rural area of Texas. All reported numerous mosquito bites. One week later several family members had headache, nausea, fever, and malaise. Two developed stiff neck and severe headache that resolved over the next 5 days, and an 8-month-old was hospitalized with diffuse encephalitis. All family members recovered completely except the infant who was left with a seizure disorder. An arbovirus was confirmed as the etiologic agent by serologic testing of the effected persons. Which of the following is the most likely etiologic agent?

a. Dengue virus
b. Lymphocytic choriomeningitis virus
c. Rubella virus
d. Western equine encephalitis virus
e. WNV

99. A 2-month-old infant was admitted to the medical center in February for treatment of bronchiolitis. An immunofluorescent assay was positive for a respiratory virus. As the infant was struggling to breathe, ribavirin treatment was started immediately. With which virus was this infant infected?

a. Coxsackievirus A
b. HBV
c. HSV
d. Parvovirus
e. Respiratory syncytial virus

100. In January, a 74-year-old woman from Iowa is brought to the emergency department by her husband. He states that she had recent onset of high fever and headache. During the last 2 days, she has been confused and cannot perform daily chores. Shortly after arrival she suffers a seizure. Her physical examination indicates some weaknesses in her left side and neck stiffness. Magnetic resonance imaging images show encephalitis localized to the right temporal lobe. What is the most likely causative agent?

a. Adenovirus
b. Coxsackievirus B
c. HSV type 1
d. *Listeria monocytogenes*
e. WNV

101. An 8-month-old girl suddenly developed a high fever (103°F). Her pediatrician examined her and found no signs of upper respiratory tract infection, meningitis, or encephalitis. Two days later, the girl's fever reached 105°F and she suffered a febrile seizure. By the time the child was brought to the pediatrician's office, her temperature had dropped. The doctor noted a generalized papular rash. What was the doctor's most likely diagnosis for this child?

a. Erythema infectiosum caused by parvovirus B19
b. Hand-foot-and-mouth disease caused by Coxsackievirus A
c. Measles caused by *Morbillivirus*
d. Roseola infantum caused by human herpes virus 6
e. Rubella caused by rubella virus

102. A 5-month-old infant, seen in the emergency room in winter, presents with fever and persistent cough with wheezing. Her mother states that the baby's older brother, age 3, had recently had a runny nose, sore throat, and fever. Physical examination of the infant revealed tachypnea and tachycardia; expiratory wheezes were heard over both lungs. The baby was cyanotic and retractions were observed and a chest x-ray showed hyperinflated lung fields. Which of the following is most likely the cause of this infection?

a. Adenovirus
b. Coxsackievirus
c. Parainfluenza virus
d. Respiratory syncytial virus
e. Rhinovirus

103. Which one of the following groups of people is most likely to be at increased risk for HIV infection?

a. Sexual partners of IV drug abusers who share needles
b. Receptionists at a hospital
c. Persons who received blood transfusions in 2013
d. Members of a household in which there is a person who is HIV-positive
e. Factory workers whose coworkers are HIV-positive

104. An obstetrician sees a pregnant patient who was exposed to rubella virus in the 18th week of pregnancy. She does not remember getting a rubella vaccination. Which of the following is the best immediate course of action?

a. Administer rubella immune globulin
b. Administer rubella vaccine
c. Order a rubella antibody titer to determine immune status
d. Reassure the patient because rubella is not a problem until after the 30th week
e. Terminate the pregnancy

105. Two viral vaccines are expected to reduce the incidence of cancers. Which vaccines are these?

a. Adenovirus and mumps virus vaccines
b. HAV and poliovirus vaccines
c. HPV 16/18 and hepatitis B vaccines
d. Measles virus and rubella virus vaccines
e. Rotavirus and VZV vaccines

106. A group of healthcare workers from the United States staffing a clinic in India were working with children admitted with acute flaccid paralysis. The illness began with fever, nausea, vomiting, and severe headache followed by neck stiffness, muscle pain and weakness, and constipation. None of the workers became ill because they had been vaccinated against this disease. Which viral vaccine protected these workers?

a. HAV
b. Measles virus
c. Poliovirus
d. Rubella virus
e. Yellow fever virus

107. A 70-year-old nursing home patient refused the influenza vaccine and subsequently developed influenza, which rapidly progressed to viral pneumonia, for which she was hospitalized. Two days later, she became profoundly worse, was hypoxemic on oxygen, and had a WBC count of 22,000/μL with 80% neutrophils. She died of acute pneumonia 1 week after contracting the flu. Which of the following microorganisms was most likely responsible for her fatal illness?

a. *Escherichia coli*
b. *Klebsiella pneumoniae*
c. *Legionella pneumophila*
d. *Listeria monocytogenes*
e. *Staphylococcus aureus*

108. Along with several children at his elementary school who had similar symptoms, a 6-year-old boy was sent home from school because his eyes were red with a watery, nonpurulent discharge. He had a fever of 102°F and complained of sore throat. A rapid test for Group A *Streptococcus* was negative and his doctor told the boy's mother that her child would recover within a week. Which of the following organisms was the most likely cause of his infection?

a. Adenovirus
b. *Chlamydia trachomatis*
c. *Haemophilus aegyptius*
d. HSV type 1
e. *Staphylococcus aureus*

109. A husband and wife performed the yearly spring cleaning of their mountain cabin, located in the southwestern part of the United States. The woman presented to her physician 2 weeks later with fever, myalgia, headache, and nausea, followed by progressive pulmonary edema and respiratory failure. How did she acquire this viral infection?

a. Contact with her husband
b. Drinking water in the cabin
c. Inhaling aerosolized rodent excreta
d. Mosquito bite
e. Tick bite

110. A 35-year-old professional businesswoman notices the appearance of several hyperkeratotic, well-demarcated growths on the palm side of her index finger and on her toe. They do not change in size and cause her only minimal discomfort. Biopsy of one of the lesions is shown at 40×. Which of the following viruses is the most likely etiologic agent?

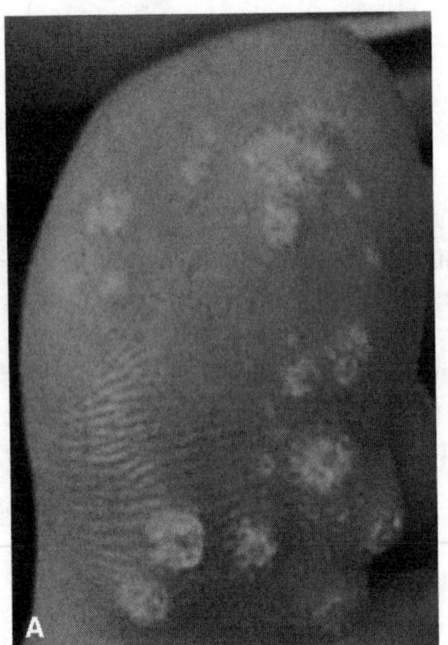

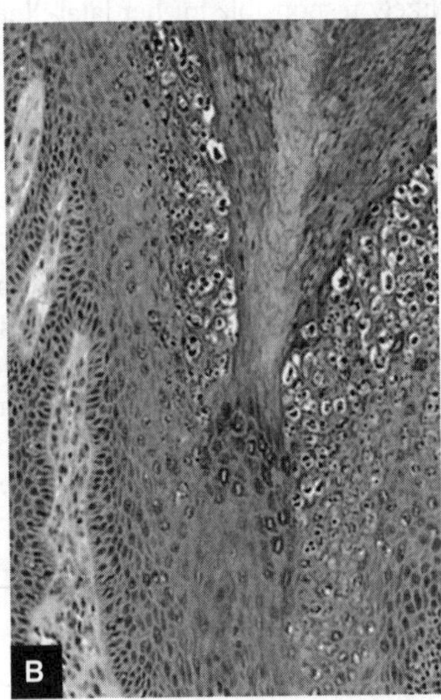

*(**A**: File in public domain; obtained from Wikimedia Commons;* **B**: H&E stain (40×) of skin biopsy. *By Nephron; permission through GNU Free Documentation License.)*

a. Adenovirus
b. HPV
c. Molluscipoxvirus
d. Echovirus
e. VZV

111. A 32-year-old gay male went to his community STD clinic, where it was found that he had perianal condyloma accuminatum. Physical removal was recommended due to the size of the sessions along with immunomodulatory therapy. Which of the following drugs was most likely selected?

a. Acyclovir
b. 5-Fluorouracil
c. Imiquimod
d. Podophyllin
e. Trichloroacetic acid

112. A 7-year-old girl with sickle cell anemia was brought to her physician by her parents who reported that she seemed to be extremely fatigued and pale-looking. They stated that several of her classmates had recently had rashes and bright red cheeks. On examination, the doctor did not see a rash, but observed that her conjunctiva, gums, and nail beds were pale and that she had tachycardia. A CBC revealed that her hemoglobin level had fallen by 2 g/dL from her last result 3 months ago; her reticulocyte count was 0.05%. From which of the following is this child suffering?

a. Aplastic crisis from parvovirus B19 infection
b. Pericarditis caused by Coxsackievirus B
c. Gastroenteritis with bleeding caused by *Norovirus*
d. Exacerbated anemia from *Coltivirus* infection
e. Hemorrhagic cystitis caused by BK polyomavirus

113. An infant who appeared healthy at birth developed sensorineural hearing loss within the first year of life. Viral culture on urine from this child is positive for a relatively slow-growing virus (3 weeks). With which virus was this infant most likely infected at birth?

a. Cytomegalovirus
b. HSV type 2
c. Rubella virus
d. Measles virus
e. VZV

114. A 6-month-old infant has had watery diarrhea for 5 days; he vomited a couple of times. The stools have no blood or pus. He is dehydrated. He has not been outside of Cincinnati, but two other toddlers who visited for a day are also sick. What is the most likely cause of this child's diarrhea?

a. Enterovirus
b. Norovirus
c. Rotavirus
d. *Salmonella enterica*
e. *Staphylococcus aureus* enterotoxin

115. Subacute sclerosing panencephalitis (SSPE) begins with mild changes in personality, behavior and memory, and seizures. The process is progressive and ends with dementia and death. Infection with which virus precedes SSPE?

a. Epstein–Barr virus
b. HIV
c. JC polyomavirus
d. Measles virus
e. Mumps virus

116. A couple who had been hiking in Utah in May developed fever, myalgias, headache, and pain behind their eyes. The fever was present for 3 days, subsided, and then recurred, lasting 3 days. Their doctor recommended antipyretic therapy and told them they should not donate blood for 6 months. With which virus was this couple most likely infected?

a. *Coltivirus*
b. Coxsackievirus B
c. Dengue virus
d. Sin Nombre hantavirus
e. Western equine encephalitis virus

117. An outbreak of disease caused by a virus occurred in Uganda, Africa. Clinical manifestations included hemoptysis and bleeding from the eyes, skin, and gastrointestinal (GI) tract. The mortality rate exceeded 70%. The virus appeared to be transmitted in the village by contact with the blood and bodily secretions of effected individuals; thus, infections rates were higher among those caring for the sick. Which viral disease occurred in this outbreak?

a. Dengue hemorrhagic fever
b. Ebola hemorrhagic fever
c. Hantavirus pulmonary syndrome
d. West Nile encephalitis
e. Yellow fever

118. A transplant patient who had serologic evidence of previous Epstein–Barr virus infection was taking high levels of immunosuppressive medications. He presents with generalized lymphadenopathy, fever, night sweats, weight loss, abdominal pain, and tonsillitis. The dosage of immunosuppressive drugs given to the patient is decreased, and the lymphadenopathy regresses. Which of the following is the best diagnosis for this patient?

a. Burkitt lymphoma
b. Hodgkin lymphoma
c. Infectious mononucleosis
d. Lymphoproliferative disorder
e. Nasopharyngeal carcinoma (NPC)

119. An infant is born to an HIV-positive mother who did not receive antiretroviral therapy during her pregnancy. The mother's HIV viral load, tested just before delivery, was 15,000 copies/mL. Both mother and baby tested positive for HIV antibodies by rapid testing. Since this infant is at risk of vertical transmission of HIV from her mother, the pediatrician decided to treat her prophylactically with a reverse transcriptase inhibitor. Which of the following is the most appropriate choice for prophylaxis?

a. Abacavir
b. Lopinavir
c. Nevirapine
d. Raltegravir
e. Zidovudine

120. A 25-year-old woman from East Texas donated blood in late July. The next day, she called the Blood Center reporting sudden onset of fever, malaise, myalgia, and backache. The staff at the Blood Center notified the woman 3 days later that her blood had tested positive for an arthropod-borne virus. With which virus was this young woman infected?

a. WNV
b. St. Louis encephalitis virus
c. Dengue virus
d. HSV
e. *Coltivirus*

121. A 25-year-old graduate student presents to the local clinic with fever, malaise, lymphadenopathy, and pharyngitis. His spleen is not enlarged and although there is a predominance of lymphocytes reported in his peripheral smear, the heterophile antibody test is negative. What is the most likely etiology of this student's infection?

a. Adenovirus
b. Cytomegalovirus
c. Epstein–Barr virus
d. Parvovirus B19
e. Hepatitis C virus (HCV)

122. A middle-aged man with a long history of multiple operations and blood transfusions was diagnosed with chronic hepatitis C. He was then treated with pegylated interferon-α (IFN-α) and weight-dosed ribavirin. How does IFN-α affect HCV?

a. Blocks viral envelope fusion with host cell membrane
b. Directly inhibits the viral RNA polymerase
c. Induces the antiviral state in host cells to prevent HCV replication
d. Inhibits the viral protease
e. Interferes with guanosine-dependent processes within the cell

123. A 35-year-old man presents with symptoms of jaundice, right upper quadrant pain, and vomiting. His ALT is elevated. He is diagnosed with HAV infection after eating at a restaurant where others were also infected. Which of the following should be done to protect his 68-year-old father and his 6-month-old son?

a. Administer IFN-α to both
b. Give each one dose of γ-globulin
c. Immunize both with one dose of hepatitis A vaccine
d. Quarantine household contacts and observe
e. No treatment is necessary

124. A 42-year-old male AIDS patient presented to the dermatology clinic for evaluation of skin lesions. He had numerous plaque-like lesions over his arms, chest, and neck. Oral examination revealed the lesion shown in the image on his palate. What is the most likely etiologic agent of these lesions?

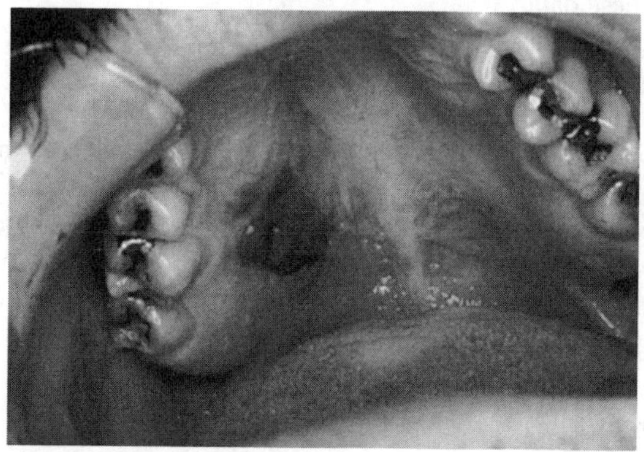

(Courtesy of CDC/Sol Silverman Jr, DDS, University of California, San Francisco 1987; ID#6070.)

a. *Bartonella henselae*
b. Human herpesvirus 8
c. HPV
d. Human T-cell leukemia virus
e. *Staphylococcus aureus*

125. Latent infection of neurons occurs with which of the following viruses?

a. Adenovirus
b. Epstein–Barr virus
c. HSV
d. Measles virus
e. Rabies virus

126. On November 6, a patient had the onset of an illness characterized by fever, chills, headache, cough, and chest pain. The illness lasted 1 week. On December 5, she had another illness very similar to the first, which lasted 6 days. She had no influenza immunization during this period. Her hemagglutination inhibition antibody titers to nH1N1 influenza virus were as follows:

November 6: 10 November 30: 10 December 20: 160

There was no laboratory error. Which of the following is the best conclusion from these data?

a. The patient was ill with influenza on November 6
b. The patient was ill with influenza on December 5
c. The patient was ill with influenza on December 20
d. It is impossible to relate either illness with the nH1N1 influenza virus

127. Recently, a new dsDNA nonenveloped virus has been associated with a human cancer. The viral genome was found to be integrated into the host chromosome of cells in an aggressive skin cancer, Merkel cell carcinoma. To which genus does this new virus belong?

a. *Alphavirus*
b. *Erythrovirus*
c. *Orthohepadnavirus*
d. *Polyomavirus*
e. *Rotavirus*

128. A tourist who recently returned from a Caribbean cruise suddenly develops fever, headache, pain behind her eyes, severe joint, bone, and muscle pain, and a maculopapular rash. The ship had made numerous stops at various islands to allow exploratory trips. The tourist reported significant encounter with mosquitoes at one of the stops. Which of the following is the most likely diagnosis?

a. Dengue
b. Hemorrhagic fever with renal syndrome
c. Hepatitis C
d. Rubella
e. Yellow fever

129. A 30-year-old female who had a history of serious illness requiring surgery and infusion of multiple blood products developed fever, nausea, and jaundice. Her condition has continued for 2 years as a clinically mild disease with fluctuating levels of bilirubin and liver enzymes. Recent blood chemistry testing showed her serum aspartate aminotransferase (AST) to be 352 U/L, ALT 512 U/L, and total bilirubin 4.5 mg/dL. Which of the following best characterizes the virus most likely causing her illness?

a. DNA virus belonging to the *Hepadnaviridae*
b. ss(+)RNA virus belonging to the *Hepeviridae*
c. ss(+)RNA virus belonging to the *Picornaviridae*
d. ss(+)RNA virus belonging to the *Flaviviridae*
e. ss(–)RNA virus known as *Deltavirus*

130. An IV-drug user discovered that a friend with whom he shared needles for injections was diagnosed with viral hepatitis. He had his blood drawn at the local public health clinic and tested for HBV. Which of the following markers is usually the first viral marker detected after infection with HBV?

a. HBcAg
b. HBeAg
c. HBsAg
d. HBeAg IgG
e. HBcAg IGM

131. A 55-year-old woman who had immigrated 30 years ago to the United States from Dominica in the Caribbean presented with cutaneous lesions and hepatosplenomegaly. She was hypercalcemic, had lymphocytosis, and bone lesions were demonstrated on x-ray. Peripheral smear showed cloverleaf lymphocytes, consistent with acute T-cell leukemia (CD4+ lymphocytes), in which a provirus was found. Which virus is most likely responsible for her disease?

a. HIV-1
b. HIV-2
c. HTLV-1
d. HTLV-2

132. A 19-year-old male presented to his family physician complaining of severe pain in his eye and intolerance to light. His eye was red and tearing. Ophthalmic visualization revealed coalescing dendritic ulcers in his right eye that were easily seen with fluorescein staining of the cornea. The patient stated that he does not wear contact lenses, and that he had never had fever blisters; his mother to corroborated this. What is the most likely etiologic agent of his ulcer?

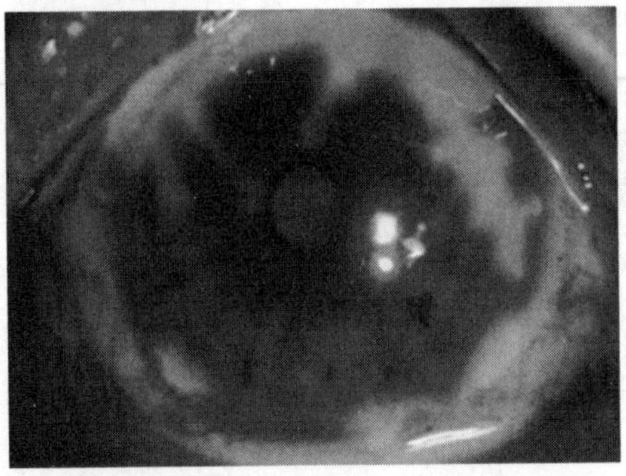

(Courtesy of HK Yang et al, Department of Ophthalmology, Seoul National University College of Medicine, Seoul, Korea, 30 August 2012. Permission licensed under the Creative Commons Attribution 2.5 Generic license.)

a. *Acanthamoeba*
b. Foreign body
c. *Fusarium*
d. HSV type 1
e. Severe allergy

133. Reactivation of VZV is known to occur in persons receiving immunosuppressive therapy. Which of the following is the best antiviral for treating this infection?

a. Amantadine
b. Boceprevir
c. Ribavirin
d. Valacyclovir
e. Zidovudine

134. An infant with microcephaly, jaundice, and hepatosplenomegaly was also small for gestation, and had thrombocytopenia. Radiology of the neonate's head revealed intracranial calcifications. Which one of the following viruses most likely caused these congenital malformations?

a. Rubella virus
b. Respiratory syncytial virus
c. HIV
d. Mumps virus
e. Cytomegalovirus

135. A 32-year-old woman who had not received the usual pediatric vaccinations developed fever, headache, malaise, and ear pain accompanied by swelling of the parotid glands. One week later, her fever subsided but she developed pelvic pain and tenderness. With which virus was she infected?

a. Cytomegalovirus
b. Mumps virus
c. Rabies virus
d. Respiratory syncytial virus
e. Rubella virus

136. Worldwide 3 to 5 million cases of severe influenza illnesses and 250,000 to 500,000 deaths occur annually. Great effort is made annually to prepare influenza vaccines against circulating strains of *Influenzavirus* A and B. Yet, in some years, the vaccine is less effective in neutralizing the virus even though the circulating strains are the same type as that from the previous year; that is, both are H1N1 or both are H2N3. Which of the following mechanisms is responsible for this problem?

a. Antigenic drift
b. Antigenic shift
c. Complementation
d. Intramolecular recombination
e. Phenotypic mixing

137. A visitor from rural Mexico visited the United States and was admitted to a hospital after being diagnosed with probable rabies. Which of the following is the best representation of his prognosis?

a. He should survive without complications
b. He should survive but have seizures for life
c. He has a 50% chance of survival if aggressive therapy is instituted
d. Rabies is almost invariably fatal

138. Although vaccination with live, attenuated, or killed viral vaccines has been the most effective way of controlling viral disease in the population, common colds remain widespread because of the multiple serotypes identified. Which of the following viruses represents this problem?

a. Cytomegalovirus
b. Mumps virus
c. Rabies virus
d. Respiratory syncytial virus
e. Rhinovirus

139. A 3-year-old girl who was in day care presented with sudden onset of fever, nausea, vomiting, and anorexia. Her sclera were yellow and her abdomen was tender to palpation. Blood chemistries showed an AST of 640 U/L and ALT was 520 U/L. Previously, two other children had had similar symptoms. Which of the following tests would be most likely to reveal the etiology of her hepatitis?

a. Viral culture of stool
b. Test for hepatitis B surface antigen
c. Electron microscopy on stool specimen
d. Detection of rotavirus antigen
e. Anti-HAV IgM

140. In January, two school districts saw a sudden increase in absences. At the same time, sales of over-the-counter medications for fever, cough, and cold symptoms increased dramatically. To determine the etiology of this outbreak of respiratory illness, the public health department conducted a survey of local physicians to see what types of patients they were currently seeing most. The doctors all reported increased numbers of patients complaining of abrupt onset of high fever, severe headache, and myalgia followed by sore throat, dry cough, weakness, and severe fatigue. The patients were ill for 3 to 5 days, but many reported persistent malaise. What is the most likely diagnosis for this outbreak?

a. Common cold
b. Hand-foot-and-mouth disease
c. Influenza
d. Pharyngitis
e. Pneumonia

141. A vaccine against *Morbillivirus* (measles virus), introduced in 1963, has decreased the incidence of measles from an expected event in the life of every child to 50 to 200 cases per year in the United States. Which of the following best characterizes the vaccine that has dramatically reduced the incidence of this disease in the United States?

a. Inactivated virus
b. Live attenuated virus
c. Recombinant viral protein
d. Virus-specific immunoglobulin
e. Wild-type live virus

142. A newlywed couple was surprised to find that both experienced genital herpes lesions in their first year of marriage. Both were given an antiviral that is activated only in infected cells. Which of the following is the viral enzyme responsible for activation of the drug of choice for this infection?

a. DNA-dependent DNA polymerase
b. Integrase
c. Protease
d. RNA-dependent RNA polymerase
e. Thymidine kinase

143. A neonate born to a woman with chronic hepatitis B infection is at great risk of contracting the virus and subsequently becoming a chronic carrier of HBV. Which of the following is the best approach to preventing the neonate becoming infected?

a. Give hepatitis B immunoglobulin (HBIg) at birth
b. Give HBIg at 6 months, when maternal antibodies have diminished
c. Immunize with recombinant HBV vaccine (rHBV) at birth
d. Immunize with rHBV at 1 year
e. Give HBIg and immunize with rHBV vaccine at birth

144. Twenty days after contact with an individual with an acute disease presentation, a 12-year-old girl has fever (low grade), malaise, and a rash composed of crops of vesicles that lasts 5 days. This common childhood disease is caused by which of the following viruses?

a. Adenovirus
b. Cytomegalovirus
c. HPV
d. Measles virus
e. VZV

145. Over 400 military recruits undergoing basic training experienced an acute respiratory disease outbreak in their second month of camp. Most had high fever and sore throats with coughing; 27 developed pneumonia, five severe enough to require intensive care, and one died. Which of the following agents is the most likely cause of this outbreak?

a. VZV
b. Rotavirus
c. Papillomavirus
d. Cytomegalovirus
e. Adenovirus

146. Which of the following genetic disorders predisposes patients to widespread HPV infection and cutaneous squamous cell carcinoma?

a. Epidermodysplasia verruciformis
b. Familial adenomatous polyposis
c. Li–Fraumeni syndrome
d. NPC
e. Xeroderma pigmentosum

147. A 9-month-old girl, who has never been vaccinated, presents with a 3-day history of fever and watery, nonbloody diarrhea. On physical examination, she appears dehydrated. Which of the following describes the genome of the most likely infecting organism?

a. Double-stranded DNA
b. Single-stranded DNA
c. Segmented single-stranded minus-sense RNA
d. Nonsegmented single-stranded plus-sense RNA
e. Segmented double-stranded RNA

148. A 20-year-old college football player presented himself to the local emergency medicine department complaining of headache, fever, and malaise for 2 weeks and now a sore throat. The physician noted enlarged lymph nodes and hepatosplenomegaly. Laboratory tests found increased number of atypical lymphocytes and a reactive heterophile antibody test. The physician advised him not to play football until his symptoms had resolved. What is the best explanation for this advice?

a. To avert heat exhaustion
b. To avoid rupture of his spleen
c. To prevent malnutrition
d. To stave off an aplastic crisis

149. A humanitarian healthcare worker deployed in emergency to Darfur, Sudan, forgot to use insect repellant. Four days after being bitten several times by mosquitoes, he developed fever, chills, headache, back ache, and muscle aches. Two days later, he suffered a nosebleed and noticed his stools were black. The next day, he was jaundiced and vomited black material. Despite supportive care, he developed organ failure and died. What was the cause of this patient's death?

a. Dengue hemorrhagic shock
b. Hantavirus cardiopulmonary syndrome
c. Hemorrhagic fever with renal syndrome
d. SARS
e. Yellow fever

150. A patient who had not been vaccinated against influenza has hemagglutination inhibition titers against influenzavirus A as follows: acute = 10, convalescent = 80. Which of the following is the correct conclusion concerning this patient?

a. No infection
b. Primary infection
c. Anamnestic response
d. Past infection

151. A 10-year-old boy in a malarial area of Africa was diagnosed with a poorly differentiated B-cell tumor of the jaw that was characterized by a translocation of the *c-myc* oncogene, t(8:14). The boy also has an elevated antibody titer to a specific viral early antigen with a restricted pattern of fluorescence. This disease is caused by which of the following?

a. *Borrelia burgdorferi*
b. *Chlamydia trachomatis*
c. *Cytomegalovirus*
d. Epstein–Barr virus
e. HSV

152. A 55-year-old Chinese man in southern China sought medical help due to a serious otitis media, which was related to obstruction of his Eustachian tubes. Medical examination and laboratory testing resulted in a diagnosis of NPC. Which of the following viruses may be detected by the PCR in a variety of cells of patients with this type of carcinoma?

a. Epstein–Barr virus
b. Measles virus
c. Mumps virus
d. Parvovirus B19
e. Rubella virus

153. A patient with HIV infection that has progressed to AIDS had been treated previously for cytomegalovirus pneumonia. For which additional CMV disease would this patient also be at risk?

a. Aplastic crisis
b. Kidney failure
c. Retinitis
d. Reye syndrome
e. SSPE

154. An estimated 6.2 million new HPV infections occur annually in the United States. The peak incidence occurs in adolescents and young adults under 25 years of age. Which of the following specimens is best for screening for the presence of HPV infection of the cervix?

a. DNA molecular probe for HPV genomes
b. HPV-specific antibodies
c. Pap smear on cells from cervix for koilocytes
d. PCR for HPV DNA
e. Viral culture for HPV

155. A business man who contracted dengue in the Philippines during a business trip in 2011 took his family to the Caribbean for a vacation in 2012. The entire family was plagued with mosquito bites while walking early one morning. Four days later, the man, his wife, and their 17-old-daughter experienced sudden onset of fever of 103 to 104°F, chills and severe head, back, and muscle aches. He had pain behind his eyes. Their 12-year-old son had similar symptoms but lessened in intensity, while their 6-year-old daughter had fever that broke and returned and a rash. Their fevers lasted 3 to 4 days with onset of rash in all. Shortly after their fevers subsided, the man and the 6-year-old developed abdominal pain, petechiae, and bleeding gums. What complication did this man and child develop?

a. Acute respiratory distress syndrome
b. Dengue hemorrhagic fever
c. Encephalitis
d. Guillain–Barré syndrome
e. Secondary bacterial infection

156. A 16-year-old male developed chest pain and dyspnea, which gradually worsened. He was examined in the Emergency Department where tachycardia and signs of heart failure were noted. Electrocardiographic changes were seen and chest x-ray revealed cardiomegaly. An enterovirus was isolated from a stool specimen. Which of the following was the agent most likely isolated?

a. Coxsackievirus A
b. Coxsackievirus B
c. Echovirus 11
d. Enterovirus 70
e. Poliovirus 3

157. A 38-year-old woman has developed crops of vesicular lesions. After 3 days, she developed pneumonia and was hospitalized. Which of the following would be most likely to be present in lung cells obtained by bronchoalveolar biopsy?

a. Cowdry A inclusion bodies
b. Guarnieri bodies
c. Koilocytes
d. Negri bodies
e. Owl's eye cells

158. A patient diagnosed with influenza reported onset of symptoms 18 hours ago. Which of the following is the most appropriate treatment for this patient?

a. Amantadine
b. Foscarnet
c. Oseltamivir
d. Ribavirin
e. Zidovudine

159. A group of 15 young college students harvested oysters from a bay near Galveston despite a warning sign that the area was contaminated with sewage. Ten ate the oysters raw. Twenty-five days later, six of them presented to their physicians with sudden onset of acute jaundice and liver function abnormalities. Which of the following is the most likely cause of their infections?

a. HAV
b. HBV
c. HCV
d. HDV
e. HEV

160. An 18-month old developed acute gastroenteritis with fever and watery diarrhea that lasted 10 days. She had been vaccinated against rotavirus at 2 and 4 months of age as recommended. Eight days later, both of her brothers, ages 3 and 6, developed acute gastroenteritis. Which of the following tests would most likely reveal the etiologic agent of their gastroenteritis?

a. Culture for *Norovirus*
b. DFA for enterovirus on intestinal biopsy
c. EIA for adenovirus 40/41
d. EM examination of stool for astrovirus
e. Serology for *Rotavirus*

161. An outbreak of diarrhea in a day care center is suspected to be of rotaviral origin. Which test is most appropriate to diagnose this outbreak?

a. Culture
b. EIA
c. Electron microscopy
d. Histologic examination of biopsy
e. Serology

162. Adults and children experienced an outbreak of diarrhea with nausea and vomiting while aboard a cruise ship in the Caribbean. The causative agent was detected by EIA testing. Which virus listed below was most likely responsible for this outbreak?

a. Adenovirus 40/41
b. *Astrovirus*
c. HAV
d. *Norovirus*
e. *Rotavirus*

163. An outbreak of diarrhea occurred among elderly patients in an assisted care facility, which had been repeatedly cited by the public health department for poor hygiene practices. The agent that caused the infections had a starlike morphology in electron micrographs. EIA tests for several agents of viral gastroenteritis were negative. Which virus was most likely responsible for this outbreak?

a. Adenovirus 40/41
b. *Astrovirus*
c. HAV
d. *Norovirus*
e. *Rotavirus*

164. A young refugee from Afghanistan developed mild fever, cervical lymphadenopathy, and a rash that began on her face and spread downward over her trunk. After 3 days, the rash disappeared. She had not been immunized against any infections except diphtheria and tetanus. What is the best diagnosis for this child?

a. Chickenpox
b. Erythema infectiosum
c. Measles
d. Hand-foot-and-mouth disease
e. Rubella

165. A 57-year-old man diagnosed previously with chronic hepatitis C is being treated for his infection. Which of the following tests is the best to evaluate his therapy for an early virologic response?

a. HCV IgG
b. HCV IgM
c. HCV RNA level
d. Liver biopsy
e. Serum ALT levels

166. A 45-year-old man with active chronic hepatitis B infection is being treated to reduce liver inflammation and fibrosis and to prevent progression to cirrhosis. He is HBeAg-positive and had begun a 48-week course of pegylated IFN-α, but he was unable to tolerate the side effects. Which of the following would be the best antiviral to treat this patient?

a. Acyclovir
b. Foscarnet
c. Ribavirin
d. Tenofovir
e. Zidovudine

167. Two weeks after a series of mid-July thunderstorms resulted in an explosion of the mosquito population, a 10-year-old boy living on a farm in southern Minnesota was brought to the emergency room by his parents. He has a 2-day history of fever, headache, and vomiting, but today he appeared confused. His cerebrospinal fluid was clear with 100 WBC (75% lymphocytes) and a head CT was normal. Enterovirus infection was quickly ruled out by PCR testing. Which of the following is the most likely cause of his symptoms?

a. La Crosse virus
b. Poliovirus
c. Rabies virus
d. St. Louis encephalitis virus
e. Venezuelan equine encephalitis virus

168. Which of the following would be present in a neonate with congenital rubella syndrome (CRS) but not in a neonate with cytomegalic inclusion disease (congenital CMV infection)?

a. Intrauterine growth retardation
b. Hepatosplenomegaly
c. Mental retardation
d. Patent ductus arteriosus
e. Sensorineural hearing loss

169. Viruses have various ways of entering the human body and producing disease. Which of the following descriptions accurately describes the route of transmission and target disease for the virus indicated?

a. Coronavirus: fecal–oral; peptic ulcers
b. Echovirus: fecal–oral; aseptic meningitis
c. HIV: respiratory droplet; anemia
d. Influenzavirus: blood-borne; maculopapular rash
e. Rabies virus: rodent-borne; pneumonia

170. A 68-year-old man from central California who liked to sit in the park and doze developed fever, headache, muscle weakness, and nausea and vomiting. His muscle weakness progressed, and he was admitted to the hospital with acute flaccid paralysis. No focal lesions were seen on MRI. After a prolonged hospital stay, he was discharged to a rehabilitation center where he regained function. With which virus was this man most likely infected?

a. WNV
b. St. Louis encephalitis virus
c. Poliovirus
d. HSV
e. *Coltivirus*

171. An immunocompromised patient presented with a progressive cerebral deterioration evidenced by difficulty speaking, memory loss, and loss of coordination that led to paralysis. An MRI revealed lesions in the white matter; brain biopsy revealed foci of demyelination, astrocytosis, and nuclear inclusion bodies within oligodendrocytes. Normal CSF findings (cell count, glucose, protein) were present, but viral DNA was found in the CSF by PCR. Which of the following viruses causes is the etiologic agent of this patient's disease?

a. HPV
b. JC polyomavirus
c. Prion variant CJD
d. Measles virus
e. WNV

172. An irritable 18-month-old toddler with fever and blister-like ulcerations on mucous membranes of the oral cavity refuses to eat (representative image, left). The symptoms worsen and then slowly resolve over a period of 2 weeks. Six months later, the child develops a single vesicular lesion that resolves in 6 days (representative image, right); she does not have fever. Which of the following scenarios is most likely?

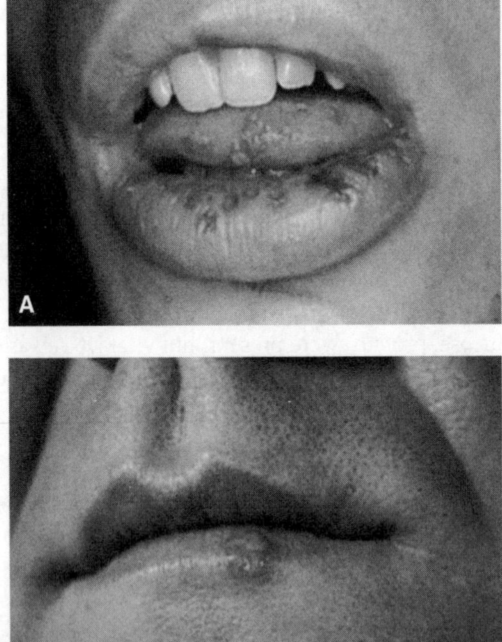

*(**A**: Courtesy of CDC/Robert E. Sumpter, 1987, ID#12616; **B**: Courtesy of CDC/Dr. Herrmann, 1964, ID#5434.)*

a. The virus will remain latent in the trigeminal ganglia
b. The vesicular lesions will not recur
c. The child will develop Guillain–Barré syndrome
d. The child will develop hepatocellular carcinoma later in life
e. The child will develop SSPE

173. A sexually active 17-year-old man presents to the local free clinic to check some small papules that appeared on his penis. The papules are small, white lesions with a central depression. There is no discharge or pain on urination. What is the virus most likely causing these lesions?

a. Adenovirus
b. Coxsackievirus A
c. HPV type 6
d. *Molluscipoxvirus*
e. Orf virus

174. A 3-month-old infant born at prematurely at 30 weeks of gestation is in the neonatal intensive care unit in November. The first cases of respiratory syncytial virus have been diagnosed in the city. Which of the following may be given to this infant as prophylaxis to prevent respiratory syncytial virus (RSV) infection?

a. IFN-α
b. Palivizumab
c. Pooled immunoglobulin
d. Ribavirin
e. Rituximab

175. Malnourished children are at risk for complications of measles, leading to greater morbidity and mortality. Which of the following should be given to children to reduce these risks?

a. Vitamin A
b. Vitamin B
c. Vitamin C
d. Vitamin D
e. Vitamin E

176. Which of the following immune responses is required to prevent target infection by poliovirus, EEEV, and La Crosse virus?

a. Complement activation
b. Cytotoxic T cells specific for the virus
c. Natural killer cells
d. Neutralizing IgG specific for the virus
e. Neutrophils

177. A 45-year-old woman living in Washington, DC, had been complaining to her landlord about mice in her apartment. A week ago, she suffered flu-like symptoms accompanied by swollen lymph nodes and a rash, which had resolved over 5 days. Four days later, she developed a severe headache and other signs of viral encephalitis. She reported no contact with mosquitoes. With which virus was she most likely infected?

a. La Crosse virus
b. Lassa fever virus
c. Lymphocytic choriomeningitis virus
d. Sin Nombre hantavirus
e. Western equine encephalitis virus

178. An elderly man had been in several military conflicts during the early 1980s and received blood transfusions for injuries. He recently consulted his physician for what was diagnosed as cryoglobulinemia and glomerulonephritis. Additional testing revealed that he was infected by a flavivirus whose transmission was bloodborne. Which of the following viruses was involved in this infection?

a. HAV
b. HBV
c. HCV
d. HDV
e. HEV

179. An outbreak of influenza occurred in a rural community. Since influenza can be treated if therapy is begun within 48 hours of onset of symptoms, specific detection of the virus is important. Which of the following tests listed is the most rapid for detection of influenza viruses?

a. Cold agglutinin test
b. Culture of respiratory secretions on monkey kidney cells
c. Detection of influenza antigen in respiratory secretions
d. Electron microscopy of sputum
e. Paired sera for specific antibody response

Virology

Answers

64. The answer is d. (*Levinson, Ch 39, 43, 45. Murray, Ch 62. Ryan, Ch 18.*) Reverse transcriptase (RT) PCR for HIV RNA (d) has recently been shown to be the most valuable test for diagnosis of acute HIV infection (acute retroviral syndrome) during the window period before antibodies can be detected. This qualitative test for detection of HIV virions is positive at the time symptoms of acute infection appear, as early as 7 days postinfection; the test is also positive in asymptomatic individuals and is used to screen donated blood. The test for HIV p24 antigen (c) is the next to become positive, 17 to 38 days after infection. Antibodies appear last at 21 to 42 days (3 to 6 weeks) postinfection. While there is some difference in the time to positivity of the various types of HIV antibody tests, the HIV antibody test by ELISA (b) would be no more likely to be positive this early than the latex aggregation test. The western blot for HIV antibodies (e) is used to confirm positive screening tests for antibodies. The CD4 T-cell count (a) is used to assess status of the immune system, determine the timing for treatment, suggest the likelihood of onset of various opportunistic infections, and monitor progress response of the immune system to treatment. The count is unlikely to be decreased at 2 weeks postinfection although a drop does coincide with the peak of viremia.

65. The answer is b. (*Levinson, Ch 38. Murray, Ch 53. Ryan, Ch 10.*) Parvovirus B19 (b) is the causative agent of erythema infectiosum (fifth disease). The infection occurs in two phases. First is the lytic, infectious phase characterized by nonspecific flulike symptoms (fever, chills, headache, and myalgia) that lasts about a week. This accompanied by a decrease in reticulocyte count and hemoglobin, which is not usually noticed in healthy children and adults. The second phase begins a week later when virus-specific IgG antibody appears and includes the characteristic "slapped cheek" appearance and lacy reticular rash. Adults often develop polyarthropathy or arthralgia. The rash and arthropathy are due to circulating antigen–antibody complexes. The rashes of rubella virus (c) and rubeola

virus (measles virus) (d) occur in conjunction with fever. The lesions produced by HSV1 (a) and VZV (e) are vesicular in nature.

66. The answer is a. (*Levinson, Ch 37. Murray, Ch 51. Ryan, Ch 10, 14.*) This patient has either primary or recurrent HSV-2. Primary infections are asymptomatic in 75% of patients making these infections responsible for the majority of the neonatal HSV infections. Women with recurrent infections who have antibodies to HSV-2 are less likely to transmit HSV to their neonates during birth. Currently (2007), the American College of Obstetricians and Gynecologists recommend that cesarean delivery (a) is indicated in women with active genital lesions at onset of labor (parturition). Additionally, such women should be offered antiviral therapy at 36 weeks of gestation or beyond. Internal fetal monitoring (b) and rupture of the membranes to speed delivery (c) should not be done when active HSV lesions are present; and if possible, vaginal delivery (d) should be avoided. If this is not possible, the pediatrician should be notified regarding the mother's active HSV.

67. The answer is b. (*Guidelines for the Use of Antiretroviral Agents in HIV-1 Infected Adults and Adolescents. Katzung, Ch 49. Levinson, Ch 39, 43, 45. Murray, Ch 62. Ryan, Ch 18. Schneider E et al.*) The image shows acute oral pseudomembranous candidiasis or thrush, one of the opportunistic infections that occur in persons with CD4 T-cell counts between 200 and 500/μL. At CD4 counts lower than 200/μL, *Candida* becomes chronic and more invasive, extending into the esophagus. The Centers for Disease Prevention and Control strongly recommends that all HIV-positive individuals be treated with highly active antiviral therapy (HAART), especially when their CD4 T-cell counts fall below 350/μL (*http://www.cdc.gov/mmwr/preview/mmwrhtml/rr5710a2.htm*) or if the patient is pregnant or has certain other concomitant conditions. The recommended regimens for treatment-naïve individuals includes two nucleoside reverse transcriptase inhibitors (NRTI) plus one nonnucleoside RTI; or two NRTI plus a ritonavir-boosted protease inhibitor (PI); or two NRTI plus one integrase inhibitor; a fifth regimen consists of three NRTI. The combination of drugs works together to forestall appearance of resistance. The combination of efavirenz plus tenofovir plus emtricitabine (b), one NNRTI plus two NRTI, respectively, meets the recommendations. Abacavir (a), a NRTI that requires HLA-B*5701 testing prior to use if at all possible; nevirapine (e), a NNRTI; and darunavir boosted with ritonavir (c), both PI, should never be used alone. Maraviroc plus enfuvirtide plus raltegravir (d), the CCR5 inhibitor, fusion inhibitor,

and integrase inhibitor, respectively, are used for salvage therapy following virologic failure or when resistance is present to many NRTI, NNRTI, and PI; although not necessarily together. The diagram shows the site of action of the available antiretrovirals.

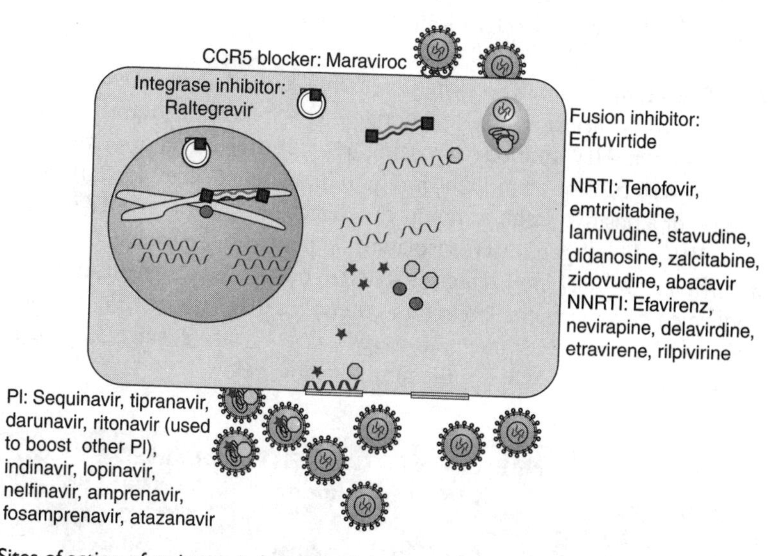

Sites of action of antiretroviral drugs and the classes to which they belong. *(Prepared by Jane Colmer-Hamood in Microsoft PowerPoint.)*

68. The answer is e. *(Beckwith. Levinson, Ch 39, 43, 45. Murray, Ch 62. Ryan, Ch 18.)* Patients often improve rapidly on appropriate HAART; their CD4 lymphocyte counts increase and their HIV viral loads are drastically reduced, often to less than 50 copies per milliliter. These two changes are indicative of the fact that the antiretroviral therapy has been effective (e). While her risk of contracting some opportunistic infections, such as esophagitis caused by *Candida albicans* or cytomegalovirus, *Cryptococcus neoformans* meningitis, *Toxoplasma gondii* encephalitis, or *Cryptosporidium parvum* diarrhea, has lessened, she is still at risk for other opportunistic infections. These include polydermatomal VZV (shingles), acquisition or reactivation of *Mycobacterium tuberculosis*, oral hairy leukoplakia caused by Epstein–Barr virus, and *C. albicans* pharyngitis (thrush), as well as recurrent bacterial pneumonia. Thus, choice (a), the patient is no longer in danger of opportunistic infections, is incorrect. While she may have an excellent

5-year prognosis (b), that cannot be stated at this time. The patient's HIV screening test (c) should remain positive until late in AIDS, when antibody levels do drop off. The patient still has viral RNA present and must be considered infectious, so choice (d) is incorrect; even if her HIV RNA drops to undetectable levels, she could still harbor the virus within macrophages, dendritic cells, or other cells within her body.

69. The answer is c. (*Beckwith. Levinson, Ch 39, 43, 45. Murray, Ch 62. Ryan, Ch 18. Schneider.*) Current criteria for HIV infection require a positive result from an HIV antibody screening test confirmed by a positive result from a western blot or indirect immunofluorescence assay for HIV antibodies; or a positive result or report of a detectable quantity of HIV nucleic acid, HIV p24 antigen, or HIV isolation (*http://www.cdc.gov/mmwr/preview/mmwrhtml/rr5710a1.htm*). Then, as stated in the revised case definitions: "A confirmed case meets the laboratory criteria for diagnosis of HIV infection and one of the four HIV infection stages (stage 1, stage 2, stage 3, or stage unknown)." The stages are outlined in the table below.

STAGES OF HIV INFECTION AS CURRENTLY DEFINED BY CDC

Stage	CD4+T-lymphocyte Count (% of Total Lymphs)	AIDS-Defining Condition[a]
HIV Infection, Stage 1	≥500 cells/μL (≥29)	None
HIV Infection, Stage 2	200-499 cells/μL (14-28)	None[a]
HIV Infection, Stage 3 (AIDS)	<200 cells/μL (<14)	None or Present[a]
HIV Infection, Stage Unknown	No information available	No information available

[a]The presence of an AIDS-defining condition moves the stage to 3 even if the CD4 count is higher. See *http://www.cdc.gov/mmwr/preview/mmwrhtml/rr57 10a2.htm* for a list of AIDS-defining conditions.

Courtesy of CDC. http://www.cdc.gov/mmwr/preview/mmwrhtml/rr5710a1.htm

70. The answer is d. (*Levinson, Ch 37. Murray, Ch 51. Ryan, Ch 10, 14.*) The patient has infectious mononucleosis (IM) caused by Epstein–Barr virus (d); the key being the positive monospot test (heterophile antibody test). CMV (b) can also cause a mononucleosis syndrome, but the monospot would be negative. In the case of heterophile (monospot)-negative

IM, tests for antibodies for CMV and for specific EBV proteins (viral capsid antigen, early antigen, and nuclear antigen) should be done. Not all persons develop heterophile antibodies, especially children and older adults; and these antibodies are transient. Adenovirus (a) is more frequently associated with pharyngoconjunctivitis or pneumonia; echovirus (c) with aseptic meningitis; and human metapneumovirus (e) with respiratory infections. The majority of infections caused by these three viruses occur in children.

71. The answer is b. (*Beckwith. Levinson, Ch 39, 43, 45. Murray, Ch 62. Ryan, Ch 18. Schneider.*) Numerous tests are now available for *screening* patients for antibodies to HIV including rapid tests performed on blood, oral secretions, and urine. The rapid tests are EIAs and latex aggregation tests that do not have to be repeated, but that require a confirmatory western blot or immunofluorescence assay. Conventional EIAs require repeat testing by the same test (b) followed by a confirmatory test if the EIA is repeatedly reactive. As screening tests, these assays have a high sensitivity, which means that false-positive results may occur. The western blot and IFA have high specificities and low false-positive rates. Key here is *screening*; diagnostic testing is different because the index of suspicion for HIV is high. In this setting, a negative EIA should be repeated in 3 months and/or a nucleic acid test be performed. The patient should not be told she is even HIV-positive, much less that she is likely to develop AIDS (d) until her positive test is confirmed. There is no reason to begin antiretroviral therapy (a) or to test the patient for *Pneumocystis jiroveci* infection (e); this infection appears in HIV-infected persons when their CD4 T-cell count drops below 200/μL.

72. The answer is e. (*Levinson, Ch 42, 43. Murray, Ch 60. Ryan, Ch 16.*) The most common arthropod-borne encephalitis viruses causing neuroinvasive disease in the United States are WNV (hundreds to thousands of cases of neuroinvasive disease per year), La Crosse virus (55-137 per year), St. Louis encephalitis virus (5-13 per year), and EEEV (4-12 cases per year). While La Crosse virus is a more common cause of neuroinvasive disease than St. Louis encephalitis virus (e), SLEV (e) is the most likely to have been responsible. LaCV (d) causes neuroinvasive disease almost exclusively in children younger than 16 years of age. See the below table for more information.

ARTHROPOD-BORNE (ARBO) VIRUSES THAT CAUSE ENCEPHALITIS IN THE UNITED STATES

Common Name	Reservoir	Vector	Distribution (Major)	Disease (Mortality)	Age; Comment
Togaviridae/Alphavirus					
Eastern equine encephalitis virus (EEEV)	Birds	*Aedes* mosquito	Atlantic Coast, Gulf Coast	Encephalitis, severe, rapidly progressing (35%)	<15, >60 years
Western EEV	Birds	*Culex* mosquito	West of Mississippi River; no cases have occurred in United States in 5 years	Encephalitis (10%)	Infants
Flaviviridae/Flavivirus					
St. Louis encephalitis virus	Birds	*Culex* mosquito	States along the Mississippi, Ohio Rivers; Gulf Coast; URBAN	Encephalitis (2% young; 20% elderly)	>70 years
West Nile virus[a]	Birds	*Aedes, Culex* mosquitoes	All states; TX, CA, LA, IL, MI, MS, OK (>100 cases in 2012)	Encephalitis (12% elderly) Meningitis	>60 years Children 10% flaccid paralysis 50% suffer sequelae
Powassan virus	Small mammals	*Ixodes* ticks	North America—northern states (MN, WI, NY, ME)	Severe encephalitis (High)	
Bunyaviridae/Bunyavirus					
LaCrosse virus	Small mammal	*Aedes* mosquito	North Central, Midwest states; RURAL (MN, WI, OH, WV)	Encephalitis (<1%)	<16 years 20% left with seizures
Reoviridae/Coltivirus					
Colorado tick fever virus	Small mammal	*Dermacentor* ticks	Rocky Mountain and Cascade Mountain regions	Colorado tick fever encephalitis rarely (low)	Mild

[a]Currently the most common cause of arthropod-borne viral encephalitis in the United States: *5890 cases 2012; 2734 cases of neuroinvasive disease; 243 deaths; ~600 asymptomatic blood donors.*

73. The answer is a. (*Levinson, Ch 44. Murray, Ch 64. Ryan, Ch 20.*) Rapidly progressive dementia and myoclonus associated with presence of 14-3-3 protein is strongly suggestive of Creutzfeldt–Jakob disease, which was confirmed by the presence of spongiform encephalopathy at autopsy. CJD occurs in four forms. Sporadic CJD (a) has a median age of onset of 62 years (60-74 for most, although cases as young as 17 have been seen) and results from spontaneous conversion of normal PrP^{C} to PrP^{SC} or spontaneous mutation of the *PRNP* gene leading to production of PrP^{SC}, the abnormal form; myoclonus is an important component of symptoms; death usually occurs within 8 months after onset of symptoms. Familial CJD (b), associated with an autosomal dominant inheritance of mutations in the *PRNP* gene, onsets between 45 and 49 years of age; progression is slower and death occurs in about 2 years. Variant CJD (d) is acquired through eating meat from cattle with bovine spongiform encephalopathy; the majority of reported cases have been linked to exposure in the United Kingdom; age of onset varies, but median is 28 years of age; psychiatric abnormalities and sensory symptoms are predominant in variant CJD; death occurs in approximately 14 months. Iatrogenic CJD (c) has occurred following corneal transplants, dura grafts, administration of human pituitary-derived gonadotropins, and use of contaminated surgical instruments and EEG electrodes; iatrogenic variant CJD has also been documented from blood transfusion.

74. The answer is b. (*Levinson, Ch 40. Murray, Ch 55. Ryan, Ch 15.*) While rhinoviruses are the major cause of the common cold (50%-80% of cases), human coronaviruses cause up to 15% of cases of common cold (b), especially in older children and adults. The coronaviruses causing severe respiratory illness have been zoonotic in origin; human coronaviruses rarely cause pneumonia (d). Coronavirus-like particles have been demonstrated by EM in stools of children and adults with diarrhea and neonates with necrotizing enterocolitis. Human coronaviruses have not been associated with vesicular lesions (e) or meningitis (c). Coxsackievirus A causes herpangina (b).

75. The answer is b. (*Levinson, Ch 41. Murray, Ch 63. Ryan, Ch 13.*) HDV, previously known as the delta agent, was first described in 1977 and has been shown to be a satellite RNA virus that requires HBsAg for encapsidation. Thus, it requires the presence of replicating HBV. It is found most often in IV drug abusers and persons who have received multiple blood transfusions. HDV can be acquired as a coinfection with HBV and follows the progress of the HBV infection. If HBV is resolved, HDV is also resolved; if HBV becomes chronic, HDV also persists. HDV can also be acquired as a superinfection in a person with chronic HBV. In these individuals, an acute hepatitis episode occurs that may progress to fulminant hepatitis described in the vignette. This situation strongly suggests that the patient contracted HDV (b). It is unlikely that a HBV mutant would develop (a). Cirrhosis (c) develops over years and is a chronic process involving fibrotic changes in the liver. It is possible that the person acquired HAV from food (d), but fulminant hepatitis is not usually seen in the United States except in those over 50; even then, it is rare (2% or less of all cases of HAV infection result in death). HEV is found in Mexico, India, parts of China and southeast Asia, and North Africa. Food in the United States would be unlikely to contain HEV (e).

76. The answer is b. (*Katzung, 49. Levinson, Ch 35. Murray, Ch 48. Ryan, Ch 8.*) Both foscarnet (b) and ganciclovir (c) are used to treat cytomegalovirus infection, but foscarnet inhibits pyrophosphate binding activity of viral DNA polymerase while ganciclovir is a nucleoside analog that prevents elongation of the DNA chain. Zidovudine (e) is a nucleoside analog that inhibits viral reverse transcriptases. Amantadine (a) blocks the M2 channel of influenzavirus A preventing release of the nucleocapsid into the cell. Ribavirin (d) targets the RNA-dependent RNA polymerases of several minus sense ssRNA viruses, especially respiratory syncytial virus and Lassa fever virus.

77. The answer is b. (*Levinson, Ch 40. Murray, Ch 54. Ryan, Ch 9, 12.*) Echoviruses were discovered accidentally during studies on poliomyelitis. On entry via ingestion or inhalation, echoviruses (and other members of the *Enterovirus* genus) replicate in the intestinal (c) and upper respiratory (e) tracts (primary replication sites). They spread to the lymphoid tissues (d) and replicate there as well (secondary replication site). From the primary and secondary replication sites, echoviruses enter the bloodstream (a) and are disseminated to the CNS (b), the TARGET tissue/organ. Infection in the intestinal tract is usually silent; virions are shed without symptoms; replication in the upper respiratory tract may produce symptoms of common cold. The TARGET disease is aseptic meningitis, described for those hospitalized. The presence of specific IgA antibody will prevent infection or modulate it by reducing the numbers of viruses that can replicate. The presence of specific IgG, either at the time of infection or prior to dissemination in the bloodstream prevents infection of target tissue/organ.

78. The answer is b. (*Levinson, Ch 37. Murray, Ch 51. Ryan, Ch 10, 14.*) The presentation of vesicular lesions in mother and severe disease in the baby suggests congenital herpes acquired in utero. Rapid diagnosis and initiation of antiviral therapy with IV acyclovir is critical for survival of the infant. Neonatal herpes is more frequently acquired during or shortly after birth and can be categorized as skin, eye, and mucous membrane (SEM) disease appearing 10 to 12 days after birth, disseminated infection apparent within the first few days of life, or CNS infection occurring at 2 to 3 weeks of age. Recognition and treatment of neonatal herpes simplex SEM is important as without treatment, many will progress to disseminated disease. When lesions are present, the most rapid test that allows *definitive* identification is the direct immunofluorescence assay on cells from the lesions (b) in which specific antisera against HSV-1 and HSV-2 are applied to the cells; the test takes as little as 30 minutes. Viral culture of the lesions (e) would also be positive, but takes 18 to 14 hours. Tzanck smear would likely be positive as well, but the test only detects the presence of multinucleated giant cells suggestive of human herpesvirus infection. As the mother most likely has a primary infection with HSV, she is unlikely to have HSV-specific IgG antibodies (a); HSV-specific IgM antibodies would not be transferred to the neonate. HSV PCR on cerebrospinal fluid (c), which takes several hours, is used to diagnosis suspected HSV meningitis or encephalitis and is often referred to specialty laboratories for testing. See below for comparison of direct IFA for HSV (in this case HSV2, A) and the Tzanck smear (B).

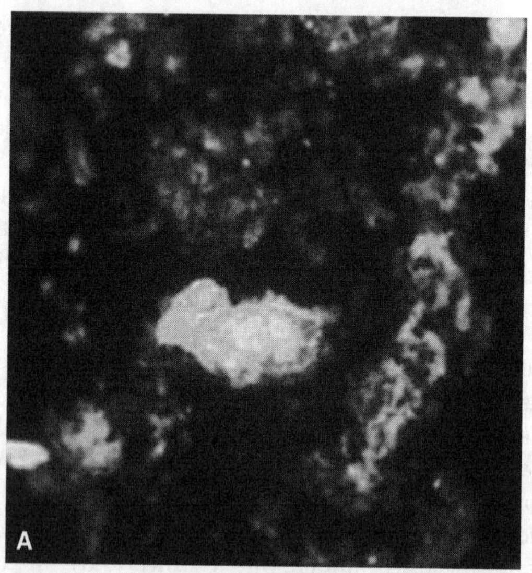

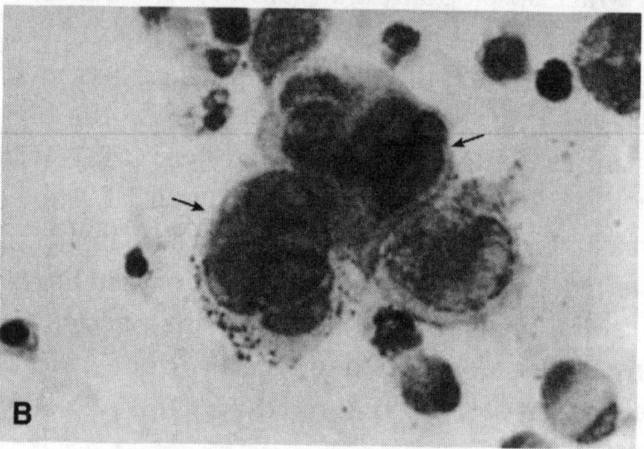

Stains for herpes simplex virus. (**A**) Direct fluorescence assay on cells obtained from lesion using antibody specific for HSV type 2. A companion test with anti-HSV type 1 was negative. (**B**) Tzanck smear on cells from lesion showing multinucleate giant cells typical of some human herpes viruses (HSV1, HSV2, and VZV). *(Courtesy of CDC and (A) Dr. Craig Lyerla, 1977, ID#3644 and (B) Joe Miller, 1975, ID#6508.)*

79. The answer is b. (*Levinson, Ch 40. Murray, Ch 54. Ryan, Ch 9, 12.*) Coxsackievirus A (b), a member of the *Enterovirus* genus, causes hand–foot–mouth disease in young children, frequently in outbreaks associated with day care centers or schools. Rhinoviruses (e) and coronavirus (a) strains endemic in the United States cause common colds; orthoreoviruses (c) are responsible for acute respiratory and gastroenteritis infections. RSV (d) causes upper respiratory tract infection in children and serious lower respiratory tract infection in infants.

80. The answer is e. (*Levinson, Ch 39, 46. Murray, Ch 56. Ryan, Ch 9, 10.*) The most common complication of mumps virus infection in postpubertal males is orchitis (e), occurring in about 33% to 50% of cases. Other complications occur at lower frequencies including myocarditis (c), meningoencephalitis, Guillain–Barré syndrome (a), mastitis, pneumonia, thyroiditis, pancreatitis, hearing loss, and immune thrombocytopenia purpura, which may be associated with hemorrhage (b). Oophoritis occurs in approximately 7% of postpubertal females.

81. The answer is f. (*Levinson, Ch 37. Murray, Ch 51. Ryan, Ch 10, 14.*) This is a classic description for a reactivation of varicella-zoster viral latent infection (f), known as herpes zoster or zoster. The geography of the lesions reflects the particular dermatome fed by the infected ganglion. Many primary infections with VZV are subclinical, yet still result in latent infections in sensory ganglion nerve tissue. Primary VZV infection (varicella or chickenpox) (e) is usually mild, and manifests as crops of lesions appearing first on the trunk and spreading to face and extremities. HSV1 primary infections (a) are most often subclinical but usually manifest as scattered lesions on lips and oral mucosa when lesions are present. HSV1 reactivation (b) produces fewer lesions than on primary infection in immunocompetent persons. EBV infection, whether primary (c) or reactivation (d), does not produce vesicular lesions. Coxsackie A viruses and orthopoxviruses (vaccinia virus, variola virus, and monkeypox virus) cause vesicular exanthems but these would appear more similar to primary infection with HSV1 and VZV, respectively.

82. The answer is d. (*Levinson, Ch 39, 46. Murray, Ch 56. Ryan, Ch 9, 10.*) Measles or rubeola characterized by the prodrome of cough, coryza, conjunctivitis, and photophobia plus the pathognomonic Koplik spots is caused by measles virus (*Morbillivirus*) (d). In industrialized countries, vaccination has reduced the importance of this childhood infection. The number of measles cases occurring annually ranges from 50 to 200, with most associated with outbreaks among groups that do not immunize their children. Adenovirus (a) may cause pharyngoconjunctivitis, an upper respiratory infection similar to the measles prodrome, but Koplik spots are not present. HSV (b), influenzavirus (c), and rubella virus (e) are not associated with the described prodrome nor with Koplik spots.

83. The answer is a. (*Levinson, Ch 38, 43. Murray, Ch 49. Ryan, Ch 19.*) HPVs cause nongenital cutaneous and anogenital or mucosal syndromes. Mucosal and anogenital syndromes include cervical intraepithelial neoplasia (CIN) and cancer; conjunctival, oral, and laryngeal papillomas, and anogenital warts or condyloma accuminatum. HPV types 16, 18, 31, and 45 are high-risk strains associated with CIN and cancer, although additional types have also been found in such lesions. HPV types 6 and 11 cause the majority of papillomas and condyloma accuminatum. HPV infect the basal keratinocytes of the epithelial layer of skin and mucous membranes. Expression of viral proteins E5, E6, and E7 stimulates cell growth and results in thickening of the layers. As the cells mature, genome replication takes place and mature virions are released at the epithelial surface. The oncogenic mechanism of HPV involves integration of the viral genome (a) into the host chromosome. This results in inactivation of genes required for viral replication (d), which does not occur in these cells, and overexpression of HPV E6 and E7 proteins, which bind p53 and p105RB cellular growth suppressor proteins, a production of a clone of replicating cells with possible progression to neoplasia. Loss of HPV E6 and E7 (b) would forestall oncogenic changes; mutation of the virus (c) is not part of the process.

84. The answer is c. (*Levinson, Ch 39, 44, 46. Murray, Ch 56. Ryan, Ch 9, 10.*) Parainfluenza viruses (genus *Respirovirus*) (c) are important causes of respiratory diseases in infants and young children. The spectrum of disease caused by these viruses ranges from a mild febrile cold to laryngotracheobronchitis (croup), and bronchitis in young children and adults to more serious bronchiolitis or pneumonia in infants. Adenovirus (a), Coxsackievirus B (b), and rhinovirus (d) cause upper respiratory tract infections that range from mild (common cold) to serious (pneumonia, ARDS), but they do not cause croup. Rotavirus (e) is a major cause of diarrheal illness in infants.

85. The answer is c. (*Andary. Levinson, Ch 41. Murray, Ch 63. Ryan, Ch 13. Weiner.*) Recognized in the 1980s, HEV, *Hepevirus*, is a ss(+)RNA nonenveloped virus placed in a new family—*Hepeviridae*. The virus is found in Southeast and Central Asia, Africa, North America (Mexico), South America, and Australia. Epidemics have been observed in Asia, Africa, India, and Mexico. Like HAV, it is enterically transmitted, often by water contaminated with human feces. Epidemics frequently affect young adults more than those of other ages. The overall fatality rate is 4%, but pregnant women more frequently develop fulminant hepatic failure (c) and 20% die from complications. Chronic hepatitis (a) does not occur in normal individuals in whom the infection resolves; there is association of HEV with chronic hepatitis in persons who already have hepatitis, liver transplantation, or who are immunocompromised in humoral immune responses. Fetal hydrops (b) may occur in women who acquire parvovirus B19 infection during pregnancy; Guillain–Barré syndrome (d) is a cluster of clinical syndromes that include acute inflammatory demyelinating polyradiculoneuropathy, acute motor axonal neuropathy, and acute motor-sensory axonal neuropathy that are associated with a number of microorganisms: *Campylobacter jejuni*, CMV, EBV, *Mycoplasma pneumoniae*, VZV, and HIV (*http://emedicine.medscape.com/article/315632-overview#a0101*; accessed 02-08-2013). Reye syndrome (e), acute noninflammatory encephalopathy and fatty degenerative liver failure, occurs primarily in children after illness with influenza A or B virus or VZV, especially in conjunction with use of aspirin to reduce fever. Numerous other viruses and some bacteria have also been implicated. However, the incidence of Reye syndrome has declined with the decrease in aspirin usage in children (*http://emedicine.medscape.com/article/803683-overview#a0101*; accessed 02-08-2013).

86. The answer is d. (*Levinson, Ch 40. Murray, Ch 54. Ryan, Ch 9, 12.*) Aseptic meningitis is characterized by a pleocytosis of mononuclear cells, usually lymphocytes, in the CSF (d). Although neutrophils may predominate during the first 12 to 24 hours, a shift to lymphocytes occurs thereafter. The cell count in aseptic meningitis is usually between 50 and 1000/μL, in contrast to the neutrophilic pleocytosis (e) of bacterial meningitis, which is usually greater than 1000/μL. The CSF persons with aseptic is free of culturable bacteria and contains normal glucose (b) and normal to slightly elevated protein levels (a). Peripheral white blood cell counts usually are normal. Although viruses are the most common cause of aseptic meningitis, spirochetes, chlamydiae, and other microorganisms also can produce the disease. Eosinophilic pleocytosis (c) is seen in some parasitic diseases, such as cysticercosis, and in disseminated *Coccidioides immitis* infection.

EXPECTED CSF FINDINGS IN MENINGITIS				
Etiology	Opening Pressure	Predominant Cells	Protein	Glucose
Bacterial	↑	Neutrophils	↑	↓
Viral	Normal/ slightly ↑	Lymphocytes	Normal/ slightly ↑	N
Fungal or tubercular	↑	Lymphocytes	↑	↓

87. The answer is b. (*Levinson, Ch 41. Murray, Ch 63. Ryan, Ch 13.*) HDV can be acquired as a coinfection—HBV and HDV acquired at the same time; or, as a superinfection—HDV acquired by a person with chronic HBV infection. Diagnosis of HDV infection may be made by detection of delta antigen, anti-HDV IgM and/or IgG, or HDV RNA. Acute, chronic, resolved, or immunized HBV status is determined by a battery of serologic tests. Superinfection with HDV is indicated by positive tests for HDV and the presence of anti-HBcAg IgG but not IgM (b). Coinfection with HDV would be indicated by the presence of anti-HBcAg IgM but not IgG (a).

INTERPRETATION OF THE HEPATITIS B STATUS FOR THE CHOICES OFFERED IN QUESTION 87					
Disease State	HBsAg	HBeAg	Anti-HBcAg-IgM	Anti-HBcAg IgG	Anti-HBsAG
Acute (a)	+	+	+	−	−
Chronic (b)	+	+	−	+	−
Resolved (c)	−	−	−	+	+
Vaccinated (d)	−	−	−	−	+

88. The answer is d. (*Levinson, Ch 41. Murray, Ch 63. Ryan, Ch 13.*) HBsAg is present in most patients before symptoms appear and remains positive during the early acute, acute, and late acute stages of disease. Near, or shortly after, the time clinical symptoms end HBsAg can no longer be detected in patients who are resolving their HBV infections. However, anti-HBsAg cannot be detected in these patients until almost a month later. The time (after the disappearance of HBsAg and before the appearance of anti-HBsAg) is known as the window period (d). During this time, diagnosis of acute hepatitis B is made by detection of anti-HBcAg IgM. The subsequent appearance of anti-HBsAg indicates resolution of infection. Resolved hepatitis B infection (b) is indicated by HBsAg –, HBeAg –, Anti-HBcAg IgM –, Anti-HBcAg IgG +, Anti-HBsAg +; chronic hepatitis B infection (c) is indicated by HBsAg +, HBeAg +, Anti-HBcAg IgM –, Anti-HBcAg IgG +, Anti-HBsAg; persons immunized against HBV (e) have only anti-HBsAg IgG. Hepatitis symptoms in the face of negative tests for viral etiology indicate another infectious agent, toxic injury to the liver, or possible disease of the biliary tract.

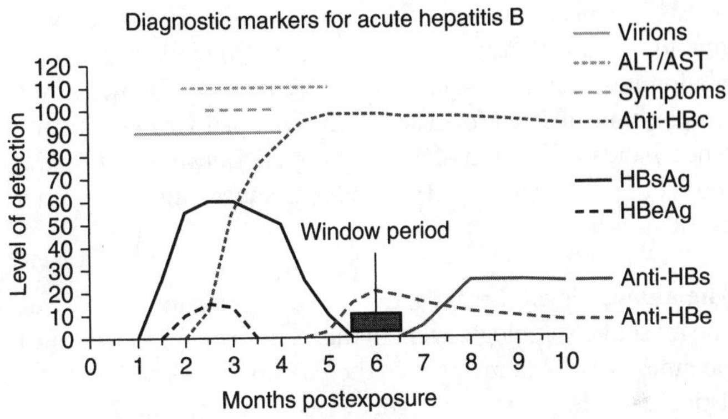

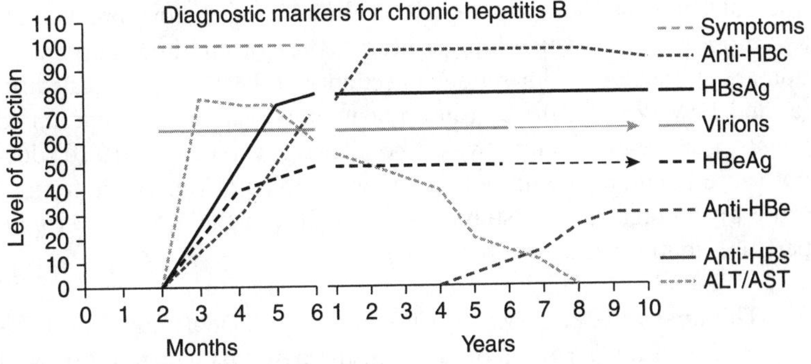

Graphs comparing symptoms, antigens, and antibodies present in acute hepatitis B and chronic hepatitis B.

89. The answer is c. (*Levinson, Ch 39, 42, 46. Murray, Ch 60. Ryan, Ch 10, 16.*) This patient has encephalitis most likely caused by the EEEV. EEEV is transmitted by mosquitoes (c) and is usually seen in the summer months. The virus is found mainly in states on the Atlantic and Gulf coasts, with Florida and Georgia recording the greatest number of cases. While the majority of those who contract EEEV are asymptomatic, those over 60 and younger than 15 years of age are at risk of developing Eastern equine encephalitis, a serious, rapidly progressing encephalitis with a poor prognosis. Birds (a) are the reservoir for EEEV. Fleas (b), sand flies (d), and ticks (e) are not vectors of EEEV. See the answer to question 72 for additional information.

90. The answer is b. (*Levinson, Ch 40. Murray, Ch 54. Ryan, Ch 9, 12.*) Rhinovirus is a major cause of the common cold. The primary mode of transmission is direct hand-to-hand contact (b), followed by transmission via fomites such as tissues, clothing or utensils, followed by respiratory droplet transmission (c). These nonenveloped viruses can survive on unwashed hands and objects for many hours. Transmission by the fecal–oral route (a), sexual contact (d), or vertical transmission (e) do not occur with rhinoviruses.

91. The answer is c. (*Levinson, Ch 39, 44, 46. Murray, Ch 56. Ryan, Ch 9, 10.*) The most likely etiologic agent of this infant's pneumonia is the human metapneumovirus (c), a member of the *Paramyxoviridae* closely related to but distinct from respiratory syncytial virus. Discovered in 2001, this virus is now known to be responsible for 5% to 15% of serious lower respiratory tract infections in young children. As with RSV, infants born prematurely and those with preexisting lung or heart disease or immunocompromisation are at greater risk for serious infection with hMPV. Cytomegalovirus (a) and HSV type 1 (b) may cause pneumonia in immunocompromised infants, but the presentation would be different. Parvovirus B19 (d) does not cause pneumonia, and only occasional strains of rhinovirus (e) may cause pneumonia as most strains prefer to grow at the much lower temperatures found in the nasal passages.

92. The answer is e. (*Levinson, Ch 46. Murray, Ch 58. Ryan, Ch 16.*) The best specimen for diagnosis of rabies in the living patient is a biopsy of skin at the back of the neck (nuchal biopsy). The finding of Negri bodies on H&E stain is pathognomonic for rabies virus (e); a positive staining reaction with rabies-specific antibodies confirms the diagnosis. Negri bodies are eosinophilic cytoplasmic inclusion bodies found within infected neurons in the hippocampus and cerebral cortex or in skin cells. The vignette describes the first phase of rabies, or entry into the CNS, which lasts from 2 to 10 days. This is followed by acute rabies, which can be paralytic or furious, and almost invariably leads to death. EEEV (b) and echovirus (c) do not produce specific inclusion bodies. HSV type 1 (d) produces eosinophilic Cowdry A inclusion bodies within the nucleus of infected cells. Cytomegalovirus (a) produces basophilic nuclear inclusion bodies that resemble owl eyes. Negri bodies of rabies virus (A), Cowdry A inclusion of HSV (B), and owl eye inclusion of CMV (C) are compared below.

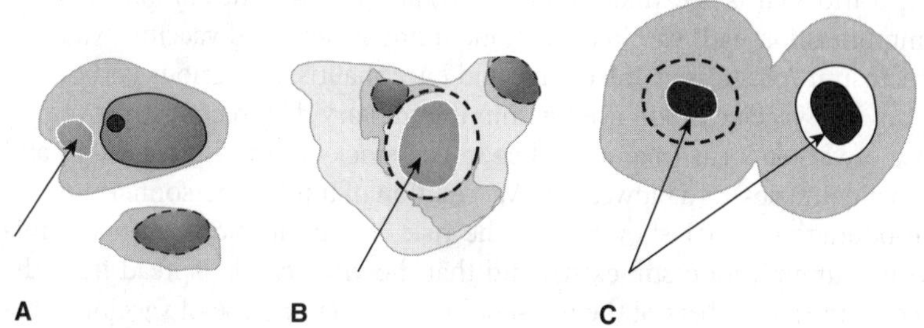

Comparison of viral inclusion bodies. Cytoplasmic Negri bodies of rabies virus (**A**), nuclear Cowdry A inclusions of HSV (**B**), and nuclear owl-eye inclusions of CMV (**C**).

93. The answer is d. (*Levinson, Ch 44. Murray, Ch 64. Ryan, Ch 20.*) Kuru and CJD are similar but not identical diseases with very different epidemiology. Kuru was prevalent among certain tribes in New Guinea who practiced ritual cannibalism by eating the brains of the departed. CJD is found worldwide in familial and sporadic forms and has been transmitted by corneal transplants and in pituitary hormone preparations (iatrogenic CJD). An infectious form—variant CJD—is associated with eating cattle with bovine spongiform encephalopathy; cases have occurred primarily in England. Prions are unconventional self-replicating proteins, sometimes called *amyloid.* It is now thought that CJD, Kuru, and animal diseases such as scrapie, visna, and bovine spongiform encephalopathy (mad cow disease) are caused by prions. Prions do not contain DNA or RNA. Bacteria, flagellates (parasites), and viruses all contain nucleic acid genomes. No apparent evidence of environmental toxins able to cause Kuru/CJD have been reported.

94. The answer is d. (*Levinson, Ch 37. Murray, Ch 52. Ryan, Ch 11.*) The description of the virus genome (dsDNA) and site of replication (cytoplasm) are characteristic of poxviruses; vaccinia virus (d) is the immunizing agent against variola virus (e). Adenovirus type 5 (a) is a dsDNA virus that replicates in the nucleus; it causes respiratory infections. Rabies virus (c) and echovirus 11 (b) are ss(−)RNA and ss(+)RNA viruses, respectively; they do replicate in the cytoplasm. None of these latter three viruses cause skin lesions like those shown in the image for question 94. Routine vaccination of the general public with vaccinia virus to prevent smallpox has been discontinued in the United States, as the risk of contracting the disease is nil (variola virus is extinct in the world) and because the complications of immunization with vaccinia virus, including generalized vaccinia, vaccinia necrosum (progressive infection), and encephalitis, are serious and can be fatal. The vaccine is still used within the military due to concerns over the use of variola virus (maintained as frozen stocks in the United States and other countries) as a bioweapon. Vaccination of military personnel and first responders in 2001 showed that the risk of complications from vaccinia virus immunization still exists, and that the virus can be spread from the recipient to members of the household. However, the use of vaccinia virus as a vector to carry the gene for the rabies glycoprotein has become common. The vector is packaged in baits designed to be eaten by raccoons and other small mammals that are known transmit rabies virus. Exposure to the vaccinia virus within the bait can lead to infection in humans, especially in immunocompromised individuals.

95. The answer is d. (*Levinson, Ch 46. Murray, Ch 58. Ryan, Ch 16.*) Rabies is caused by a rhabdovirus, a minus-sense, single-stranded, nonsegmented RNA virus with an enveloped, bullet-shaped virion). The virus infects a wide range of warm-blooded animals, including humans. The virus is widely disseminated within the infected animals, with high levels in saliva. If the animal is captured or killed, examination of its brain for rabies virus can be done in time to determine whether rabies prophylaxis is necessary. The best means to prevent rabies begins with scrupulous wound care, including washing and probing for any foreign bodies (eg, broken teeth) in the wound. If the animal is not available, or tests positive for rabies, and if the person has not been immunized with rabies vaccine, the treatment of choice is to give human rabies immunoglobulin (HRIg) plus rabies vaccine at separate sites (d). The HRIg should be infused into the wound and the remainder given as a deep IM injection. After onset of symptoms, neither of these should be given. Broad-spectrum antibiotics (a) may be given as part of wound care to prevent bacterial infection, but they will not prevent rabies. Acyclovir (b) and ribavirin (c), regardless of dosage or route of administration, have no role in rabies prophylaxis. Tetanus immune globulin and/or tetanus toxoid vaccine (e) may also be part of the wound care regimen, but are given to prevent tetanus, not rabies.

96. The answer is a. (*Levinson, Ch 38. Murray, Ch 50. Ryan, Ch 9, 15.*) Mild ocular involvement often occurs as part of the respiratory syndromes caused by adenoviruses. Adenovirus (a) also can cause severe keratitis that can lead to permanent eye damage. These infections may occur in outbreaks in industrial, hospital, or clinic settings through exposure of groups of workers/patients to contaminated fomites. The workers involved in this cluster of infections had shared eye drops due to the dusty environment in which they were working. EBV (b), parvovirus (c), RSV (d), and VZV (e) are not routinely reported as causing this type of illness. HSV-1, which was not among the choices, can cause keratoconjunctivitis and keratitis. Dendritic or coalescing (geographic) ulcers can be visualized in HSV-1 keratitis.

97. The answer is b. (*Levinson, Ch 41. Murray, Ch 63. Ryan, Ch 13.*) As can be seen in the figure found in the answer to Question 88, HBsAg and infectious virions are shed over the same course of time, with HBeAg appearing in the bloodstream at the height of viral replication. Thus, the presence of HBeAg indicates the individual is highly contagious (b). Although HBsAg can be shed after infectious virions are no longer being produced, the patient is still considered contagious, but to a lesser degree (c) than when HBeAg is present. The person is considered infectious as long as HBsAg persists, so answers d (not contagious) and e (resolved) are incorrect. The incidence of false-positive results for HBeAg is low (a), with specificities ranging from 98.6% to 99% reported, depending on the product used.

98. The answer is d. (*Levinson, Ch 39, 42, 46. Murray, Ch 60. Ryan, Ch 10, 16.*) Western equine encephalitis virus (d) is the only virus on the list likely to cause encephalitis in an infant. It is also found mainly west of the Mississippi River; states with the highest number of reported cases include Colorado, Texas, North Dakota, and California. Rubella virus (c) can cause encephalitis, but this virus is extremely uncommon in the United States because of the successful vaccine developed to prevent rubella. WNV (e) is more likely to cause meningitis in a child and encephalitis in a person over 60. Dengue virus (a) infection rarely leads to encephalitis. Lymphocytic choriomeningitis virus (b) is rodent-borne rather than arthropod-borne. See the table accompanying the answer to question 72. Note, according to the Centers for Disease Prevention and Control, WEEV activity has been absent from the United States for the past 5 years.

99. The answer is e. (*Levinson, Ch 39, 44, 46. Murray, Ch 56. Ryan, Ch 9, 10.*) Ribavirin, a guanosine analog, is approved for aerosol treatment of respiratory syncytial virus infections (e) in premature or immunocompromised infants who are likely to have a more severe clinical course. Currently, aerosol treatment of children is no longer standard treatment. Ribavirin is approved for oral treatment of HCV infection (in combination with IFN-α) and for IV treatment of Lassa fever and other viral hemorrhagic fevers. It is not used for treatment of Coxsackievirus A (a), HBV (b), HSV (c), or parvovirus (d) infections.

100. The answer is c. (*Levinson, Ch 37. Murray, Ch 51. Ryan, Ch 10, 14.*) HSV type 1 (c) encephalitis (HSE), which usually involves the temporal lobe, is the most common cause of sporadic (nonepidemic) encephalitis and is often lethal. Severe neurologic sequelae are seen in surviving patients. Most HSE cases occur in adults over 50, but a first peak of infections occurs in those younger than 20 years of age. PCR amplification of viral DNA from CSF has replaced viral isolation. Coxsackievirus B (and A) strains (b) cause aseptic meningitis, as well as other conditions. Adenoviruses (a) are primarily known for causing pharyngoconjunctivitis in children; they rarely cause encephalitis. *Listeria monocytogenes* is a bacterium that can cause meningoencephalitis primarily in immunocompromised patients; it infects the brain parenchyma, especially the brainstem. WNV (e) causes encephalitis associated with mosquito transmission, so it is more common in summer and early fall. Localized lesions are not seen with West Nile encephalitis.

101. The answer is d. (*Levinson, Ch 37. Murray, Ch 51. Ryan, Ch 10, 14.*) Roseola infantum caused by human herpes virus 6 (d) leads to seizures in 15% of symptomatic infants. In healthy infants, the infection is asymptomatic or follows the course described in the vignette. In immunocompromised children, the abrupt onset includes CNS and other organ system involvement. Following infection, the virus remains latent in lymphocytes and monocytes. Infection in adults or reactivation in adulthood may produce a mononucleosis-like syndrome with lymphadenopathy and hepatitis. In immunocompromised patients such as bone marrow, kidney, and liver transplant patients, much more serious infections/reactivations occur that may lead to organ rejection and death. Erythema infectiosum (a), hand-food-and-mouth disease (b), measles (c), and rubella (d) (caused by the viruses indicated in the choices) each present differently: "slapped cheek" reticular rash 7 to 10 days following a nonspecific prodrome; vesicles appearing on the hands, and disseminated maculopapular rashes beginning on the neck, respectively.

102. The answer is d. (*Levinson, Ch 39, 44, 46. Murray, Ch 56. Ryan, Ch 9, 10.*) The vignette describes an infant with severe bronchiolitis caused by respiratory syncytial virus (*Pneumovirus*) (d). RSV is the most common cause of bronchiolitis and pneumonia in infants less than 1 year of age. The infection is localized to the respiratory tract. The virus can be detected rapidly by immunofluorescence on respiratory epithelia cells obtained by nasopharyngeal suction. In older children, the infection resembles the common cold. Adenovirus (a) and cytomegalovirus (b) can cause pneumonia in infants, but the presentation does not usually include bronchiolitis. Parainfluenza virus (*Respirovirus*) (c) infection may present as bronchiolitis, but it is less common than RSV, especially in winter. Rhinovirus (e) rarely causes pneumonia as most strains cannot replicate at core body temperature.

103. The answer is a. (*Levinson, Ch 39, 43, 45. Murray, Ch 62. Ryan, Ch 18.*) The risk of acquiring HIV infection is increased in persons who have multiple sexual partners, especially sexual partners who inject drugs using shared needles (a). Hospital receptionists (b), members of a household in which there is a person who is HIV-positive (d), and factory workers with HIV-positive coworkers (e) have little to no risk for contracting HIV in their normal and usual interactions with people around them. The risk of HIV acquired through blood products began dropping in 1985 with the development of tests for HIV p24 antigen and HIV antibodies. Since the advent of nucleic acid amplification testing for HIV, the risk for acquiring HIV through blood or blood products (in the United States) has dropped further to 1/1,000,000 units. Persons who receive blood now (2013) (c) are at little risk. Risks associated with HIV transmission are shown in the table from the Centers for Disease Prevention and Control.

AIDS DIAGNOSES BY TRANSMISSION CATEGORY

	Estimated Number of Diagnoses of HIV Infection, 2010		
Transmission Category	**Adult and Adolescent Males**	**Adult and Adolescent Females**	**Total**
Male-to-male sexual contact	28,782	—	28,782
Injection drug use	2,373	1,393	3,766
Male-to-male sexual contact and injection drug use	1,443	—	1,443
Heterosexual contact[a]	4,416	8,459	12,875
Other[b]	31	16	47

[a]Heterosexual contact with a person known to have, or to be at high risk for, HIV infection.

[b]Includes hemophilia, blood transfusion, perinatal exposure, and risk not reported or not identified.

Printed with permission from CDC. http://www.cdc.gov/hiv/topics/surveillance/basic.htm#exposure

104. The answer is c. (*Levinson, Ch 39, 42, 46. Murray, Ch 60. Ryan, Ch 10, 16.*) The highest risk of teratogenic effects from fetal infection with rubella occurs during the first 20 weeks of gestation; therefore, answer d, which states rubella is not a problem until the 30th week, is incorrect. In seronegative patients, the risk of infection exceeds 90%. However, before other measures (such as termination of pregnancy [e]) are considered, a rubella antibody titer to determine immune status (c) must be performed. Rubella immune globulin (a) is not available, and IV pooled immune globulin injected into the mother would be unlikely to protect the fetus against rubella because viremia occurs at the time symptoms appear. Immunizing the mother against rubella (b) would not protect the fetus for the same reason—antibodies that develop would be too late to prevent transplacental spread. And, while inadvertent administration of rubella vaccine to pregnant women did not result in neonates with congenital syndrome, it is generally unwise to give a live attenuated vaccine to a pregnant woman.

105. The answer is c. (*Levinson, Ch 36. Murray, Ch 11, 49-51, 54, 56, 59, 60, 63.*) HPV 16/18 and HBV (c) are implicated in cervical (and other genital) cancer and hepatocellular carcinoma, respectively. Thus, the vaccines against these agents are expected to reduce the incidence of these cancers. This has been seen in regions of the world where routine HBV vaccine is used at birth or shortly thereafter. The other viruses—adenovirus/mumps virus (a), HAV/poliovirus (b), measles virus/rubella virus (d), and rotavirus/VZV (e)—are not associated with cancers in humans, although adenoviruses cause cancer in some animals.

106. The answer is c. (*Levinson, Ch 40. Murray, Ch 54. Ryan, Ch 9, 12.*) The disease described in the vignette is poliomyelitis (or polio), which is still present in India, Pakistan, Afghanistan, and several countries in Africa. The workers from the United States had received either the Salk killed poliovirus vaccine or the Sabin live attenuated poliovirus vaccine (c) depending on their ages. Because the polioviruses have been eradicated from the Northern Hemisphere and the live attenuated poliovirus vaccine strains have been associated with CNS infection in some recipients, the killed vaccine is the only one used in the United States today. The workers most likely had also received the measles (b), mumps, and rubella (d) virus vaccines and the HAV (a) vaccine, but those would not protect them from polio. The yellow fever virus (e) vaccine is generally given only to those traveling to an endemic area.

107. The answer is e. (*Levinson, Ch 39. Murray, Ch 57. Ryan, Ch 9.*) *Staphylococcus aureus* (e) is one of the most common causes of secondary bacterial pneumonia following influenza. The others are *Streptococcus pneumoniae* and *Haemophilus influenzae*. *Escherichia coli* (a) and *Klebsiella pneumoniae* (b) may also cause postinfluenza secondary bacterial pneumonia, but the numbers of cases are much lower. Primary influenza pneumonia is a serious complication of influenza in its own right, most often affecting elderly persons in nursing homes, persons with cardiovascular disease, and pregnant women in their third trimester. *S. aureus* secondary bacterial pneumonia develops rapidly, within 2 to 3 days of primary influenza pneumonia; secondary bacterial pneumonia caused by *S. pneumoniae* or *H. influenzae* occurs 2 to 3 weeks after the initial symptoms of influenza. *Legionella pneumophila* is usually the primary cause of lung disease. *Listeria monocytogenes* (d) is acquired via ingestion of contaminated food, spreading from the GI tract to the joints or CNS in immunocompromised individuals or to the placenta in pregnant women.

108. The answer is a. (*Levinson, Ch 38. Murray, Ch 50. Ryan, Ch 9, 15.*) Conjunctivitis is seen in many childhood infections. When accompanied by fever and sore throat, pharyngoconjunctival fever is most often caused by adenovirus (a). HSV type 1 (d) eye infections usually present as keratitis (corneal ulcer). The remaining choices are bacteria, which usually cause purulent drainage rather than watery. *Chlamydia trachomatis* (b) is associated with eye infections in neonates born to mothers with genital infections. *C. trachomatis* also causes trachoma, a slowly progressive disease that begins as follicular inflammation of the eyelid and can lead to scarring and blindness; trachoma occurs primarily in Africa, the Middle East, and northern India. *Haemophilus aegyptius* (c) causes epidemic purulent conjunctivitis, often known as "pink-eye." This species of *Haemophilus* is found more frequently in tropical climates and is now uncommon in the United States where *Haemophilus influenzae* is encountered more frequently. *Staphylococcus aureus* (e) usually causes blepharitis, or inflammation of the eyelids.

109. The answer is b. (*Levinson, Ch 39, 42, 46. Murray, Ch 61. Ryan, Ch 16.*) The vignette describes hantavirus pulmonary syndrome (HPS) (also known as hantavirus cardiopulmonary syndrome), which is acquired by inhaling aerosolized rodent excreta (c). The first cases of HPS recognized in the modern era occurred in 1993, when an outbreak of a fatal respiratory disease occurred in the southwestern United States. Deer mice were the vectors in that outbreak caused by a *Hantavirus* given the name "Sin Nombre." At least 24 different types of New World hantaviruses, distributed throughout the Americas, are now known; each has a different rodent vector and all cause HPS. The mortality rate for HPS is high, 80% in the 1993 outbreak, but with development of aggressive interventions, it is now 30% to 40%. Members of the *Bunyavirus* genus, also of the *Bunyaviridae*, are arthropod-borne, with the species found in the Americas transmitted by mosquitoes (d) and the African species transmitted by ticks (e) or flies. Human-to-human transmission by contact (a) occurs with some South American strains of *Hantavirus*, but is not common. Drinking water (b) is not implicated in the spread of *Hantavirus* infections.

110. The answer is b. (*Levinson, Ch 38, 43. Murray, Ch 49. Ryan, Ch 19.*) The vignette describes common warts caused by HPV (b) and the accompanying image shows koilocytes in hyperplastic skin, which are pathognomonic for HPV infection. HPVs cause nongenital cutaneous and anogenital or mucosal syndromes. Nongenital cutaneous syndromes include common warts, flat warts, plantar warts, and epidermodysplasia verruciformis. The HPV types associated with these lesions are different from the types that cause mucosal syndromes (6, 11, 16, 18, 31, and 45) except for type 2 that can cause common warts, plantar warts, and oral papillomas. Adenovirus (a) does not cause skin lesions; *Molluscipoxvirus* (c) causes pearly lesions with dimpled centers from which white material can be extruded. When it causes skin lesions, echovirus (d) is associated with a maculopapular rash. VZV (e) causes vesicular lesions.

111. The answer is c. (*Levinson, Ch 38, 43. Murray, Ch 49. Ryan, Ch 19.*) Of the choices listed, only imiquimod (c) is an immunomodulatory agent. It is an inducer of cytokines of innate immunity, stimulating production of IFN-α, tumor necrosis factor, interleukin-1, and interleukin-8. It can be used in conjunction with physical removal of HPV outgrowths to prevent viral replication in any remaining infected cells. Acyclovir (a) is an antiviral specific for HSVs and VZVs, which have viral thymidine kinases to activate the drug. 5-Fluorouracil (b) is a cytotoxic agent that interferes with RNA and DNA synthesis, podophyllin (d) is a cytotoxic agent that is antimitotic, and trichloroacetic acid (e) is a keratolytic agent that chemically cauterizes skin, keratin, and other tissues. The latter three agents can all be used in treating condyloma accuminatum, but they are not immunomodulatory.

112. The answer is a. (*Levinson, Ch 38. Murray, Ch 53. Ryan, Ch 10.*) Parvovirus B19 causes erythema infectiosum in previously well children and adults that often results in a drop in hemoglobin level that is not noticed. In children with chronic hemolytic anemias, such as sickle cell disease, parvovirus B19 infection can result in aplastic crisis (a) associated with a drop in the hemoglobin level of 2 g/dL or more. This can necessitate hospitalization in these children. The virus preferentially infects erythroid precursors. The child has tachycardia from the anemia. There is nothing in the history to suggest Coxsackievirus B pericarditis (b), *Norovirus* gastroenteritis (c), or BK polyomavirus hemorrhagic cystitis (e); nor is there any reason to suspect *Coltivirus* infection (d), which would be associated with location, season, and tick bite. *Norovirus* gastroenteritis is not associated with bleeding. Additional complications of parvovirus B19 infection include maternal transplacental infection of the fetus with resultant fetal hydrops related to anemia in the fetus, unremittent anemia in immunosuppressed persons such as transplant recipients, and polyarthropathy/arthritis in adults.

113. The answer is a. (*Levinson, Ch 37. Murray, Ch 51. Ryan, Ch 10, 14.*) Approximately 40,000 infants (out of 4 million births) are born with congenital CMV infections. Of these, 10% will be symptomatic and considered to have cytomegalic inclusion disease; and 90% of these infants will suffer neurologic sequelae such as hearing loss at birth, microcephaly, mental retardation, and developmental disabilities. The remaining 36,000 will have asymptomatic CMV (a) infection and approximately 15% will develop neurological sequelae, including sensorineural hearing loss. HSV type 2 (b) congenital infection presents as vesicular lesions or as disseminated infection or CNS disease, both of which can be lethal. Congenital varicella syndrome caused by VZV (e) is associated with microcephaly, skin lesions, and limb and eye defects. Rubeola virus (measles virus) (d) infection in the mother leads to spontaneous abortion or preterm birth of the fetus. CRS caused by rubella virus (d) led to abortion, stillbirth, and serious defects including sensorineural hearing loss, ocular abnormalities, and congenital heart defects. CRS has been virtually eliminated in the United States by the use of the live attenuated rubella vaccine since 1969.

114. The answer is c. (*Levinson, Ch 40. Murray, Ch 59. Ryan, Ch 9, 15.*) The symptoms of rotavirus (c) infection last longer than those of norovirus (b), which generally runs its course in 72 hours or less. The rotavirus vaccine has greatly reduced the numbers of cases of rotavirus infection and the morbidity associated with it in those who develop the infection despite vaccination. However, no vaccine is 100% effective and some infants will still develop full-blown rotavirus enteritis. Enteroviruses (a) do not cause gastroenteritis. *Salmonella enterica* (a) in diarrhea is characterized by the presence of WBC in the stool and sometimes blood. *Staphylococcus aureus* enterotoxin (e) would be unlikely in an infant 6 months old, but would present within 1 to 6 hours of ingestion with nausea and vomiting the major symptoms. A number of viruses that cause gastroenteritis have been recognized. The following table summarizes the characteristics of these viruses.

CHARACTERISTICS OF VIRUSES THAT CAUSE GASTROENTERITIS[a]

Family	*Reoviridae*	*Caliciviridae*	*Astroviridae*	*Adenoviridae*
Virus	*Rotavirus*	*Norovirus*, *Sapovirus*	*Mamastrovirus*	*Mastadenovirus*
Genome[b]	dsRNA	(+)ssRNA	(+)ssRNA	dsDNA
Serotypes	5	More than 4	8 or more	2 (40/41)
Epidemicity	Sporadic, outbreak, epidemic	Epidemic, outbreak	Sporadic, epidemic	Sporadic
Season	Nov–Apr	Summer (ships)	Peak in winter	None
Risk for clinical disease	Infants <2 years; all ages mild	Adults; all ages	Infants <2 years; all ages	Infants; all ages
Incubation period	1-3 days	12-48 hours	1-2	8-10
Major symptoms	Fever, vomiting, watery diarrhea, abdominal pain	Vomiting, nausea, watery diarrhea, stomach pain, fever	Diarrhea followed by nausea, vomiting, fever	Fever, watery diarrhea, vomiting
Duration of symptoms	3-8 days	24-72 hours	3-4 days (?)	7-14 days
Diagnosis	EIA	EIA	EM	EIA

[a]All are transmitted via the fecal–oral route; *Norovirus* can be transmitted in food, water, and via close personal contact with an infected person or fomites.

[b]All are naked capsid virions.

Compiled from information provided in references listed and from *http://viralzone.expasy.org/*. and *http://www.cdc.gov/ncidod/dvrd/revb/gastro/faq.htm*.

115. The answer is d. (*Levinson, Ch 39, 44, 46. Murray, Ch 56, 64. Ryan, Ch 9, 10, 20.*) SSPE, a very late and rare sequela of infection with *Morbillivirus* (measles virus) (d), occurs approximately 10 years after measles. It is a degenerative CNS infection resulting from a persistent infection caused by a defective virus that spreads cell to cell but does not produce cell-free mature virions. Measles can also result in acute encephalitis in 1/1000 cases, often resulting in permanent brain damage and 10% fatality; delayed acute encephalitis that occurs 1 to 6 months later and is invariably fatal; or acute disseminated encephalomyelitis (postinfectious encephalitis), a demyelinating condition affecting the brain and spinal cord. Epstein–Barr virus (a) can cause neurologic complications in 1% of infections, including acute encephalitis or meningitis, Guillain–Barré syndrome, Bell palsy, and transverse myelitis. HIV (b) can cause HIV dementia, while the JC polyomavirus causes progressive multifocal leukoencephalopathy in persons who are profoundly immunosuppressed, including those with AIDS and those on immunosuppressive therapy. The mumps virus (*Rubulavirus*) (e) involves the CNS in 50% of cases, 10% of whom develop aseptic meningitis; 1 in 200 of these patients develop encephalitis as well. Mumps can also result in hearing loss.

116. The answer is a. (*Levinson, Ch 40. Murray, Ch 59. Ryan, Ch 9, 16.*) *Coltivirus* (a), a member of the Reoviridae, is a double-stranded RNA virus with a segmented genome. It causes Colorado tick fever as described in the vignette. The virus circulates in red blood cells, which have an average life span of 120 days; thus, the recommendation to avoid donating blood for 6 months. CTF is usually a mild disease with episodes of fever interspersed with afebrile periods, the "saddle-back" fever pattern. The virus is limited to the mountainous regions of the Northwest United States and Canada and is found at elevations of 4000 feet or higher, the range of the rodent reservoir and the *Dermacentor andersoni* tick vector. The infection is common; several hundred cases occur each year. Western equine encephalitis virus (e) usually presents as encephalitis; no cases have been recorded in the United States for the past 5 years. Dengue virus (c) may begin with a similar presentation but would be associated with travel in subtropical or tropical regions. Coxsackievirus B (b) causes nonspecific symptoms that are mild followed by target organ disease such as myositis or pleurodynia. The presentation of Sin Nombre hantavirus (d), which overlaps the range of *Coltivirus*, causes hantavirus pulmonary syndrome.

117. The answer is b. (*Levinson, Ch 46. Murray, Ch 58. Ryan, Ch 16.*) The vignette describes viral hemorrhagic fever transmitted by contact with blood. Of the three hemorrhagic fevers given as choices, only Ebola hemorrhagic fever (b), caused by the *Filovirus* Ebola, is transmitted by contact with blood and body fluids. The filoviruses are also acquired by collecting bush meat (dead carcasses of primates), and epidemiologic studies suggest that bats may also serve as vector. Dengue hemorrhagic fever (a) and yellow fever (e) are caused by arthropod-borne flaviviruses, as is West Nile encephalitis (d). Hantavirus pulmonary syndrome is acquired through inhalation of aerosolized excreta from infected rodents.

118. The answer is d. (*Levinson, Ch 37. Murray, Ch 51. Ryan, Ch 10, 14.*) All of the choices are associated with EBV. The patient most likely has lymphoproliferative disorder (posttransplant) (d), a polyclonal response to reactivation or acquisition of EBV in persons on immunosuppressive therapy to prevent transplant rejection. The disorder responded to reduction of the immunosuppressive agent, a response not expected if the patient had Burkitt lymphoma (a) or Hodgkin lymphoma (b), more aggressive monoclonal B-cell lymphomas that often require antilymphoma treatment. Infectious mononucleosis (c) occurs in immunocompetent individuals. NPC (e) does not fit the vignette.

119. The answer is e. (*Katzung, Ch 49. Levinson, Ch 39, 45. Murray, Ch 62. Ryan, Ch 18.*) The replication of a retroviral genome is dependent on the reverse transcriptase enzyme, which performs a variety of functions—RNA-dependent DNA polymerase, RNase, and DNA-dependent DNA polymerase. Abacavir (a), nevirapine (c), and zidovudine (e) are reverse transcriptase inhibitors. However, only zidovudine (e) is used alone for prophylaxis to prevent perinatal transmission of HIV during the first 6 weeks of life. Abacavir should not be used without testing the infant for HLA-B*5701, a mutation that renders the individual hypersensitive to this drug. Raltegravir (d), the integrase inhibitor, and lopinavir (b), a PI, are not used alone at any time—prophylactically or therapeutically. Two regimens are currently recommended for children younger than 3 years of age: nevirapine plus two NRTIs (abacavir, didanosine or zidovudine plus lamivudine, or emtricitabine) or lopinavir/ritonavir plus two NRTIs (same choices as for nevirapine).

120. The answer is a. (*Levinson, Ch 42, 43. Murray, Ch 60. Ryan, Ch 16.*) The widespread distribution of WNV (a) across the United States and the high incidence of infections, most of which are asymptomatic or only mildly symptomatic, has led centers that collect blood for transfusion to test all donors for the virus. This is done by nucleic acid amplification tests (NAAT) on pools of donors. If a positive pool is found, each donor is tested individually. For 2012, the Centers for Disease Prevention and Control recorded 5890 cases of WNV illness, of which 2734 were neuroinvasive. Among those with neuroinvasive disease, 243 died (~9%). Almost 600 asymptomatic blood donors were reported. The incidence of St. Louis encephalitis is too low to warrant testing the blood supply at this time. Dengue virus (c) rarely causes encephalitis and is currently transmitted endogenously only in Florida. *Coltivirus* (e) may be transmitted to recipients of blood from donors infected with the virus, but this virus is restricted to the Rocky Mountain states and is not routinely tested for in other states. Travel history would exclude dengue virus and *Coltivirus*. HSV (d) is not transmitted by arthropods. See the table accompanying answer to question 72 for additional information.

121. The answer is b. (*Levinson, Ch 37. Murray, Ch 51. Ryan, Ch 10, 14.*) While the majority of CMV (b) infections acquired in young adulthood are asymptomatic, some may develop heterophile-negative mononucleosis syndrome, described in the vignette. Generally, the lymphadenopathy and pharyngitis are less severe than that seen with infectious mononucleosis caused by EBV (c). Adult primary CMV infection may also manifest as hepatitis, but tests for HAV, HBV, and HCV would be negative. Adenovirus (a), parvovirus B19 (d), and HCV (e) do not cause mononucleosis syndrome.

122. The answer is c. (*Levinson, Ch 41. Murray, Ch 63. Ryan, Ch 13.*) IFN-α and IFN-β are proteins that alter cell metabolism to inhibit viral replication. They activate 2′-5′-oligoadenylate synthase, which in turn activates RNase L to degrade poly(A) mRNA transcripts. Together with dsRNA intermediates produced during replication of RNA viruses, IFN activates protein kinase R, which then phosphorylates eukaryotic initiation factor-2, rendering it nonfunctional. The activation of these cellular proteins is known as the antiviral state (c). Ribavirin directly inhibits the viral RNA polymerase (b) and interferes with guanosine-dependent processes within the cell (e). Neither IFN nor ribavirin blocks viral envelope fusion with host cell membrane (a) or inhibits viral proteases (d).

123. The answer is b. (*Levinson, Ch 41. Murray, Ch 63. Ryan, Ch 13.*) Since this was diagnosed and confirmed as a Hepatitis A infection, there is little likelihood of long-term sequelae. However, persons over 40 and those younger than 12 months are more likely to have severe manifestations. One dose of standard γ-globulin (b), which contains antibodies from a series of normal population individuals, will provide passive protection to the family members for several weeks due to the presence of antibodies against HAV. Vaccination with the killed HAV vaccine (c), which is recommended by CDC (*http://www.cdc.gov/hepatitis/HAV/HAVfaq.htm#general*), is for those in the 12 months to 40 years age bracket. IFN-α (a) treatment is approved only for HBV and HCV infections. HAV transmits readily, so the quarantine and observe approach (d) and the no-treatment option (e) will not guarantee that transmission will not occur within the family.

124. The answer is b. (*Levinson, Ch 37, 39, 43, 45. Murray, Ch 51, 62. Ryan, Ch 10, 1, 18.*) The lesions described and shown are characteristic of Kaposi sarcoma caused by human herpesvirus 8 (b). This is the most common opportunistic skin disease seen in males with AIDS. Bacillary angiomatosis, caused by *Bartonella henselae* (a) or *B. quintana*, is the second most common; it is characterized by vascular blood-filled nodules. Human T-cell leukemia virus (d) may cause nodular, indurated, or exfoliative skin lesions associated with acute T-cell leukemia. HTLV infections are seen most frequently in persons originating from or having lived in certain parts of Japan, the Caribbean, Central or West Africa, or South America, or who is a Native American Indian. HPV (c) causes papillomatous, or wartlike, outgrowths of the skin and mucous membranes. *Staphylococcus aureus* (e) causes abscesses in the skin characterized by swelling, redness, warmth, and pain; such lesions do not usually appear in the oral cavity.

125. The answer is c. (*Levinson, Ch 32. Murray, Ch 45, 46. Ryan, Ch 7.*) A latent infection is usually manifested by persistence of viral genomes, expression of none or a few viral genes, and survival of the infected cells. Reactivation with shedding of infectious virions may occur sporadically or not at all, usually dependent on immune competence. HSV (b) becomes latent in neurons. Adenovirus (a) can form latent infection of lymphoid tissue (tonsils, adenoids, Peyer patches). Epstein–Barr virus (c) becomes latent in B cells in the presence of immunocompetent T cells. All three viruses can be reactivated by loss of immunocompetence, infection with another agent, and other triggers, depending on the virus. Measles virus (d) can develop defective mutants, which cause persistent infection of the brain resulting in SSPE approximately 10 years after primary measles. Rabies virus (e) has a long incubation time with the virus replicating slowly in muscle cells and then peripheral nerves at the site of entry for 60 to 365 days after the bite. These latter two infections are persistently replicative rather than latent.

126. The answer is b. (*Levinson, Ch 34. Murray, Ch 47. Ryan, Ch 6.*) The symptoms described for her illnesses on both November 6 and December 5 are consistent with influenza. However, the November 6 illness (a) was not caused by nH1N1 influenza virus; the low titers (10 on November 6 and 10 on November 30) most likely represent cross-reacting antibodies from the agent that caused her first illness. The greater than fourfold rise in titer from 10 on November 30 (baseline) to 160 on December 20 reflects a definitive diagnostic rise in antibody against nH1N1 influenza virus. Thus, her December 5 illness (b) was influenza. There is enough serologic evidence to make the diagnosis (choice e is incorrect).

127. The answer is d. (*Levinson, Ch 31. Murray, Ch 44, 49. Ryan, Ch 7.*) The description of the viral genome as dsDNA and the virion as nonenveloped fits *Mastadenovirus* (human adenoviruses), *Papillomavirus* (HPV), and *Polyomavirus* (d), which is the only one of the three given as a choice. The new virus has been given the name Merkel cell polyomavirus, or *Polyomavirus* type MCPyV. It is the first *Polyomavirus* associated with a human cancer; general scientific opinion suggests that MCPyV causes most Merkel cell cancers. *Orthohepadnavirus* (HBV) (c) is enveloped and partially dsDNA; it is associated with hepatocellular carcinoma. *Erythrovirus* (parvovirus B19) (b) is nonenveloped, but is ssDNA. *Alphavirus* (togavirus) (a) is a (+) ssRNA enveloped virus, and *Rotavirus* (e) is a dsRNA nonenveloped virus. *Erythrovirus*, *Alphavirus*, and *Rotavirus* have not been associated with cancer in humans or animals.

128. The answer is a. (*Levinson, Ch 42, 43. Murray, Ch 60. Ryan, Ch 16.*) The illness described in the vignette is dengue (breakbone fever) (a) is the most common arthropod-borne infection among humans. There are four serotypes of dengue virus, which belong to the *Flaviviridae*, each causing the same type of symptoms. Yellow fever (e), caused by the yellow fever virus, is another flavivirus; it is characterized by fever with hemorrhage and hepatitis. Hepatitis C (c) is caused by another flavivirus, the HCV, but this infection manifests as hepatitis, rather than fever and bone pain; HCV is not spread by mosquitoes. Hemorrhagic fever with renal syndrome (b) is caused by the Old World strains of *Hantavirus* (*Bunyaviridae*), and is spread by rodents; the disease is seen in East Asia, Eastern Europe, western Russia, and Japan. Rubella (d), a very mild disease, is caused by *Rubivirus*, a member of the *Togaviridae*; unlike the *Alphavirus* genus, *Rubivirus* is not spread by arthropods.

129. The answer is d. (*Levinson, Ch 31, 41. Murray, Ch 44, 63. Ryan, Ch 6, 13.*) The vignette describes a patient with chronic hepatitis most likely acquired by blood transfusion, which could be caused by HBV or HCV. HCV infection is far more likely to lead to chronic hepatitis (approximately 85% in adults) than HBV (about 5% in adults); and HCV infection leads to a chronic illness characterized by fluctuating levels of liver enzymes and bilirubin, with normal results obtained at times. Acquisition of HDV leads to exacerbation of HBV if superinfection occurs or as acute infection if coinfection occurs; if the HBV infection continues as a chronic infection, HDV may become chronic as well. The answer requires knowledge of the families of viruses in which the hepatitis viruses reside as well as those that are bloodborne (HBV, HDV, and HCV) versus those that are fecal-orally transmitted (HAV and HEV), which do not lead to chronic infection. HCV is a ss(+)RNA virus belonging to the *Flaviviridae* (d). HBV is a partially dsDNA virus belonging to the *Hepadnaviridae* (a); HDV, which can only be acquired when HBV is present, is a ss(−)RNA virus known as *Deltavirus* (e); HAV is a ss(+)RNA virus belonging to the *Picornaviridae* (c); and HEV is a ss(+)RNA virus belonging to the new family *Hepeviridae* (b).

130. The answer is c. (*Levinson, Ch 41. Murray, Ch 63. Ryan, Ch 13.*) The markers of HBV infection, in order of appearance, are hepatitis B surface antigen (c), hepatitis e antigen (b), anti-hepatitis B core antigen IgM (e), and anti-hepatitis B e antigen (d), followed by anti-hepatitis B surface antigen IgG if the infection resolves. Hepatitis B core antigen (a) is found only in the nuclei of infected hepatocytes and not free in the bloodstream, although it is present in circulating intact hepatitis B virions (originally called "Dane particles").

131. The answer is c. (*Levinson, Ch 39, 43, 45. Murray, Ch 62. Ryan, Ch 18.*) After a long incubation period (up to 30 years), HTLV-1 (d) can cause either acute T-cell leukemia, a disease of CD4+ T lymphocytes, or HTLV-associated myelopathy/tropical spastic paresis. The virus is distributed worldwide, but found in concentrations in Southwest Japan, the Caribbean basin, some Sub-Saharan African countries, and South America, especially countries abutting the Caribbean Sea. In the United States, HTLV-1 is found mainly in immigrants from endemic areas, children of immigrants, sex workers, and IV drug users. HTLV-2 (d) causes hairy cell leukemia, a disease of CD8 T lymphocytes. It is found in high concentrations among indigenous peoples in Central, South, and North America (Native Americans) and in Europe among IV drug users. HIV-1 (a) is the causative agent of acute retroviral syndrome and AIDS. HIV-2 (b) causes a less-aggressive infection similar to that caused by HIV-1. HIV-2 is rare in the developed world; most cases are found in West Africa.

132. The answer is d. (*Levinson, Ch 37. Murray, Ch 51. Ryan, Ch 10, 14.*) All of the choices listed can cause corneal ulceration. However, HSV type 1 (d) is the most likely etiologic agent, in part because of the dendritic ulcers, which are characteristic of HSV corneal infection. Fungal infection (*Fusarium*, c) is frequently associated with a history of outdoor trauma involving plant material; an outbreak of fungal keratitis was associated with contaminated contact lens moistening solution, but has resolved. *Acanthamoeba* keratitis (a) occurs most frequently in contact lens wearers and is associated with water exposure. Foreign bodies (b) may cause abrasions, but these would not appear dendritic. Allergies (e) are not as likely to cause ulceration; nor does the young man give a history of connective tissue disease such as rheumatoid arthritis or SLE, which can be associated with ophthalmic pathology.

133. The answer is d. (*Katzung, Ch 49. Levinson, Ch 37. Murray, Ch 51. Ryan, Ch 10, 14.*) Acyclovir and its derivatives valacyclovir (d), famciclovir, and penciclovir all are effective in treating active herpes zoster (shingles). There is some evidence that valacyclovir and famciclovir are better in speeding cutaneous healing and resolving pain than acyclovir. Only acyclovir may be used in children. Amantadine (a) blocks the M2 channel of influenza A virus, although the vast majority of strains circulating currently are resistant; boceprevir (b) is an inhibitor of HCV NS3/4A protease; ribavirin (c) is used in the treatment of HCV and respiratory syncytial virus; and zidovudine (e) is a nucleoside reverse transcriptase inhibitor used in the treatment of HIV.

134. The answer is e. (*Levinson, Ch 37. Murray, Ch 51. Ryan, Ch 10, 14.*) The vignette describes cytomegalic inclusion disease (CID) caused by CMV (e). Seizures, deafness, jaundice, and purpura can also occur. CID is also one of the leading causes of mental retardation in the United States. Rubella virus (a) causes CRS, which has some similarities to CID, but differs in ophthalmic and cardiac manifestations are part of the syndrome. Mumps virus (d) and respiratory syncytial virus (b) do not cross the placenta. HIV (c) can cross the placenta but does not produce the symptoms/findings described in the vignette.

135. The answer is b. (*Levinson, Ch 39, 46. Murray, Ch 56. Ryan, Ch 9, 10.*) The vignette describes an adult woman with mumps virus (*Rubulavirus*) (b) infection, or mumps, who develops oophoritis, a complication that occurs in postpubertal females. Cytomegalovirus (a), rabies virus (c), respiratory syncytial virus (d), and rubella virus (e) do not cause this clinical picture.

136. The answer is a. (*Levinson, Ch 30, 39. Murray, Ch 44, 57. Ryan, Ch 6, 9.*) Antigenic drift (a) in which point mutations gradually change the antigenic structure of the hemagglutinin (H) and neuraminidase (N) proteins of *Influenzavirus* A, making an antibody developed against the original strain less neutralizing for the drifted strain. Antigenic shift (b) is another name for reassortment recombination that occurs in segmented RNA viruses. With *Influenzavirus* A, two different HN types infect the same cell, usually in a pig; during packaging, the H (and/or N) segments are packaged in different combinations than the original viruses; that is H1N1 becomes H2N1. Intramolecular recombination (d) occurs by homologous recombination in DNA viruses or strand switching in nonsegmented RNA viruses. Complementation (c) results when a protein from a wild type virus allows a replication-defective virus to be replicated and packaged into infectious virions; it does not repair the genetic defect. Phenotypic mixing occurs when two or more viruses of the same genus but different serotypes replicate in the same cell; for example, poliovirus type 1 and type 2 replicating together could produce virions with capsids containing both type 1 and type 2 proteins.

137. The answer is d. (*Levinson, Ch 46. Murray, Ch 58. Ryan, Ch 16.*) Very few persons have survived symptomatic rabies when untreated; of the first six recorded cases, three had received rabies vaccine before onset of clinical symptoms. In 2009, a regimen of aggressive therapy involving ribavirin, amantadine, and a ketamine–midazolam-induced coma was successful in saving the first patient on whom it was used. The original protocol and variations have been used since with little success; therefore, (c) is incorrect. Thus, rabies should be considered almost invariably fatal (d) once clinical symptoms begin. Adult patients recover from some forms of viral encephalitis, such as western equine and eastern equine encephalitis without complications (a), whereas children often suffer seizure disorders (b) and other complications; this is reversed with St. Louis and West Nile encephalitis.

138. The answer is e. (*Levinson, Ch 40. Murray, Ch 54. Ryan, Ch 9, 12.*) Rhinoviruses (e) are the most common cause of common colds. They can be recovered from people with mild upper respiratory illness. Their preference for growth at 33°C confines rhinoviruses to the nasopharynx and oropharynx; thus, serious infection caused by rhinoviruses is rare. Neutralizing IgG and IgA antibodies form but last only about 18 months. More than 100 serotypes are known, each requiring specific neutralizing antibody. For these reasons, development of a vaccine against rhinoviruses would be difficult, if not impossible; nor is such a vaccine necessary due to the mild nature of the illnesses caused. Excellent vaccines are available against mumps virus (b) and rabies virus (c). A passive vaccine, the monoclonal antibody palivizumab, is available for premature infants for prophylaxis against RSV (d). No vaccine is available for CMV (a).

139. The answer is e. (*Levinson, Ch 41. Murray, Ch 63. Ryan, Ch 13.*) The diagnosis of hepatitis begins with the clinical symptoms and is confirmed by the results of specific serologic tests, in this case the detection of anti-HAV IgM (e). The case presentation does not suggest hepatitis B (longer incubation, insidious onset), so HBsAg (b) is unlikely to be helpful. Viral culture (a) is not routinely done for any of the hepatitis viruses, although some will grow in cell culture. Electron microscopy on stool (c) might be positive, but would not be specific and is not generally available for clinical diagnosis. Rotavirus (d) causes gastroenteritis, not hepatitis.

140. The answer is c. (*Levinson, Ch 39. Murray, Ch 57. Ryan, Ch 9.*) The symptoms described by the physicians are those of classic uncomplicated influenza (c), which usually occurs in successive waves of infection (outbreaks) with peak incidences during the winter months in temperate climates. The abrupt onset of systemic symptoms (fever, chills, head, and muscle aches) followed by respiratory symptoms is typical of influenza. Neither the common cold (a) or pharyngitis (d) takes into account the whole group of symptoms. Some patients may develop primary viral pneumonia or secondary bacterial pneumonia, but the symptoms are not characteristic of pneumonia (e). Hand-foot-and-mouth disease (b) is not as severe and includes vesicular lesions.

141. The answer is b. (*Levinson, Ch 39, 46. Murray, Ch 56. Ryan, Ch 9, 10.*) Live, attenuated measles virus (b) vaccine given at 15 months to 2 years of age effectively prevents measles in 95% of children. Revaccination at 4 to 6 years or 11 to 15 years is recommended to maintain immunity. Inactivated virus (a) does not provide sufficient protection. Recombinant viral protein (c) may be used when neutralizing IgG is sufficient to prevent target infection, which is not the case with measles virus. Pooled immunoglobulin is used for passive immunization postexposure in the immunocompromised; virus-specific immunoglobulin (d) is not available. Wild-type live viruses (e) are never used as vaccines.

142. The answer is e. (*Katzung, Ch 49. Levinson, Ch 37. Murray, Ch 51. Ryan, Ch 10, 14.*) Acyclovir is an analog of guanosine or deoxyguanosine that strongly inhibits HSV but has little effect on other DNA viruses. It also has few side effects because the drug is activated only within HSV-infected cells by the viral enzyme thymidine kinase (e). HSV does encode a DNA-dependent DNA polymerase (a) which recognizes acyclovir triphosphate and incorporates the activated drug into the growing nucleotide chain, ending DNA synthesis; but this enzyme does not activate acyclovir. Integrase (b) and protease (c) are drug targets for antiretroviral therapy; proteases of HCV and influenza virus (neuraminidase) are also targeted by specific antivirals. Ribavirin targets the RNA-dependent RNA polymerases (d) of several minus sense ssRNA viruses, especially respiratory syncytial virus and Lassa fever virus.

143. The answer is e. (*Levinson, Ch 41. Murray, Ch 63. Ryan, Ch 13.*) The best approach to prevent HBV infection in a neonate born to an HBV-positive mother is to give HBIg and immunize with rHBV vaccine at birth (e). A person with chronic hepatitis B infection develops antibodies to HBcAg, and sometimes to HBeAg, neither of which is protective (neutralizing). Therefore, waiting until maternal antibodies diminish (b) would leave the baby unprotected. HBIg alone (a) does not provide immunity later and administration of HBV vaccine alone at birth (c) or at 1 year (d) will not provide the necessary immediate protection.

144. The answer is e. (*Levinson, Ch 37. Murray, Ch 51. Ryan, Ch 10, 14.*) VZV (e) is a herpesvirus that causes chickenpox, a highly contagious disease of childhood that used to occur in outbreaks in late winter and early spring. It is characterized by a fever, malaise, and generalized vesicular eruption with relatively insignificant systemic manifestation in immunocompetent children. Advent of an effective live attenuated vaccine in 1995 has reduced the number of cases of chickenpox by 90% and mortality has decreased 66%. Adults and immunocompromised individuals have more severe disease. Measles virus (d) produces a maculopapular rash. Adenovirus (a), CMV (b), and HPV (c) do not produce maculopapular or vesicular rashes.

145. The answer is e. (*Levinson, Ch 38. Murray, Ch 50. Ryan, Ch 9, 15.*) Adenovirus (e) has been associated with acute respiratory disease in adults, frequently among newly enlisted military troops. Close living conditions and strenuous exercise may account for the severe infections seen in this otherwise healthy group. VZV (a) often causes pneumonia in adults with chickenpox; the typical crops of vesicular skin lesions would usually be present as an aid to this diagnosis. Cytomegalovirus (d) causes pneumonia in persons immunocompromised by loss of T-cell function (AIDS, organ transplant recipients, persons undergoing chemotherapy for cancer). Papillomavirus (c) may cause papillomas in the respiratory tract (oral, laryngeal) but does not cause the symptoms described or pneumonia. Rotavirus (b) does not infect the respiratory tract.

146. The answer is a. (*Kumar, Ch 5. Levinson, Ch 38, 43. Murray, Ch 49. Ryan, Ch 19.*) Epidermodysplasia verruciformis (EV) (a), an inherited disorder most commonly autosomal recessive, has been linked to defective cell-mediated immunity due to mutations in *EVER1* and *EVER2*, although their exact mechanism of pathogenesis in EV is not known. EV leads to widespread HPV infection that manifests as flat warts distributed over the entire body. The disorder leads to cutaneous squamous cell carcinoma in 30% to 70% of the patients. NPC (d) is linked to Epstein–Barr virus infection, primarily in persons of Southeast Asian and North African descent. Familial adenomatous polyposis (b), Li–Fraumeni syndrome (c), and xeroderma pigmentosum (e) are inherited disorders in the *APC* gene, *p53* gene, and mechanisms of DNA repair, respectively. They are not associated with viral infections.

147. The answer is e. (*Levinson, Ch 40. Murray, Ch 59. Ryan, Ch 9, 15.*) Rotaviruses cause the major portion of diarrheal illness in infants and children worldwide but not in adults. They are nonenveloped RNA viruses containing 11 segments of double-stranded RNA genome (e) within a double-shelled capsid. Rotaviruses, like the influenzaviruses that have a segmented genome, can undergo genetic reassortment. Other viruses that cause gastroenteritis are represented by adenovirus 40/41, double-stranded DNA (a) and norovirus, nonsegmented single-stranded plus-sense RNA (d). Segmented single-stranded minus-sense RNA viruses (c) and single-stranded DNA viruses (b) do not cause gastroenteritis. See the table in answer to question 114 for additional information.

148. The answer is b. (*Levinson, Ch 37. Murray, Ch 51. Ryan, Ch 10, 14.*) Young athletes with splenomegaly from infectious mononucleosis are at risk of splenic rupture (b). They should be advised to refrain from contact sports until their symptoms have resolved. Heat exhaustion (a) could occur in any athlete and is not a consequence of EBV infection; malnutrition (c) is unlikely to occur in an IM patient in the United States. Aplastic crisis (d) is not a result of EBV infection but a complication of parvovirus B19 infection in persons with anemia or hemoglobinopathy such as sickle disease.

149. The answer is e. (*Levinson, Ch 42, 43. Murray, Ch 60. Ryan, Ch 16.*) The vignette describes classic yellow fever (e), which is endemic in the tropical regions of Africa, South America, and Central America. There is a vaccine against yellow fever, and travelers to endemic regions are advised to obtain immunization 9 months in advance. In 2012, there was an outbreak of yellow fever in Darfur that resulted in 849 cases with 171 deaths. Dengue hemorrhagic fever (a) is a possibility, but this is preceded by typical dengue and is not accompanied by jaundice, nor does it proceed as quickly. Hantavirus cardiopulmonary syndrome (b) is caused by New World hantaviruses and is seen in North and South America. Hemorrhagic fever with renal syndrome (c) is caused by Old World hantaviruses and is seen mainly in Eastern Asia, Eastern and Northern Europe, and Japan. SARS (d), caused by the novel SARS coronavirus, appeared in China in 2002, became pandemic, and then disappeared; a new outbreak occurred in 2004, but did not spread. In 2012, another novel coronavirus that causes a SARS-like illness appeared in Saudi Arabia; cases have occurred in Saudi Arabia, Qatar, and Britain.

150. The answer is b. (*Levinson, Ch 34. Murray, Ch 47. Ryan, Ch 6.*) Antibody measurements against viruses may be a useful diagnostic tool if two serum samples are collected from the patient. The acute serum is collected as early in the illness as possible, and the convalescent serum is collected 7 days to 2 weeks later. Both are included in the same test run against the viral antigen. The sera are diluted in a twofold manner beginning with a 1:2 or 1:10 dilution, depending on the virus. A fourfold or greater rise in titer between the acute and convalescent sera indicates recent primary infection (b). Titers that are equal or only twofold different (up or down) indicate past infection (d). In an anamnestic response (c), the titers are usually the same, but are much higher than the peak titer observed during primary infection; for example, 2560, 5120, or 10,240. However, such a response is usually detected only during epidemiologic studies as the patient is unlikely to symptomatic during a second infection with the same virus. See the figure for comparison of antibody response to primary infection and re-exposure.

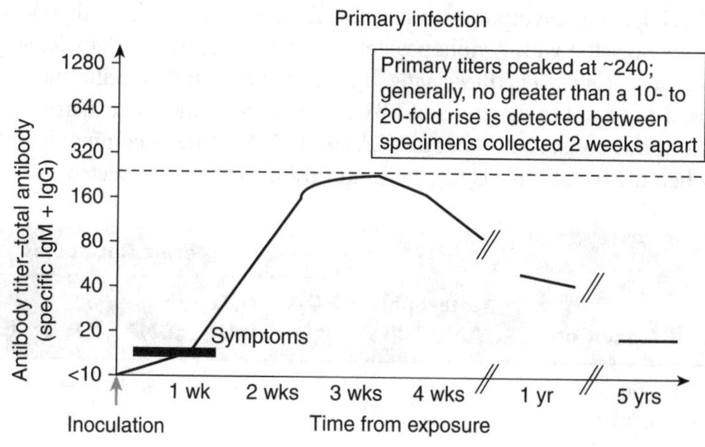

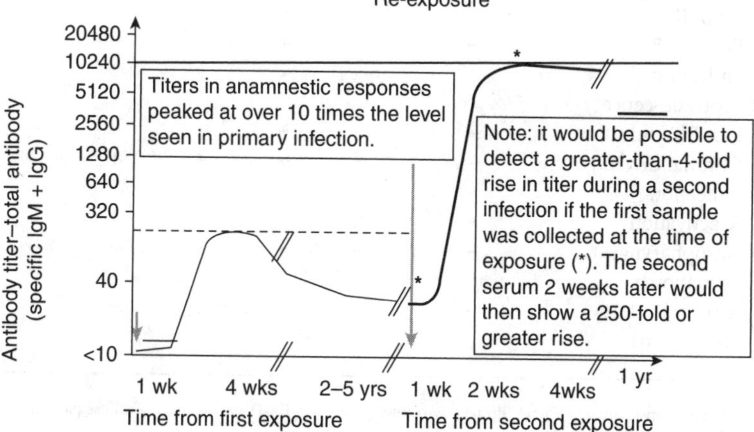

Graphs comparing the antibody responses to primary infection to influenza A virus (*top*) and re-exposure to the same virus (*bottom*).

151. The answer is d. (*Levinson, Ch 37, 43. Murray, Ch 51. Ryan, Ch 10, 14.*) Epstein–Barr virus (d), more commonly known for causing infectious mononucleosis, has been associated with several lymphomas, the first of which was Africa Burkitt lymphoma, described in the vignette. More recently, Burkitt lymphoma (outside of Africa) and Hodgkin lymphoma were added to the list. In males with congenital T-cell defects, overwhelming

B-cell leukemia/lymphoma can occur. Cytomegalovirus (c) and HSV (e) are not associated with lymphoproliferative disorders; nor are *Borrelia burgdorferi* (a) or *Chlamydia trachomatis* (b). Antibodies to EBV-specific antigens are used as an aid to diagnosis of EBV-related conditions other than infectious mononucleosis. Antibodies to VCA and EBNA are more commonly ordered when the heterophile is negative and EBV infection is suspected.

		EBV-Specific Antibodies				
Condition	**Heterophile Antibodies**	**VCA IgM**	**VCA IgG**	**EBNA**	**EA-D**	**EA-R**
Susceptible	−	−	−	−	−	−
Acute infectious mononucleosis	+	+	+	−	+	−
Acute EBV infection (not IM)	−	+	+	−	+	−
Recent EBV infection, convalescence	−	±	+	±	−	−
Past EBV infection	−	−	+	+	−	−
Chronic EBV infection	−	−	+	+	+	−
Reactivation	−	±	+	+	+	−
Nasopharyngeal carcinoma	−	−	+	+	+[a]	−
African Burkitt lymphoma	−	−	+	+	−	+

VCA, viral capsid antigen; EBNA, Epstein–Barr nuclear antigen; EA-D, early antigen—diffuse pattern; EA-R, early antigen—restricted pattern.

[a]The majority of patients with types 2 or 3 NPC have positive EA-D while only 35% of those with type 1 NPC have a positive EA-D.

152. The answer is a. (*Levinson, Ch 37, 43. Murray, Ch 51. Ryan, Ch 10, 14.*) Epstein–Barr virus (a) causes a variety of syndromes other than infectious mononucleosis, including an association with NPC, a disease commonly seen in adults in Asia, although the development of NPC after EBV infection is not limited to persons of Asian descent. EBV components have been detected in cells from patients with NPC by PCR. No such evidence of the presence of mumps virus, parvovirus B19, rubeola virus, or rubella virus within NPC has been observed. See the above table.

153. The answer is c. (*Levinson, Ch 37. Murray, Ch 51. Ryan, Ch 10, 14.*) CMV, which is usually asymptomatic or causes mild symptoms in immunocompetent persons, can cause a variety of devastating diseases in patients with AIDS, including retinitis (c), esophagitis, colitis, and encephalitis. Aplastic crisis (a) is associated with parvovirus B19 infection in persons with sickle cell anemia and other hemoglobinopathies; kidney failure (b) can result from CMV infection of a transplanted kidney; Reye syndrome (d) occurs mainly in children associated with VZV and other viral infections if aspirin is used to reduce fever; SSPE (e) is an uncommon, lethal, late complication of measles virus infection.

154. The answer is c. (*Levinson, Ch 38, 43. Murray, Ch 49. Ryan, Ch 19.*) The diagnosis of a viral infection is made easier by the creation of a greater number of diagnostic virology laboratories during the last few decades. In order for viral diagnosis to be successful, the most appropriate specimen must be collected for the disease in question. The best screening test for cervical HPV infection is a Pap smear on cells from the cervix for the presence of koilocytes (c), which are pathognomonic for HPV infection in any site. DNA molecular probe for HPV genomes (in situ hybridization) (a) and PCR for HPV DNA (d) are used to determine the type of HPV infection. HPV does not grow in viral culture (e) and HPV-specific antibodies (b) are not helpful for determining cervical infection.

155. The answer is b. (*Levinson, Ch 42, 43. Murray, Ch 60. Ryan, Ch 16.*) The entire family experienced dengue (breakbone fever). The man, who had previously been infected with one dengue virus, and the 6-year-old suffered dengue hemorrhagic fever (b). This complication is seen primarily in children younger than 15 years of age and in some who have been infected with one serotype of dengue virus and are subsequently infected with another. Nothing in the vignette suggests acute respiratory distress syndrome (a), encephalitis (b), Guillain–Barré syndrome (d), or a secondary bacterial infection (e).

156. The answer is b. (*Levinson, Ch 40. Murray, Ch 54. Ryan, Ch 9, 12.*) Coxsackievirus B (b) is the major cause of viral myocarditis; this group also causes pleurodynia, pancreatitis, orchitis, CNS disease, and respiratory infections. Strains of Coxsackievirus A (a) cause CNS disease, herpangina, hand-foot-and-mouth disease, acute hemorrhagic conjunctivitis, and respiratory tract infections. Echovirus 11 (c) is primarily associated with CNS disease, rashes, and respiratory tract infections. Enterovirus 70 (d) causes acute hemorrhagic conjunctivitis. Poliovirus 3 (e) causes aseptic meningitis and paralytic poliomyelitis. Enteroviruses are shed during the first days of infection and may be isolated from the respiratory tract during acute infection; they are shed from the intestinal tract for up to 30 days after symptoms appear. The best specimen for diagnosis is tissue/fluid from the target, in this case the heart, but that is not always possible. Characterization of an enterovirus isolated from the stool as the etiologic agent can be corroborated by serology in the case of viral myocarditis because the number of serotypes is limited.

157. The answer is a. (*Levinson, Ch 37. Murray, Ch 51. Ryan, Ch 10, 14.*) The vignette describes an adult with chickenpox. Adults who contract VZV have an increased risk for varicella pneumonia (the majority of VZV pneumonia occur in adults) and other complications, including VZV encephalitis. H&E staining of cells obtained by bronchoalveolar biopsy would show cells with eosinophilic intranuclear Cowdry A inclusion bodies (a) and multinucleated giant cells, both typical of HSV and VZV infections. Guarnieri bodies (b) indicate poxvirus infection; koilocytes (c) are seen in HPV infected cells; Negri bodies (d) are produced by rabies virus; and owl's eye cells (e) with basophilic intranuclear inclusions are typical of cytomegalovirus infection. See the diagram in answer to question 92.

158. The answer is c. (*Katzung, Ch 49. Levinson, Ch 39. Murray, Ch 57. Ryan, Ch 9.*) Oseltamivir (c) and zanamivir are the current drugs of choice to treat influenza. Both drugs inhibit the neuraminidase of *Influenzavirus* A and *Influenzavirus* B. Amantadine (a) and its analog rimantadine, drugs that block the M2 channel of *Influenzavirus* A only, are no longer recommended due to widespread resistance among circulating influenzaviruses. Foscarnet (b) is used to treat cytomegalovirus infection, ribavirin (d) is used to treat respiratory syncytial virus infection, and zidovudine (e) is an antiretroviral drug used to treat HIV infection.

159. The answer is a. (*Levinson, Ch 41. Murray, Ch 63. Ryan, Ch 13.*) The most likely hepatitis virus involved in a particular illness or outbreak can be postulated by the route of transmission, the incubation period, and the type of onset.

	HAV (a)	HBV (b)	HDV[a] (d)	HCV (c)/ HGV	HEV (e)
Incubation period	Short (15-45 days)	Long (30-180 days)	Long[b]	Long (15-150 days)	Short (21-56 days)
Onset	Sudden	Slow	Varies[b]	Insidious	Sudden
Transmission	Fecal–oral	Parenteral/ sexual	Parenteral/ sexual	Parenteral/ sexual	Fecal–oral

[a]Requires HBV—already present, or coinfection.

[b]Depends on whether acquired as coinfection (long) or superinfection (shorter).

160. The answer is c. (*Levinson, Ch 38. Murray, Ch 50. Ryan, Ch 9, 15.*) The lack of vomiting, duration of her symptoms, and timing of onset of her brothers' symptoms described in the clinical vignette, and her up-to-date immunization against rotavirus strongly suggest that adenovirus is the etiologic agent. Therefore, an EIA for adenovirus types 40/41 (c) is the best test. *Rotavirus* and *Norovirus* infections can also be diagnosed by EIA; however, culture for *Norovirus* (a) is not available and serology for *Rotavirus* (e) would be expected to be positive due to her immunizations. An EM examination of stool for astrovirus (d) would not likely be available in most clinical settings, although EM can also reveal *Rotavirus*, *Norovirus* and other caliciviruses, and adenovirus. Enteroviruses, although they infect cells of the intestinal tract, do not usually cause acute gastroenteritis. A DFA for enterovirus on intestinal biopsy (b) would not likely be helpful in establishing the etiologic agent. See the table in the answer to question 114 for additional information.

161. The answer is b. (*Levinson, Ch 40. Murray, Ch 59. Ryan, Ch 9, 15.*) EIA (b) is the best test for clinical diagnosis of rotavirus infection. Culture (a) is now possible, but is not routinely done. Electron microscopy (c) detects rotavirus infection as well as other viruses that cause gastroenteritis, but EM is not routinely available for clinical diagnosis. Histologic examination of biopsy (d) would show characteristic changes in the small intestine caused by rotavirus but the changes are similar to those caused by noroviruses; such an invasive test is unnecessary. Serology (e) is used for epidemiologic purposes only. See the table in the answer to question 114 for additional information.

162. The answer is d. (*Levinson, Ch 40. Murray, Ch 55. Ryan, Ch 15.*) A number of viruses that cause gastroenteritis have been recognized. The table in the answer to question 160 summarizes the characteristics of these viruses. *Norovirus* (d) has been associated with outbreaks in healthcare settings (hospitals, nursing homes), leisure settings (resorts, cruise chips), schools, and restaurants. Often the source is an infected food handler who fails to use good hand washing protocol. *Rotavirus* (e) and adenovirus 40/41 (a) cause infections primarily in infants, although all ages can be affected; both can be diagnosed by EIA. *Astrovirus* (b) has been demonstrated by EM in stools of young children and elderly nursing home residents during outbreaks of diarrhea. HAV (c) does not cause gastroenteritis. See the table in the answer to question 114 for additional information.

163. The answer is b. (*Levinson, Ch 40. Murray, Ch 55. Ryan, Ch 15.*) A number of viruses that cause gastroenteritis have been recognized. The table in the answer to question 160 summarizes the characteristics of these viruses. *Astrovirus* (b) has been demonstrated by EM in stools of young children and elderly nursing home residents during outbreaks of diarrhea. EIA tests are available to detect adenovirus 40/41 (a), *Norovirus* (d), and *Rotavirus* (e), so these cannot be the causative agents. HAV (c) does not cause gastroenteritis. See the table in the answer to question 114 for additional information.

164. The answer is e. (*Levinson, Ch 39, 42, 46. Murray, Ch 60. Ryan, Ch 10, 16.*) Rubella (e), also called German measles or 3-day measles, is an acute febrile illness characterized by a maculopapular rash and lymphadenopathy that affects children and young adults. It is the mildest of the viral exanthems. Chickenpox (a) is characterized by vesicular lesions appearing in crops beginning on the trunk and spreading to the extremities. Lesions of hand-foot-and-mouth disease (d) are also vesicular in nature with the majority of the lesions seen in the sites named. In erythema infectiosum (b), the rash on the face is red and distributed on the cheeks, while the rash on the body is lacy or reticular; the rash blanches and returns. Measles (c), also called rubeola or hard measles, is a much more severe illness characterized by prodrome of cough, coryza, and conjunctivitis. The prodrome is followed by the appearance of Koplik spots on the buccal mucosa. The maculopapular rash then appears beginning on the neck and spreading downward. Measles lasts much longer than rubella.

165. The answer is c. (*Levinson, Ch 41. Murray, Ch 63. Ryan, Ch 13.*) HCV is treatable with combinations of drugs, although whether treatment should be offered and the type of treatment given must be determined on an individual case basis. In general, those considered for treatment should have elevated serum alanine aminotransferase (ALT) levels, positive HCV antibody, and positive HCV RNA by PCR. Additional criteria, such as genotyping of the virus, or presence of coinfection with HIV or HBV, may be needed. The types of antivirals available for HCV infection include IFN-α, pegylated-IFN-α, ribavirin, and PIs. The goals of antiviral therapy are to attain sustained eradication of the virus and to prevent progression to cirrhosis, severe liver disease requiring liver transplantation, or hepatocellular carcinoma. Treatment spans from 24 weeks to 1 year depending on the drug(s) used and the genotype of the virus. The test used to monitor therapy for early virologic response, and for sustained virologic response, is the HCV RNA level (c). The patient already has antibodies to HCV, so testing for antibodies, whether IgG (a) or IgM (b), would not determine effectiveness of therapy. Serum ALT levels (e) may be monitored, but are liable to fluctuate and normalization of ALT is not proof of cure. Liver biopsy (d) is used in some cases to determine whether antiviral treatment should be initiated, but is not used to follow therapy.

166. The answer is d. (*Levinson, Ch 41. Murray, Ch 63. Ryan, Ch 13.*) Antiviral treatment for HBV infection was greatly enhanced by the recognition that the viral polymerase has reverse transcriptase functions. Since 1998, numerous antiretroviral reverse transcriptase inhibitors have been tried and two were found to be effective against HBV as well—lamivudine and tenofovir (d). Additional antivirals specific for the HBV DNA polymerase have been developed: adefovir in 2002, entecavir in 2005, and telbivudine in 2006. The antiretroviral zidovudine (e) has not been effective against HBV. Acyclovir (a) is specific for HSVs 1 and 2; foscarnet (b) for cytomegalovirus; and ribavirin (c) for severe respiratory syncytial virus infection, HCV infection, and viral hemorrhagic fever caused by Lassa fever virus.

167. The answer is a. (*Levinson, Ch 39, 42, 46. Murray, Ch 61. Ryan, Ch 16.*) La Crosse virus (a), an arthropod-borne *Bunyavirus* that causes viral encephalitis, is the most likely etiologic agent. This virus is found throughout the eastern half of the United States from Minnesota south to Louisiana and all states to the east. The majority of cases have been documented from rural areas of Minnesota, Wisconsin, Illinois, Indiana, and Ohio; and most occur in children younger than 16 years of age. In contrast, St. Louis encephalitis virus (d) is distributed through the entire United States, with the majority of cases occurring in persons older than 70 years of age, and in urban areas. Symptoms of viral encephalitis are not sufficient to determine the etiologic agent, but geographic distribution and age are good guides to the presumptive agent. Serologic studies, PCR, or viral isolation are needed to confirm the diagnosis. Venezuelan equine encephalitis virus (e) is rarely encountered in the United States, and is restricted to south Florida and south Texas. Rabies virus (c) does not cause the symptoms described and would be associated with animal bite or exposure to bats. Poliovirus (b), which is an enterovirus, was ruled out by the negative PCR. See the table accompanying answer to question 72 for additional information.

168. The answer is d. (*Levinson, Ch 37, 39, 42, 46. Murray, Ch 51, 60. Ryan, Ch 10, 14, 16.*) CRS includes several signs and symptoms that overlap with cytomegalic inclusion disease. These are intrauterine growth retardation (a), hepatosplenomegaly (b), microcephaly (c), mental retardation and developmental delays, sensorineural hearing loss (e), and skin lesions known as "blueberry muffin spots," although the etiology of the lesions is different in the two infections. CRS is different in that congenital heart defects such as patent ductus arteriosus (d) and pulmonary artery stenosis, and eye defects such as cataracts and infantile glaucoma also occur. Blueberry muffin spots in CRS are due to dermal erythropoiesis. Cytomegalic inclusion disease is characterized by the presence of intercerebral calcifications, cerebral atrophy, ventriculomegaly, hematologic abnormalities including thrombocytopenia, and chorioretinitis; the blueberry muffin spots are usually smaller than those seen in CRS and represent petechiae and purpura due to low platelets. Previously very common, CRS has been virtually eliminated in the United States with the use of rubella vaccine.

169. The answer is b. (*Levinson, Ch 32. Murray, Ch 45, 46. Ryan, Ch 7.*) Echovirus, an enterovirus, is spread via the fecal–oral route and causes aseptic meningitis (b). Coronaviruses (a) are more commonly spread via respiratory droplets and cause the common cold. HIV (c), the causative agent of AIDS, is spread via blood and sexual contact. Influenzavirus (d) is spread by respiratory droplets and causes influenza and sometimes primary viral pneumonia. Rabies virus (e) is spread by bites of mammals and causes the CNS disease rabies.

170. The answer is a. (*Levinson, Ch 42, 43. Murray, Ch 60. Ryan, Ch 16.*) The vignette describes WNV (a) encephalitis presentation in a person over 60. Although prevalent in Europe, Africa, and the Middle East, it was not seen in the United States until the summer of 1999. Since then, the virus has spread across the United States and is now endemic in all 48 continental states. It is transmitted by mosquitoes and birds, especially crows, are the reservoir. WNV infection ranges from asymptomatic, to a febrile illness with headache, to neuroinvasive disease, which ranges from meningitis in children to encephalitis in adults; it is especially severe in persons over 60 year of age and in the immunocompromised. Up to 10% of the encephalitis patients suffer acute flaccid paralysis. The mortality rate can be as high as 12%, almost all in the elderly. Since 2007, a number of neuroinvasive cases reported to CDC have varied from a low of 386 in 2009 to 2779 in 2012. St. Louis encephalitis virus is also more likely to cause encephalitis in the elderly (most in persons over 70), but this infection is less likely to occur than WNV; and acute flaccid paralysis is not part of the presentation. Poliovirus (c), the classic cause of acute flaccid paralysis, or poliomyelitis is not present in the United States. HSV (d) encephalitis is not associated with acute flaccid paralysis and is characterized by focal lesions in the temporal or occipital lobes on one side of the brain. *Coltivirus* (e) is confined to the Rocky Mountain region and rarely causes encephalitis. See the table accompanying the answer to question 72 for additional information.

171. The answer is b. (*Levinson, Ch 38, 44. Murray, Ch 49. Ryan, Ch 19.*) JC virus, a polyomavirus, was first isolated from the diseased brain of a patient with Hodgkin lymphoma who was dying of progressive multifocal leukoencephalopathy (PML), which is described in the vignette. This demyelinating disease occurs almost exclusively in immunosuppressed persons (AIDS, leukemia, tumors, and organ transplants). Recently, PML has occurred in patients receiving natalizumab and rituximab immune therapy. PML is the result of abortive infection of astrocytes and productive infection of oligodendrocytes by JC virus (b). HPVs cause cutaneous and mucosal infections. Prion variant CJD (c) manifests similarly to PML, but brain biopsy or section at autopsy shows amyloid plaques and spongiform vacuoles. SSPE caused by rubeola (measles) virus (d) and occurs about 10 to 11 years after clinical measles; symptoms include changes in behavior and intellect and seizures. WNV (e) causes acute encephalitis with symptoms that include headache, fever, and decreased consciousness.

172. The answer is a. (*Levinson, Ch 37. Murray, Ch 51. Ryan, Ch 10, 14.*) While primary HSV-1 infections are usually asymptomatic, symptomatic disease occurs most frequently in small children (1-5 years old). Buccal and gingival mucosa are most often involved, and lesions, if untreated, may last 2 to 3 weeks. Reactivation results in sporadic vesicular lesions that heal more quickly than the primary lesions. Following primary oral infection, whether symptomatic or asymptomatic, the virus enters the trigeminal ganglia and remains latent there throughout life (a). The virus may reactivate under conditions of physical, emotional, or mental stress and if the individual becomes immunocompromised from other infections or medical conditions. Each individual is unique regarding reactivation of HSV (type 1 or type 2), with some having no symptomatic reactivation, some one or two, and some multiple instances throughout their lives; therefore, one cannot say that the vesicular lesions will not recur (b). Guillain–Barré syndrome (c) is more with other human herpes viruses (VZV, CMV, and EBV) and bacterial infections (*Campylobacter jejuni* and *Mycoplasma pneumoniae*). Hepatocellular carcinoma (d) is seen in some patients with chronic hepatitis due to HCV or HBV; and SSPE (e) is a rare complication of measles virus infection.

173. The answer is d. (*Levinson, Ch 37. Murray, Ch 52. Ryan, Ch 11.*) The disease described in the vignette is molluscum contagiosum, caused by *Molluscipoxvirus* (d), a member of the *Poxviridae*. This self-limiting disease is more common in children than adults and is spread by direct contact (including sexual activity) and fomites such as towels. Biopsy of the lesions differentiates them from condyloma accuminatum caused by HPV types 6 and 11 (c). Molluscum bodies, similar to Guarnieri bodies observed with other poxviruses, are present in molluscum contagiosum and koilocytes are seen in HPV infections. Coxsackievirus A (b) can cause skin lesions, but these are vesicular; while the lesions caused by orf virus (e) are pustular in nature. Adenovirus (a) does not cause skin lesions.

174. The answer is b. (*Levinson, Ch 39, 46. Murray, Ch 56. Ryan, Ch 9, 10.*) The recently developed monoclonal antibody palivizumab (b) is recommended for prophylaxis of RSV infection in premature infants who are less than 12 months of age at the onset of RSV season. Pooled immunoglobulin (c) does not contain sufficient anti-RSV antibodies to be effective. IFN-α (a) is used to treat acute hepatitis C, chronic hepatitis B, condyloma accuminatum, and some cancers. Ribavirin (d) is administered as an aerosol to treat RSV infection but is not used for prophylaxis. Rituximab is a monoclonal antibody that reacts with CD20 on B cells and is used to reduce their numbers.

175. The answer is a. (*Levinson, Ch 39, 44, 46. Murray, Ch 56. Ryan, Ch 9, 10.*) High-dose vitamin A (a) given to malnourished children and anyone with vitamin A deficiency reduces the risk of mortality. The World Health Organization recommends that all children with measles receive vitamin A supplementation (not necessarily high-dose). The remaining vitamins listed do not have any effects on the outcome of measles.

176. The answer is d. (*Levinson, Ch 32, 33. Murray, Ch 10, 45, 46. Ryan, Ch, 33.*) Natural killer cells function in innate immunity to kill virus-infected cells (c); they may be sufficient to eradicate all infected cells, but usually some infectious particles escape from the site of primary replication to the reticuloendothelial system to undergo secondary replication. Neutralizing IgG specific for the virus (d) that is circulating prior to infection (from immunization or past infection) or that develops before the onset of dissemination by viremia prevents these viruses from reaching their target organ, in this case the meninges and/or brain. Antibody against these viruses develops rapidly; thus, many persons have only nonspecific symptoms or remain asymptomatic. Only in those in whom the virus replication outstrips host defense does meningitis, encephalitis, or meningoencephalitis occur. Cytotoxic T cells (a) are necessary to destroy all virus-infected cells and are responsible for part of the damage at target sites, but they cannot prevent the virus from reaching the target. Complement (b) and neutrophils (e) play little to no role in the host responses to these viruses.

177. The answer is c. (*Levinson, Ch 39, 46. Murray, Ch 61. Ryan, Ch 16.*) Biphasic illness culminating in encephalitis is characteristic of infection with the *Arenavirus* lymphocytic choriomeningitis virus (c), which is transmitted in rodent excreta; in this case, the common gray house mouse. Lassa fever virus is also an *Arenavirus* transmitted by rodents, but is found in Africa and causes hemorrhagic fever. Sin Nombre hantavirus (d) is also transmitted by rodents, but causes hantavirus pulmonary syndrome. La Crosse virus (a) and western equine encephalitis virus (e) cause encephalitis but are transmitted by mosquitoes.

178. The answer is c. (*Levinson, Ch 41. Murray, Ch 63. Ryan, Ch 13.*) HCV is a flavivirus that is transmitted by parenterally or sexually in the majority of cases; unlike the other members of the *Flaviviridae* known to infect humans, it is not transmitted by arthropods. Most new HCV infections are subclinical, and 70% to 90% develop into chronic hepatitis. Most HCV chronic cases remain without symptoms but 10% to 20% may develop to chronic active hepatitis and cirrhosis or hepatocellular carcinoma. Mixed cryoglobulinemia and glomerulonephritis complications are not uncommon with HCV (c). HAV (a) is a member of the *Enterovirus* genus; transmitted fecal-orally, it produces only acute disease. HBV (b), a member of the *Hepadnaviridae*, is transmitted similarly to HCV; it can produce acute or chronic infections. HDV (d) is a minus-sense RNA virus that can only cause infection in HBV-infected individuals. HEV is a member of the new family *Hepeviridae*; transmission and disease caused by HEV is similar to that of HAV, although the mortality is higher, especially in pregnant women.

179. The answer is c. (*Levinson, Ch 39. Murray, Ch 57. Ryan, Ch 9.*) During the influenza season, diagnosis is usually based on clinical presentation and detection of influenza antigens in respiratory secretions (c), which is the most rapid test available. However, influenza-like illness presenting out of season, infections strongly suspected to be influenza but for which the rapid test is negative, and sporadic cases should be tested for influenzaviruses and other respiratory viruses by other types of testing, including culture (b), immunofluorescence assays for multiple viruses, or RT-PCR and PCR. Testing of paired sera (e) is more frequently used epidemiologically to determine the extent of the outbreak or epidemic, the number of asymptomatic cases (if any), the effectiveness of detection methods, and vaccine efficacy. Electron microscopy (d) is rarely done. The cold agglutinin test (a) is used to diagnose *Mycoplasma pneumoniae* infection.

Bacteriology

Questions

180. A 65-year-old man presents to an emergency room in the United States. He complains of a 6-month history of night sweats, fever, and cough with the production of sputum. He also states that he has lost about 30 pounds in the last year. He denies illegal drug use, but admits to having sex with men. He demonstrated positive immunodeficiency virus serology and a low $CD4^+$ lymphocyte count. Gram stain of his sputum demonstrated thin rods that did not stain. When these organisms were stained with the acid fast stain, they took up the stain. He is most likely to be infected with which of the following organisms?

a. *Mycobacterium avium*-complex
b. *Mycobacterium scrofulaceum*
c. *Mycobacterium tuberculosis*
d. *Mycoplasma hominis*
e. *Mycoplasma pneumoniae*

181. A 40-year-old woman who has lived in southwest Louisiana all her life presents to the emergency room. She has strange-looking, raised areas on her face, arms, and legs. She also complains that she is losing feeling in her fingers and toes. She says that when she cuts or burns herself, she does not feel it and that makes the injury even greater because she does not know to pull away from the injuring source. A Gram stain of scrapings from the raised areas on her skin shows thin bacterial rods that do not take up the stain. However, an acid fast stain of the same material shows numerous bacilli. What disease is the woman most likely to have?

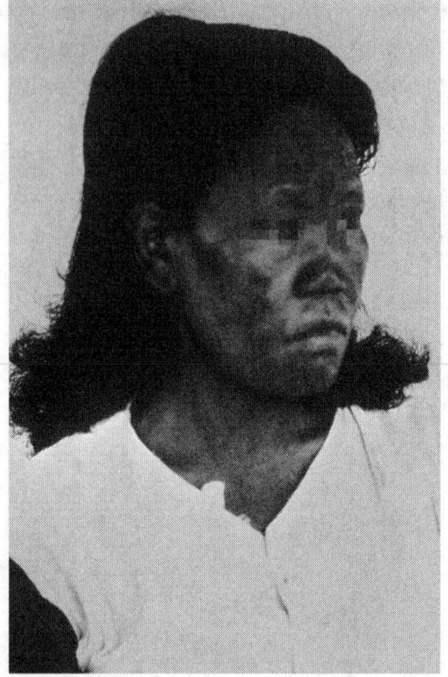

(Courtesy of Dr. Charles C. Shepard, Public Health Image Library, Centers for Disease Control and Prevention.)

a. Borderline tuberculoid leprosy
b. Lady Windermere syndrome
c. Lepromatous leprosy
d. Scrofula
e. Tuberculoid leprosy

182. An 85-year-old homeless man is brought to the emergency room. He says that he has been living on the street for the past 10 years. There is a strong smell of alcohol on his clothing and you suspect he is an alcoholic. He says he has constant headaches, and a fever that comes and goes about every 5 days. He also complains of great pains in his legs. The nurses say that when they cut off his clothes, they found lice. You suspect that he has trench fever caused by which organism?

a. *Bacillus anthracis*
b. *Brucella abortis*
c. *Bartonella bacilliformis*
d. *Bartonella henselae*
e. *Bartonella quintana*

183. A 45-year-old man goes to his family doctor complaining of a constant, non-productive cough. The man also has severe chest pains which he says have bothered him for the past week. The man also says that this is unusual for him because it is summer and he usually gets his "colds" in the winter and not in July. When the physician examines the man's chest, he hears an abnormal or pathological sound upon auscultation. The man had pneumonia with consolidation in both lobes. No organism was isolated from his sputum on blood agar, but the physician gave him a shot of penicillin "just in case". As it turned out, the penicillin shot did nothing to relieve the man's distress. After 96 hours, a Gram-negative bacterium from the man's sputum did grow on buffered charcoal yeast extract. What disease did this man have?

a. Legionnaires' disease
b. Lobar pneumonia caused by *Klebsiella pneumoniae*
c. Lobar pneumonia caused by *Streptococcus pneumoniae*
d. Psittacosis
e. Tuberculosis

184. At a state dinner, the menu included steak or fried chicken, baked potato or homemade potato salad, green beans, and a "green" salad. The salad dressing was either Italian or Russian. Dessert included either chocolate cake or apple pie. The beverage was water, iced tea, or coffee. After 3 hours, only the diners who had eaten the potato salad, became violently ill with vomiting, stomach cramps, and/or diarrhea. It became immediately obvious that the source of the food poisoning was the potato salad. When the potato salad was sent to a clinical microbiology lab, which of the following bacteria was isolated in large numbers?

a. *Bacillus cereus*
b. *Clostridium botulinum*
c. *Escherichia coli*
d. *Staphylococcus aureus*
e. *Staphylococcus epidermidis*

185. A young boy, 9 years of age, is outside playing in the summer in Texas and steps on a board with a rusty nail in it. The nail goes right through his gym shoe and enters his right foot. He does not tell his parents about it because he is sure his mother will yell at him because she is always telling him not to do what he just did. He is also afraid she will curtail his playing outside privileges. Besides, it did not bleed much and the bleeding stopped before he went in for supper. Besides, the boy's family did not believe in going to the doctor for every little thing. In fact, the boy cannot remember the last time he saw a doctor. About a week later, the boy developed a sore throat and then 4 days later his parents did take him to the hospital (reluctantly) with difficulty in swallowing, talking, and breathing. Also, the boy began to experience muscle spasms. The hospital doctor recognized the signs of tetanus and immediately administered tetanus immune globulin. The doctor asked the parents when the last time the boy had received a tetanus shot and they replied that they did not know. After being in the hospital for a week, the boy unfortunately died of respiratory failure. This unfortunate incident occurred because which of the following facts represents the best answer?

a. The causative organism, *Clostridium tetani*, is a strict anaerobe
b. The causative organism, *Clostridium tetani*, is a strict aerobe
c. The causative organism, *Clostridium tetani*, produces a potent heat-labile neurotoxin
d. The causative organism, *Clostridium tetani*, is a spore producer, a strict anaerobe, and produces a potent heat-labile neurotoxin
e. The causative organism, *Clostridium tetani*, is a spore former, a strict aerobe, and produces a potent heat-labile neurotoxin

186. A 6-year-old girl in Russia developed a sore throat and was taken to the doctor by her parents. The doctor diagnosed a "strep throat" and gave her a shot of penicillin. The penicillin shot did not help, and the child's health worsened and she was brought back to the doctor. Now the child complained of more than a sore throat. Now she refused to eat and was very lethargic. She also had a fever of 40°C. When the doctor reexamined the child, he observed a normal chest sound, a productive pharyngitis, and inflamed cervical lymph nodes. A throat culture did not reveal any Group A streptococci, and the child was becoming increasingly lethargic. The doctor then noticed a structure in the back of the child's throat that looked like a leather membrane. The parents told the doctor when he asked that the girl had received no vaccinations. The doctor then knew what disease he was observing. The organism most likely to be the causative agent of this infection was which of the following?

a. *Bacillus anthracis*
b. *Clostridium botulinum*
c. *Clostridium perfringens*
d. *Clostridium tetani*
e. *Corynebacterium diphtheriae*

187. A patient with a burning epigastric pain is admitted to the hospital, and a gastric biopsy is performed. The tissue is cultured on chocolate agar incubated in a microaerophilic environment at 98.6°F (37°C) for 5 to 7 days. On fifth day of incubation, colonies appear on the plate and curved, gram-negative, oxidase-positive rods are observed. Which of the following is the most likely identity of this organism?

a. *Campylobacter fetus*
b. *Campylobacter jejuni*
c. *Haemophilus influenzae*
d. *Helicobacter pylori*
e. *Vibrio parahaemolyticus*

188. A 2-year-old boy who missed several scheduled immunizations presents to the emergency room with a high fever, irritability, and a stiff neck. Fluid from a spinal tap reveals 20,000 white blood cells per milliliter with 85% polymorphonuclear cells. Gram stain evaluation of the fluid reveals small pleomorphic gram-negative rods that grow on chocolate agar. If an inhibitor is designed to block its major virulence, which of the following would be the most likely major virulence factor?

a. Capsule formation
b. Endotoxin assembly
c. Exotoxin liberator
d. Flagella synthesis
e. IgA protease synthesis

189. A local community is in distress due to a natural disaster. After consuming contaminated water, many individuals experience nausea, vomiting, and diarrhea that produce stools resembling rice water. An experimental compound is discovered that prevents the activation of adenylate cyclase and the resulting increase in cyclic adenosine monophosphate (AMP). The toxic effects of which of the following bacteria would most likely be prevented with the use of this experimental compound?

a. *Brucella abortus*
b. *Corynebacterium diphtheriae*
c. *Listeria monocytogenes*
d. *Pseudomonas aeruginosa*
e. *Vibrio cholerae*

190. A single, 30-year-old woman presents to her physician with vaginitis. She complains of a slightly increased, malodorous discharge that is gray-white in color, thin, and homogenous. Clue cells are discovered when the discharge is examined microscopically. Which of the following organisms is the most likely cause of her infection?

a. *Candida albicans*
b. *Trichomonas vaginalis*
c. *Escherichia coli*
d. *Gardnerella vaginalis*
e. *Staphylococcus aureus*

191. A 12-year-old girl begins to limp while playing soccer. She has pain in her right leg and upper right thigh. Her temperature is 102°F. X-ray of the femur reveals that the periosteum is eroded. Assuming that this case is managed as an infectious disease, which of the following is the most likely etiologic agent?

a. *Listeria monocytogenes*
b. *Salmonella enteritidis*
c. *Staphylococcus saprophyticus*
d. *Staphylococcus aureus*
e. *Streptococcus pneumoniae*

192. A scraping from a painful, inflamed wound is found to contain numerous gram-negative bacteria. Upon questioning, the feverish patient states that he was bitten by a cat while trying to rescue it from a storm drain earlier in the day. Given these observations, which of the following organisms is the most likely cause of infection?

a. *Aeromonas* species
b. *Campylobacter jejuni*
c. *Pasteurella multocida*
d. *Pseudomonas aeruginosa*
e. *Yersinia enterocolitica*

193. A 40-year-old male, who was in good health earlier, begins experiencing a chronic cough. Over the following 6 weeks, the cough gradually worsens and becomes productive. He is also coughing up blood, and notes weight loss, fever, and night sweats. A sputum sample is positive for acid-fast bacilli. Which of the following pathogenic mechanisms can be primarily attributed to the etiologic agent involved in this disease?

a. Cell-mediated hypersensitivity
b. Clogging of alveoli by large numbers of acid-fast mycobacteria
c. Humoral immunity
d. Specific cell adhesion sites
e. Toxin production by the mycobacteria

194. A person living on streets is infected with an invasive salmonella organism that is resistant to most of the antibiotics that could be considered for treatment. It did show sensitivity to quinolones that are bacteriocidal. Which of the following is the best explanation of their mode of action on growing bacteria?

a. Inactivation of penicillin-binding protein II
b. Inhibition of β-lactamase
c. Inhibition of DNA gyrase
d. Inhibition of reverse transcriptase
e. Prevention of the cross-linking of glycine

195. A high school student with a natural immunodeficiency is treated aggressively with a variety of potent antibiotics to overcome several bacterial infections. The most recent problem is caused by *S. aureus*, which is reported to be vancomycin-indeterminate (VISA). Which of the following statements concerning VISA is correct?

a. Patients with VISA isolates need not be isolated
b. Minimum inhibitory concentration (MIC) for vancomycin is at least 1.0 mcg/mL
c. VISAs have emerged because of the extended use of vancomycin for methicillin-resistant *Staphylococcus aureus* (MRSA)
d. VISA isolates are infrequent, so surveillance at the present time is not warranted
e. VISA isolates are usually methicillin susceptible

196. A 3-year-old girl, who has missed several scheduled immunizations, presents to the emergency room with a fever and troubled breathing. A sputum sample is brought to the laboratory for analysis. Gram stain reveals the following: rare epithelial cells, 8 to 10 polymorphonuclear leukocytes per high-power field, and pleomorphic gram-negative rods. As a laboratory consultant, which of the following interpretations is correct?

a. The appearance of the sputum is suggestive of *H. influenzae*
b. The patient has pneumococcal pneumonia
c. The patient has Vincent disease
d. The sputum specimen is too contaminated by saliva to be useful
e. There is no evidence of an inflammatory response

197. A 25-year-old medical student presents with a ruptured appendix. A peritoneal infection develops, despite prompt removal of the organ and extensive flushing of the peritoneal cavity. An isolate from a pus culture reveals a gram-negative rod identified as *Bacteroides fragilis*. Anaerobic infection with *B. fragilis* is best characterized by which of the following?

a. A black exudate in the wound
b. A foul-smelling discharge
c. A heme-pigmented colony formation
d. An exquisite susceptibility to penicillin
e. Severe neurologic symptoms

198. Several days after an unprotected sexual encounter, a healthy 21-year-old male develops pain and pus on urination. A Gram stain reveals gram-negative diplococci. Which of the following structures is responsible for adherence of the offending microbe to the urethral mucosa?

a. Capsule
b. Fimbriae
c. Flagella
d. F pili
e. Peptidoglycan
f. Lipopolysaccharide (LPS)

199. A 1-week-old newborn develops meningitis. Short, gram-positive rods are isolated. History reveals that the mother had eaten unpasteurized cheese from Mexico during pregnancy, and she recalled having a flu-like illness. Which of the following is the most likely etiologic microorganism?

a. *Corynebacterium diphtheriae*
b. *Escherichia coli*
c. Group B streptococci
d. *Listeria monocytogenes*
e. *Streptococcus pneumoniae*

Questions 200 to 203

200. A 30-year-old male patient is seen by the emergency service and reports a 2-week history of a penile ulcer. He notes that this ulcer did not hurt. Which of the following conclusions/actions is most valid?

a. Draw blood for a herpes antibody test
b. Even if treated, the lesion will remain for months
c. Failure to treat the patient will have no untoward effect, as this is a self-limiting infection
d. Perform a dark-field examination of the lesion
e. Prescribe acyclovir for primary genital herpes

201. The laboratory reports that the Venereal Disease Research Laboratory (VDRL) test performed on the above patient is reactive at a dilution of 1:4 (4 dils). The patient also reports to you that he has recently been diagnosed with hepatitis A. Which one of the following is most appropriate next step in management?

a. Order a confirmatory test such as the fluorescent treponemal antibody (FTA) test
b. Order a rapid plasma reagin (RPR) test
c. Perform a spinal tap to rule out central nervous system (CNS) syphilis
d. Repeat the VDRL test
e. Report this patient to the health department, as he has syphilis

202. In the same patient from the previous vignette, which of the following test combinations for syphilis is most appropriate?

a. FTA-Abs (IgG)/FTA-Abs (IgM)
b. RPR/culture of the lesion
c. RPR/FTA-Abs
d. *Treponema pallidum* hemagglutination (TPHA)/microhemagglutination—*Treponema pallidum* (MHTP) tests
e. VDRL/RPR

203. Assume that the same patient from the previous vignette absolutely denies any contact, sexual or otherwise, with a person who had syphilis. Also assume that both the RPR and the FTA-Abs are positive on this patient. Which of the following tests could be used to show that this patient probably does not have syphilis?

a. Frei test
b. MHTP test
c. Quantitative RPR
d. *Treponema pallidum* immobilization (TPI) test
e. VDRL

204. A patient is hospitalized after an automobile accident. The wounds become infected, and the patient is treated with tobramycin, carbenicillin, and clindamycin. Five days after antibiotic therapy was initiated, the patient develops severe diarrhea and pseudomembranous enterocolitis. Antibiotic-associated diarrhea and the more serious pseudomembranous enterocolitis can be caused by which of the following organisms?

a. *Bacteroides fragilis*
b. *Clostridium difficile*
c. *Clostridium perfringens*
d. *Clostridium sordellii*
e. *Staphylococcus aureus*

205. A 2-year-old child has a fever, stiff neck, and is irritable. Gram stain smear of spinal fluid reveals gram-negative, small pleomorphic coccobacillary organisms. What is the most appropriate procedure to follow in order to reach an etiological diagnosis?

a. Culture the spinal fluid in chocolate agar, and identify the organism by growth factors
b. Culture the spinal fluid in mannitol-salt agar
c. Perform a catalase test of the isolated organism
d. Perform a coagulase test with the isolate
e. Perform a latex agglutination (LA) test to detect the specific antibody in the spinal fluid

206. A patient complains to his dentist about a draining lesion in his mouth. A Gram stain of the pus shows a few gram-positive cocci, leukocytes, and many-branched gram-positive rods. Branched yellow sulfur granules are observed by a microscope. Which of the following is the most likely cause of the disease?

a. *Actinomyces israelii*
b. *Actinomyces viscosus*
c. *Corynebacterium diphtheriae*
d. *Propionibacterium acnes*
e. *Staphylococcus aureus*

207. A 39-year-old primigravid Caucasian female lawyer develops premature rupture of membranes at 35 weeks of gestation. She develops fever up to 103°F, and the amniotic fluid reveals a group B *Streptococcus*. Which of the following is the best option to reduce Group B streptococcal infection in her fetus?

a. Identification of possible high-risk births
b. Intravenous penicillin administered at least 4 hours before delivery
c. Screening of pregnant female at the first office visit, usually during the first trimester
d. Screening of pregnant female in the last trimester
e. Use of a polysaccharide vaccine

208. A 1-week-old neonate presents to the pediatric emergency room with fever, irritability, poor feeding, and a bulging anterior fontanelle. Lumbar puncture is performed, and the cerebrospinal fluid (CSF) grows group B *Streptococcus*. Which of the following is the most likely pathogenic mechanism?

a. Complement C5a, a potent chemoattractant, activates polymorphonuclear neutrophils (PMNs)
b. In the absence of a specific antibody, opsonization, phagocyte recognition, and killing do not proceed normally
c. The alternative complement pathway is activated
d. The streptococci are resistant to penicillin

209. A man who has a penile chancre appears in a hospital's emergency service. The VDRL test is negative. Which of the following is the most appropriate course of action?

a. Perform dark-field microscopy for treponemes
b. Perform a Gram stain on the chancre fluid
c. Repeat the VDRL test in 10 days
d. Send the patient home untreated
e. Swab the chancre and culture on Thayer-Martin (TM) agar

210. A clinically depressed farmer complains of extreme weakness, a daily rise and fall in fever, and night sweats. Small gram-negative rods are isolated from blood cultures after a 2-week incubation period. Which of the following organisms is the most likely etiologic agent?

a. *Brucella melitensis*
b. *Campylobacter jejuni*
c. *Francisella tularensis*
d. *Salmonella enteritidis*
e. *Serratia marcescens*

211. An outbreak occurs in a community where the water supply is contaminated. Multiple patients experience nausea and vomiting as well as profuse diarrhea with abdominal cramps; stools are described as "rice water." Curved, gram-negative rods are isolated on a sulfate-citrate-bile-sucrose agar. In the treatment of patients who have cholera, the use of a drug that inhibits adenyl cyclase would be expected to have which of the following characteristics?

a. Block the action of cholera toxin
b. Eradicate the organism
c. Increase fluid secretion
d. Kill the patient immediately
e. Reduce intestinal motility

212. A box of ham sandwiches with mayonnaise, prepared by a person with a boil on his neck, is left out of the refrigerator for the on-call interns. Three doctors become violently ill approximately 2 hours after eating the sandwiches. Which of the following is the most likely cause?

a. *Clostridium perfringens* toxin
b. Coagulase from *S. aureus* in the ham
c. Penicillinase given to inactivate penicillin in the pork
d. *Staphylococcus aureus* enterotoxin
e. *Staphylococcus aureus* leukocidin

213. A 34-year-old diabetic truck driver notices maceration of the web space of his toes on the right foot. Two days later he has a temperature of up to 100°F, exquisite tenderness, erythema, and swelling of the right leg. Culture exudate from the foot yields *S. aureus*. Which of the following often complicates treatment of *S. aureus* infection with penicillin?

a. Allergic reaction caused by staphylococcal protein
b. Inability of penicillin to penetrate the membrane of *S. aureus*
c. Lack of penicillin-binding sites on *S. aureus*
d. Production of penicillin acetylase by *S. aureus*
e. Production of penicillinase by *S. aureus*

214. Two of 3 family members have dinner at a local restaurant and, within 48 hours, start experiencing double vision, difficulty in swallowing and speaking, and breathing problems. These symptoms are consistent with which of the following?

a. Activation of cyclic AMP
b. Endotoxin shock
c. Ingestion of a neurotoxin
d. Invasion of the gut epithelium by an organism
e. Secretion of an enterotoxin

215. A clinical research group attempting to develop an improved *Neisseria meningitidis* vaccine is granted approval to gather volunteers for a clinical trial. Part of the volunteer evaluation is to sample bacteriologically for normal oral flora *Neisseria.* They find that almost all of the participants have several commensal species as part of their upper respiratory tract (URT) flora. Which of the following statements accurately describes the significance of these bacteria?

a. As a part of the normal flora, *Neisseria* provide a natural immunity in local host defense
b. As a part of the respiratory flora, they are the most common cause of acute bronchitis and pneumonia
c. Commensal bacteria stimulate a cell-mediated immunity (CMI)
d. Commensal *Neisseria* in the upper respiratory tract impede phagocytosis by means of lipoteichoic acid
e. Normal flora, such as nonpathogenic *Neisseria*, provides effective nonspecific B-cell-mediated humoral immunity

216. A family routinely consumes unpasteurized milk, claiming "better taste." Several members experience a sudden onset of crampy abdominal pain, fever, and profuse bloody diarrhea. *Campylobacter jejuni* is isolated and identified from all patients. Which of the following is the treatment of choice for this type of enterocolitis?

a. Ampicillin
b. *Campylobacter* antitoxin
c. Ciprofloxacin
d. Erythromycin
e. Pepto-Bismol

217. An unimmunized, 2-year-old boy presents with drooling from the mouth, elevated temperature, and enlarged tonsils. During attempts at intubation, no gray-white membrane is observed but the epiglottis appears "beefy" red and edematous. Which of the following is the most likely organism?

a. *Haemophilus haemolyticus*
b. *Haemophilus influenzae*
c. *Klebsiella pneumoniae*
d. *Mycoplasma pneumoniae*
e. *Neisseria meningitidis*

Questions 218 to 220

218. A 70-year-old female patient is readmitted to a local hospital with fever and chills following cardiac surgery at a major teaching institution. A gram-positive coccus grows within 24 hours from blood taken from the patient. Initial tests indicate that this isolate is resistant to penicillin. Which of the following is the most likely identification?

a. *Enterococcus species*
b. Group A *Streptococcus*
c. Group B *Streptococcus*
d. *Neisseria* species
e. *Streptococcus pneumoniae*

219. Further testing of the patient in the previous question reveals that the isolate possesses the group D antigen, and is not β-lactamase-positive, but is resistant to vancomycin. Which of the following is the most likely identification of this isolate?

a. *Enterococcus casseliflavus*
b. *Enterococcus durans*
c. *Enterococcus faecalis*
d. *Enterococcus faecium*
e. *Streptococcus pneumoniae*

220. Which of the following is the treatment of choice for the isolate in Question 219?

a. Ciprofloxacin
b. Gentamicin
c. Gentamicin and ampicillin
d. Rifampin
e. No available treatment

221. A young man crashes his bicycle, injuring one leg. Bacteria from the wound and a subsequent blood culture are isolated and identified, and an acute hematogenous osteomyelitis is diagnosed. Which organism listed below most often causes this type of infection?

a. *Escherichia coli*
b. *Proteus mirabilis*
c. *Staphylococcus aureus*
d. *Staphylococcus epidermidis*
e. *Streptococcus faecalis*

222. A 3-year-old girl, with no history of vaccination, is brought to the hospital with a sore throat, fever, malaise, and difficulty in breathing. Physical examination reveals a gray membrane covering the pharynx. Growth of the etiologic agent on cysteine-tellurite agar forms gray-to-black colonies with a brown halo. The major virulence factor of this organism is only produced by those strains that will most likely have which of the following characteristics?

a. Encapsulated
b. Endotoxin
c. Glucose fermenters
d. Lysogenic for β-prophage
e. Sucrose fermenters

Questions 223 to 225

A 28-year-old menstruating woman appears in the emergency room with the following signs and symptoms: fever, 104°F (40°C); WBC, 16,000/μL; blood pressure, 90/65 mm Hg; a scarlatiniform rash on her trunk, palms, and soles; extreme fatigue; vomiting; and diarrhea.

223. Which of the following is the most likely diagnosis?

a. Chicken pox
b. Guillain–Barré syndrome
c. Scalded skin syndrome
d. Staphylococcal food poisoning
e. Toxic shock syndrome (TSS)

224. Culture of the menstrual fluid in this case cited would most likely reveal a predominance of which of the following?

a. *Clostridium difficile*
b. *Clostridium perfringens*
c. *Gardnerella vaginalis*
d. *Staphylococcus aureus*
e. No organisms isolated

225. Which of the following is the most likely source and characteristic finding not yet revealed in the case just presented?

a. A meal of chicken in a fast-food restaurant
b. A retained tampon
c. Heavy menstrual flow
d. Recent exposure to rubella
e. Travel to Vermont

Questions 226 and 227

A severe URT outbreak occurs in the residence of students of a private school, resulting in several cases of otitis media and acute sinusitis. Some students do not have any clinical evidence of infection. The state public health laboratory receives and evaluates a new LA reagent for *H. influenzae* polysaccharide capsular antigen in urine (intact antigen elimination). The results, shown below, are compared with the isolation of *H. influenzae* from pharyngeal swabs.
LA POS, CULT POS: 25
LA POS, CULT NEG: 5
LA NEG, CULT POS: 5
LA NEG, CULT NEG: 95

226. Which of the following best indicates the sensitivity of LA?

a. 0%
b. 30%
c. 85%
d. 95%
e. 100%

227. Which of the following best indicates the specificity of LA?

a. 0%
b. 30%
c. 80%
d. 95%
e. 100%

228. A severely burned firefighter develops a rapidly disseminating bacterial infection while hospitalized. "Green pus" is noted in the burned tissue, and cultures of both the tissue and blood yield small, oxidase-positive, gram-negative rods. Which of the following statements best describes this organism?

a. Endotoxin is the only virulence factor known to be produced by these bacteria
b. Humans are the only known reservoir hosts for these bacteria
c. The bacteria are difficult to culture because they have numerous growth requirements
d. These are among the most antibiotic resistant of all clinically relevant bacteria
e. These highly motile bacteria can "swarm" over the surface of culture media

229. Several hours after dining on sweet and sour chicken and pork fried rice at the home of an Asian friend, a 34-year-old car salesman exhibits abdominal discomfort, nausea, and vomiting. In the middle of the night he awakens with watery diarrhea. Which of the following pairs of organisms is routinely responsible for food poisoning?

a. *Clostridium botulinum* and *Bacillus anthracis*
b. *Clostridium difficile* and *C. botulinum*
c. *Clostridium perfringens* and *B. cereus*
d. *Clostridium tetani* and *B. anthracis*
e. *Clostridium tetani* and *B. cereus*

230. MRSA is isolated from seven patients in a 14-bed intensive care unit. All patients are isolated and the unit closed to any more admissions. Which of the following best explains these rigorous methods to control MRSA?

a. MRSA causes TSS
b. MRSA is inherently more virulent than other staphylococci
c. MRSA is resistant to penicillin
d. MRSA spreads more rapidly from patient to patient than antibiotic-susceptible staphylococci do
e. The alternative for treatment of MRSA is vancomycin, an expensive and potentially toxic antibiotic

231. A 2-year-old infant is brought to the emergency room with hematuria, fever, and thrombocytopenia. Which one of the following bacteria would most likely be isolated from a stool specimen?

a. *Aeromonas* species
b. *Enterobacter aerogenes*
c. *Escherichia coli* 0157/H7
d. *Salmonella enteritidis*
e. *Shigella flexneri*

232. A 65-year-old healthy, retired female executive goes to Mexico on her yearly vacation. Unlike her previous trips, she decides to use the local water to make her favorite punch. Thirty-six hours later, she develops profuse watery diarrhea, severe cramping, and abdominal pain. She is diagnosed with *Escherichia coli*-related diarrhea. Which of the following *E. coli* types is characterized by the presence of heat-labile (LT) and heat-stable (ST) toxin proteins?

a. Enteroinvasive (EIEC)
b. Enterotoxigenic (ETEC)
c. Enterohemorrhagic (EHEC)
d. Enteropathogenic (EPEC)

233. A 48-year-old farmer in New Mexico is bitten by a flea and, 5 days later, develops a sudden onset of fever, chills, weakness, and headache. A few hours later he develops swollen, necrotic lymph nodes (buboes) in the right axilla and groin, which are intensely painful. This patient is subsequently diagnosed with bubonic plague and does not develop any pneumonic features of the disease. Human plague can be bubonic or pneumonic. Which of the following is the primary epidemiologic difference between the two clinical forms of plague?

a. Age of the patient
b. Geographic location of the animal vector
c. Health of the animal vector
d. Route of infection
e. Season of the year

234. A 9-year-old child is brought to the emergency room with the chief complaint of enlarged, painful axillary lymph nodes. The resident physician also notes a small, inflamed, dime-sized lesion surrounding what appears to be a small scratch on the forearm. The lymph node is aspirated and some pus is sent to the laboratory for examination. A Warthin-Starry silver impregnation stain reveals many highly pleomorphic, rod-shaped bacteria. Which of the following is the most likely cause of this infection?

a. *Bartonella henselae*
b. *Brucella canis*
c. *Mycobacterium scrofulaceum*
d. *Yersinia enterocolitica*
e. *Yersinia pestis*

235. A sixth-grade boy returns from a summer camp with several minor cuts and abrasions. Within a week, extensive cellulitis develops, and it is apparent that subcutaneous tissue is involved, requiring surgical removal of nonviable tissue. Antibiotics are used aggressively. Cellulitis is usually caused by which of the following?

a. *Bacillus cereus*
b. *Clostridium tetani*
c. Group A streptococci
d. *Micrococcus* species
e. *Staphylococcus aureus*

236. A 40-year-old female reports chronic gastritis. She tests positive for *H. pylori*. After a course of the appropriate antibiotic therapy, her symptoms subside. Which of the following is the most effective noninvasive test for the diagnosis of *Helicobacter*-associated gastric ulcers?

a. Culture of stomach contents for *H. pylori*
b. Detection of *H. pylori* antigen in stool
c. Growth of *H. pylori* from a stomach biopsy
d. Growth of *H. pylori* in the stool
e. IgM antibodies to *H. pylori*

237. The following examination and test results are observed in a woman tested in November who reports being in the woods in Pennsylvania during the last summer. While there, she was bitten by a tick, and now has a flattened red area near the bite with central clearing. She also has flu-like illness with fever, myalgia, and headache. Which of the following is the most appropriate course of action?

a. Ask the patient if she has a severe headache
b. Do a spinal tap for CSF
c. Observe the lesion
d. Order a Lyme disease antibody titer
e. Start treatment with tetracycline

238. Several white male patients, over 50 years of age and suffering from cavitary pulmonary disease, being followed and treated at a university AIDS clinic are found to be infected by *Mycobacterium avium*, a major opportunist pathogen. *M. avium* from these patients is best characterized by which one of the following statements?

a. Few isolates from AIDS patients are acid-fast.
b. Most isolates from AIDS patients are sensitive to isoniazid and streptomycin
c. *M. avium* can be isolated from the blood of many AIDS patients
d. *M. avium* isolates from AIDS patients are of multiple serovars
e. The majority of *M. avium* isolates from AIDS patients are nonpigmented

239. A 12-year-old girl experiences a group A streptococcus pharyngitis and, within 3 weeks, has chest pain and develops new murmurs of mitral regurgitation. Which of the following statements best typifies the disease she is suffering from?

a. It is a complication of group A streptococcal skin disease but usually not of pharyngitis
b. It is characterized by inflammatory lesions that may involve the heart, joints, subcutaneous tissues, and CNS
c. It is very common in developing countries but extremely rare and decreasing in incidence in the United States
d. Prophylaxis with benzathine penicillin is of little value
e. The pathogenesis is related to the similarity between a staphylococcal antigen and a human cardiac antigen

240. After extraction of a wisdom tooth, an 18-year-old male student is diagnosed with subacute bacterial endocarditis (SBE). He has a congenital heart disease that has been under control. Which of the following is the most likely organism causing the infection?

a. *Staphylococcus aureus*
b. *Staphylococcus epidermidis*
c. *Streptococcus pneumoniae*
d. *Streptococcus viridans*
e. *Enterococcus faecalis*

241. A 70-year-old male is taken to the emergency room with a history of "cold-like" symptoms for at least 3 days. At the time of the visit, his temperature is 102°F and he experienced shaking, chills, chest pain, and a productive cough with bloody sputum. Blood agar culture reveals gram-positive α-hemolytic colonies. If a quellung test was done on the colonies, which of the following bacteria would most likely be positive?

a. *Corynebacterium diphtheriae*
b. *Enterobacter* species
c. *Haemophilus parainfluenzae*
d. *Neisseria gonorrhoeae*
e. *Streptococcus pneumoniae*

242. A 6-month-old infant is admitted to the hospital with acute meningitis. The Gram stain reveals gram-positive, short rods, and the mother indicates that the child has received "all" of the meningitis vaccinations. Which of the following is the most likely cause of the disease?

a. *Haemophilus influenzae*
b. *Listeria monocytogenes*
c. *Neisseria meningitidis*, group A
d. *Neisseria meningitidis*, group C
e. *Streptococcus pneumoniae*

243. A 40-year-old man presents to the emergency medicine department 1 week following a foot injury. He is experiencing intense pain in the area of injury and the muscles of the jaw. Which of the following is the most common portal of entry for the etiologic organism?

a. Gastrointestinal (GI) tract
b. Genital tract
c. Nasal tract
d. Respiratory tract
e. Skin

244. A 22-year-old homeless person with a known drug abuse problem and multiple opportunistic infections has a positive PPD (purified protein) test. Which of the following is the most common way this infection is acquired?

a. GI tract
b. Genital tract
c. Nasal tract
d. Respiratory tract
e. Skin

245. A 31-year-old school teacher returns from foreign travel and experiences a sudden (1-2 days) onset of abdominal pain, fever, and watery diarrhea, caused by a heat-labile exotoxin that affects both the gut and the CNS. This infection is caused by an etiologic agent commonly acquired through which of the following routes?

a. GI tract
b. Genital tract
c. Nasal tract
d. Respiratory tract
e. Skin

246. A college student is surprised one morning by painful urination and a cream-colored exudate. Any person who acquires the gram-negative microbe that causes this infection is most likely to have acquired it via which of the following?

a. GI tract
b. Genitourinary tract
c. Nasal tract
d. Respiratory tract
e. Skin

247. A 25-year-old college student with no history of allergic rhinitis has a 12-day history of facial pain, clear rhinorrhea, fever, headache, and back pain. Her symptoms do not respond to over-the-counter medication. Culture of the fluid from the sinus reveals *Moraxella (Branhamella) catarrhalis*. Which of the following best characterizes *M. catarrhalis?*

a. A gram-negative, pleomorphic rod that can cause endocarditis
b. A gram-negative rod, fusiform-shaped, that is associated with periodontal disease but may cause sepsis
c. The causative agent of rat-bite fever
d. The gram-negative diplococcus, which is the causative agent of sinusitis, bronchitis, and pneumonia
e. The causative agent of trench fever

248. A 16-year-old Hispanic female with poor oral hygiene and severe gingivitis presents with a temperature of 103.5°F and hypotension. Blood culture is positive for *Capnocytophaga*. Which of the following best characterizes *Capnocytophaga*?

a. A gram-negative, pleomorphic rod that can cause endocarditis
b. A gram-negative rod, fusiform-shaped, that is associated with periodontal disease but may cause sepsis
c. The causative agent of rat-bite fever
d. The causative agent of sinusitis, bronchitis, and pneumonia
e. The causative agent of trench fever

249. Several employees in a veterinary facility experience a mild influenza-like infection after working on six sheep with an undiagnosed illness. The etiologic agent causing the human disease is most often transmitted to humans by which of the following methods?

a. Fecal contamination from flea deposits on the skin
b. Inhalation of infected particles or aerosols from the suspected animal urine and feces
c. Lice feces scratched into the broken skin during the louse's blood feeding
d. Tick saliva during feeding on human blood
e. Urethral discharge from infected humans

250. An endocarditis patient under a physician's care develops a urinary tract infection (UTI). A group D enterococcus (*Enterococcus faecium*) is isolated but the UTI does not respond to ampicillin and gentamicin treatments. Which of the following options would be considered the most clinically appropriate action?

a. Consider vancomycin as an alternative drug
b. Determine if fluorescent microscopy is available for the diagnosis of actinomycosis
c. Do no further clinical workup
d. Suggest to the laboratory that low colony counts may reflect infection
e. Suggest a repeat antibiotic susceptibility test

251. A patient with symptoms of a UTI has a culture taken, which grows 5×10^3 *E. coli.* The laboratory reports it as "insignificant." Which of the following is the most appropriate next step in management?

a. Consider vancomycin as an alternative drug
b. Determine if fluorescent microscopy is available for the diagnosis of actinomycosis
c. Do no further clinical workup
d. Suggest to the laboratory that low colony counts may reflect infection; follow up with culture
e. Suggest a repeat antibiotic susceptibility test

252. A patient appears in the emergency room with a submandibular mass. A smear is made of the drainage and a bewildering variety of bacteria are seen, including branched, gram-positive rods. Which of the following is the most clinically appropriate action?

a. Consider vancomycin as an alternative drug
b. Determine if fluorescent microscopy is available for the diagnosis of actinomycosis
c. Do no further clinical workup
d. Suggest to the laboratory that low colony counts may reflect infection
e. Suggest a repeat antibiotic susceptibility test

253. A 55-year-old male develops malaise, fever up to 103.5°F, non-productive cough, headache, and shortness of breath a few days after he repaired the cooling system of an old hotel. A chest x-ray reveals fluid in his lungs. From a sputum sample, a gram-negative rod grew slowly on a buffered cysteine containing charcoal-yeast agar. Which of the following antibiotic therapies is most appropriate for treating this patient?

a. Ampicillin
b. Ceftriaxone
c. Erythromycin
d. Penicillin
e. Vancomycin

254. A 60-year-old male resident from a nursing home presents to the emergency room with a fever of 105.8°F (41°C), shaking chills, severe pain to the right side of his chest that worsens with breathing, and a productive cough with blood-tinged sputum. During the previous 3 days, he noted cold-like symptoms. Gram stain evaluation of the sputum reveals gram-positive diplococci that grow into α-hemolytic colonies on blood agar. Which of the following antibiotic therapies is the most appropriate treatment for this patient?

a. Ampicillin
b. Ceftriaxone
c. Erythromycin
d. Penicillin
e. Vancomycin

255. A 12-year-old boy, after a camping trip near a wooded area in Northern California, is taken to the emergency room after complaining of a headache. He has an erythema migrans rash around what appears to be a tick bite. Which of the following is the antibiotic of choice for treating this patient?

a. Ampicillin
b. Ceftriaxone
c. Erythromycin
d. Penicillin
e. Vancomycin

256. A 6-year-old girl presents to her pediatrician with fever, headache, and a sore throat. She has swollen, tender cervical lymph nodes, and her oropharynx is red with a gray-white exudate covering both her tonsils. A rapid strep test of her throat swab is positive, and the culture subsequently grows β-hemolytic *Streptococcus*. Which of the following antibiotic therapies is most appropriate for treating this patient?

a. Ampicillin
b. Ceftriaxone
c. Erythromycin
d. Penicillin
e. Vancomycin

257. A young woman being treated with a broad-spectrum antimicrobial develops endoscopically observed microabscesses and diarrhea. Which of the following is the therapy of choice for this form of enterocolitis?

a. Ampicillin
b. Ceftriaxone
c. Erythromycin
d. Penicillin
e. Vancomycin

258. Although cholera, a *Vibrio* infection, has rarely been seen in the United States, there have been recent outbreaks of classic cholera associated with shellfish harvested from the Gulf of Mexico. Vibrios are shaped like curved rods, and infections more common than cholera may be caused by a variety of curved-rod bacteria. Which of the following best describes *C. jejuni?*

a. Cause of gastroenteritis; reservoir in birds and mammals, optimal growth at 107.6°F (42°C)
b. Human pathogen, halophilic, lactose-negative, sucrose-negative; causes GI diseases primarily from ingestion of under-cooked seafood
c. Human pathogen, halophilic, lactose-positive; produces heat-labile, extracellular toxin wound infections
d. Organisms are susceptible to acid; not an invasive organism
e. Urease-positive; cause of fetal distress in cattle

259. *Vibrio cholerae* is worldwide in distribution and continues to expand as water sources become polluted. Which of the following best describes this organism?

a. Cause of gastroenteritis; reservoir in birds and mammals, optimal growth at 107.6°F (42°C)
b. Human pathogen, halophilic, lactose-negative, sucrose-negative; causes GI diseases primarily from ingestion of under-cooked seafood
c. Human pathogen, halophilic, lactose-positive; produces heat-labile, extracellular toxin, wound infections
d. Organisms susceptible to acid; not an invasive organism
e. Urease-positive; cause of fetal distress in cattle

260. A 20-year-old female in post-Katrina New Orleans eats poorly cooked seafood (oysters, clams, and mollusks) for her birthday dinner. Twenty-four hours later, she develops explosive watery diarrhea and abdominal cramps. She is positive for *V. parahaemolyticus*. Which of the following best describes this organism?

a. Cause of gastroenteritis; reservoir in birds and mammals, optimal growth at 107.6°F (42°C)
b. Human pathogen, halophilic, lactose-negative, sucrose-negative; causes GI diseases primarily from ingestion of under-cooked seafood
c. Human pathogen, halophilic, lactose-positive; produces heat-labile, extracellular toxin, wound infections
d. Organisms susceptible to acid; not an invasive organism
e. Urease-positive; cause of fetal distress in cattle

261. A 25-year-old male, with a history of hepatitis C, has to wade through brackish water in post-Katrina New Orleans. He develops worsening abdominal pain and jaundice. Regarding *Vibrio vulnificus*, which of the following best describes this organism?

a. Cause of gastroenteritis; reservoir in birds and mammals, optimal growth at 107.6°F (42°C)
b. Human pathogen, halophilic, lactose-negative, sucrose-negative; causes GI diseases primarily from ingestion of under-cooked seafood
c. Human pathogen, halophilic, lactose-positive; produces heat-labile, extracellular toxin, wound infections
d. Organisms susceptible to acids; not an invasive organism
e. Urease-positive; cause of fetal distress in cattle

262. *Yersinia enterocolitica*, formerly a *Pasteurella*, has more than 50 serotypes that can be isolated from rodents, sheep, cattle, swine, dogs, and cats and water contaminated by them, and is best described by which of the following?

a. Commonly inhabits the canine respiratory tract and is an occasional pathogen for humans; strongly urease-positive
b. Gram-negative bipolar stained bacilli that cause diarrhea by means of a heat-stable enterotoxin, with abdominal pain that may be mistaken for appendicitis
c. Pits agar, grows both in carbon dioxide and under anaerobic conditions, and is part of the normal oral cavity flora
d. Typically infects cattle, requires 5% to 10% carbon dioxide for growth, and is inhibited by the dye thionine
e. Typically is found in infected animal bites in humans and can cause hemorrhagic septicemia in animals

263. Four weeks after assisting in several calf deliveries, a farmer develops fever, weakness, muscle aches, and sweats. The fever rises in the afternoon and falls during the night. *Brucella abortus* is isolated. Which one of the three *Brucella* species is a possible bioterrorism agent and is best described by one of the following?

a. Commonly inhabits the canine respiratory tract and is an occasional pathogen for humans; strongly urease-positive
b. Gram-negative bipolar stained bacilli that cause diarrhea by means of a heat-stable enterotoxin, with abdominal pain that may be mistaken for appendicitis
c. Pits agar grows both in carbon dioxide and under anaerobic conditions, and is part of the normal oral cavity flora
d. Typically infects cattle, requires 5% to 10% carbon dioxide for growth, and is inhibited by the dye thionine
e. Typically is found in infected animal bites in humans and can cause hemorrhagic septicemia in animals

264. *Bordetella bronchiseptica* could be confused with the agent of whooping cough since it occasionally causes chronic respiratory tract infections in humans, but has less intensive symptoms (rhinitis and cough). It is best described by which of the following?

a. Commonly inhabits the canine respiratory tract and is an occasional pathogen for humans; strongly urease-positive
b. Gram-negative bipolar stained bacilli that cause diarrhea by means of a heat-stable enterotoxin, with abdominal pain that may be mistaken for appendicitis
c. Pits agar grows both in carbon dioxide and under anaerobic conditions, and is part of the normal oral cavity flora
d. Typically infects cattle, requires 5% to 10% carbon dioxide for growth, and is inhibited by the dye thionine
e. Typically is found in infected animal bites in humans and can cause hemorrhagic septicemia in animals

265. *Pasteurella* species can produce a range of human diseases and formerly included all *yersiniae* and *francisellae* organisms. *Pasteurella multocida* occurs worldwide in the URT and GI tracts of domestic and wild animals. It is best described by which of the following?

a. Commonly inhabits the canine respiratory tract and is an occasional pathogen for humans; strongly urease-positive
b. Gram-negative bipolar stained bacilli that cause diarrhea by means of a heat-stable enterotoxin, with abdominal pain that may be mistaken for appendicitis
c. Pits agar grows both in carbon dioxide and under anaerobic conditions, and is part of the normal oral cavity flora
d. Typically infects cattle, requires 5% to 10% carbon dioxide for growth, and is inhibited by the dye thionine
e. Typically is found in infected animal bites in humans and can cause hemorrhagic septicemia in animals

266. A 26-year-old male presents to his family physician with complaints of painful burning during urination and a milky discharge. The purulent discharge reveals many neutrophils with intracellular gram-negative diplococci. Which of the following mediums would most likely be used for isolating *Neisseria gonorrhoeae*, the suspected organism?

a. Löffler medium
b. Löwenstein–Jensen medium
c. Sheep blood agar
d. TM agar
e. Thiosulfate citrate bile salts sucrose medium

267. Twenty-four hours after returning from a short trip to Asia, a 35-year-old female has a sudden onset of vomiting and massive watery diarrhea that is colorless, odorless, and contains flecks of mucus. Which of the following mediums would most likely be used for isolating *V. cholerae*, the suspected organism?

a. Löffler medium
b. Löwenstein–Jensen medium
c. Sheep blood agar
d. TM agar
e. Thiosulfate citrate bile salts sucrose medium

268. A 32-year-old female prostitute is seen at the public health clinic with fever, night sweats, and reports coughing up blood. Her medical history reveals that she is HIV positive and has lost 20 lbs over the past month. Acid-fast bacilli are observed in the sputum. After digestion of the sputum, isolation of the suspected organism is best accomplished by using which one of the following media?

a. Löffler medium
b. Löwenstein–Jensen medium
c. Sheep blood agar
d. TM agar
e. Thiosulfate citrate bile salts sucrose medium

269. *Bacillus* and *Clostridium* species are spore-forming bacilli and can survive in the environment for years. Several species cause important disease in humans, although most will respond quickly to appropriate antibiotic therapy. However, which organism listed below would not benefit from such prompt antibiotic treatment?

a. *Bacillus anthracis*
b. *Clostridium botulinum*
c. *Clostridium difficile*
d. *Clostridium perfringens*
e. *Clostridium tetani*

270. A 12-year-old boy has sudden onset of fever, headache, and stiff neck. Two days earlier, he swam in a lake that is believed to have been contaminated with dog excreta. Leptospirosis is suspected. Which of the following laboratory tests is most appropriate to determine whether he has been infected with leptospira?

a. Agglutination test for leptospiral antigen
b. Counterimmunoelectrophoresis of urine sample
c. Gram stain of urine specimen
d. Spinal fluid for dark-field microscopy and culture in Fletcher serum medium
e. Urine culture on EMB and TM agar

271. A 60-year-old female complains of tenderness and pain around a peritoneal catheter. Blood cultures reveal gram-positive, catalase-positive cocci. Which of the following is the most likely organism that is also considered a predominant organism on skin?

a. α-Hemolytic streptococci
b. *Bacteroides fragilis*
c. *Escherichia coli*
d. *Lactobacillus* species
e. *Staphylococcus epidermidis*

272. A healthy 45-year-old female had root canal treatment about 3 weeks ago. She now presents with a new heart murmur, fever, painful skin nodules, abdominal pain, and an abnormal liver function test. Which of the following organisms would mostly likely cause endocarditis and is implicated in dental caries or root canal infections?

a. α-Hemolytic streptococci
b. *Bacteroides fragilis*
c. *Escherichia coli*
d. *Lactobacillus* species
e. *Staphylococcus epidermidis*

273. A 17-year-old man is hospitalized with trauma to the abdomen following a gang-related fight. He develops an intraabdominal abscess, which is drained and sent to the laboratory. A mixture of gram-negative anaerobes is detected. Which of the following microorganisms is the most likely and is also the most prevalent bacterium in the gut?

a. α-Hemolytic streptococci
b. *Bacteroides fragilis*
c. *Escherichia coli*
d. *Lactobacillus* species
e. *Staphylococcus epidermidis*

274. A 25-year-old female is treated with a course of broad-spectrum antibiotics for severe pelvic inflammatory disease. She now reports a thick milky white pruritic vaginal discharge. Which of the following is the most prevalent microorganism in the vagina and may also be protective?

a. α-Hemolytic streptococci
b. *Bacteroides fragilis*
c. *Escherichia coli*
d. *Lactobacillus* species
e. *Staphylococcus epidermidis*

275. Viridans streptococci (*S. mutans, S. mitis*) usually have α-hemolysis and are optochin-resistant. They are becoming increasingly important as causes of endocarditis and abscesses (mixed infections). Which of the following best describes *S. mutans?*

a. An anaerobic, filamentous bacterium that often causes cervicofacial osteomyelitis
b. A β-hemolytic organism that causes a diffuse, rapidly spreading cellulitis
c. A facultative anaerobe that is highly cariogenic and sticks to teeth by synthesis of a dextran
d. A facultative anaerobe that often inhabits the buccal mucosa early in a neonate's life and can cause bacterial rheumatic fever (RF)
e. A facultatively anaerobic, rod-shaped bacterium that sticks to teeth and is cariogenic, commonly involved in problems involving dental procedures, trauma, surgery, or aspiration

276. *Streptococcus salivarius*, a common isolate, which is considered as normal, nonpathogenic flora in the clinical laboratory, is best described by which of the following?

a. An anaerobic, filamentous bacterium that often causes cervicofacial osteomyelitis
b. A β-hemolytic organism that causes a diffuse, rapidly spreading cellulitis
c. A facultative anaerobe that is highly cariogenic and sticks to teeth by synthesis of a dextran
d. A facultative anaerobe that often inhabits the buccal mucosa early in a neonate's life and can cause bacterial RF
e. A facultatively anaerobic, rod-shaped bacterium that sticks to teeth and is cariogenic, commonly involved in problems involving dental procedures, trauma, surgery, or aspiration

277. *Actinomyces* species are a large, diverse group of gram-positive bacilli. *Actinomyces israelii* is an organism that causes pyogenic lesions with interconnecting sinus tracts that contain granules of microcolonies embedded in the tissues. It is best described by which of the following?

a. An anaerobic, filamentous bacterium that often causes cervicofacial osteomyelitis
b. A β-hemolytic organism that causes a diffuse, rapidly spreading cellulitis
c. A facultative anaerobe that is highly cariogenic and sticks to teeth by synthesis of a dextran
d. A facultative anaerobe that often inhabits the buccal mucosa early in a neonate's life and can cause bacterial RF
e. A facultatively anaerobic, rod-shaped bacterium that sticks to teeth and is cariogenic, commonly involved in problems involving dental procedures, trauma, surgery, or aspiration

278. *Actinomyces viscosus*, a ubiquitous actinomycete, grows under microaerophilic or strict anaerobic conditions and produces a yellow-orange granule in the typical tissue exudates. It is best described by which of the following?

a. An anaerobic, filamentous bacterium that often causes cervicofacial osteomyelitis
b. A β-hemolytic organism that causes a diffuse, rapidly spreading cellulitis
c. A facultative anaerobe that is highly cariogenic and sticks to teeth by synthesis of a dextran
d. A facultative anaerobe that often inhabits the buccal mucosa early in a neonate's life and can cause bacterial RF
e. A facultatively anaerobic, rod-shaped bacterium that sticks to teeth and is cariogenic, commonly involved in problems involving dental procedures, trauma to or surgery of the oral cavity, or aspiration

279. A 3-year-old girl from a family that does not believe in immunization presents to the emergency room with a sore throat, fever, malaise, and difficulty breathing. A gray membrane covering the pharynx is observed on physical examination. Which of the following best describes *C. diphtheriae*, the etiologic agent?

a. It produces at least one protein toxin consisting of two subunits, A and B, that cause severe spasmodic cough, usually in children
b. It produces a toxin that blocks protein synthesis in an infected cell and carries a lytic bacteriophage that produces the genetic information for toxin production
c. It secretes an erythrogenic toxin that causes the characteristic signs of scarlet fever
d. It secretes an exotoxin that has been called "verotoxin" and "Shiga-like toxin"; infection is mediated by specific attachment to mucosal membranes
e. It requires cysteine for growth

280. A 4-year-old boy is taken to see his pediatrician because of a persistent cough that gradually worsened over a 12-day period. On the day of the examination, the cough is so severe that it is frequently followed by vomiting. A blood cell count shows marked leukocytosis with a predominance of lymphocytes. Which of the following best characterizes this microorganism?

a. It produces a toxin that increases cAMP levels, resulting in increased mucus production
b. It produces a toxin that blocks protein synthesis in an infected cell and carries a lytic bacteriophage that produces the genetic information for toxin production
c. It secretes an erythrogenic toxin that causes the characteristic signs of scarlet fever
d. It secretes an exotoxin that has been called "verotoxin" and "Shiga-like toxin"; infection is mediated by specific attachment to mucosal membranes
e. It requires cysteine for growth

281. A 48-year-old deer hunter presents to the emergency room with lymphadenopathy and a skin lesion, which started as a painful papule at the site of a tick bite. The papule then ulcerates with a necrotic center and raised border. Aspirate of the ulcer is positive for *F. tularensis*. Which one of the following best characterizes this bacterium?

a. It produces at least one protein toxin consisting of two subunits, A and B, that cause severe spasmodic cough, usually in children
b. It produces a toxin that blocks protein synthesis in an infected cell and carries a lytic bacteriophage that produces the genetic information for toxin production
c. It secretes an erythrogenic toxin that causes the characteristic signs of scarlet fever
d. It secretes an exotoxin that has been called "verotoxin" and "Shiga-like toxin"; infection is mediated by specific attachment to mucosal membranes
e. It requires cysteine for growth

282. Ten boy scouts are hospitalized with bloody diarrhea and severe hematological abnormalities. An investigation establishes that all of the boys developed symptoms following consumption of hamburgers from the same fast-food restaurant chain. Which of the following best describes *E. coli 0157/H7*, the etiologic bacterium responsible for the outbreak?

a. It produces at least one protein toxin consisting of two subunits, A and B, that cause severe spasmodic cough, usually in children
b. It produces a toxin that blocks protein synthesis in an infected cell and carries a lytic bacteriophage that produces the genetic information for toxin production
c. It secretes an erythrogenic toxin that causes the characteristic signs of scarlet fever
d. It secretes an exotoxin that has been called "verotoxin" and "Shiga-like toxin"; infection is mediated by specific attachment to mucosal membranes
e. It requires cysteine for growth

283. A 4-year-old girl awakens at midnight complaining of a sore throat and headache, and she has a fever of 101°F. Physical examination reveals an erythematous throat. A rapid strep test is positive. A throat swab is sent to the laboratory for further testing. Which of the following best characterizes *S. pyogenes* as the presumed etiologic agent?

a. It produces at least one protein toxin consisting of two subunits, A and B, that cause severe spasmodic cough, usually in children
b. It produces a toxin that blocks protein synthesis in an infected cell and carries a lytic bacteriophage that produces the genetic information for toxin production
c. It secretes an erythrogenic toxin that causes the characteristic signs of scarlet fever
d. It secretes an exotoxin that has been called "verotoxin" and "Shiga-like toxin"; infection is mediated by specific attachment to mucosal membranes
e. It has capsules of polyglutamic acid, which is toxic when injected into rabbits

284. A 19-year-old military recruit who lives in the barracks develops a macular papular skin rash, severe headache, photophobia, fever, stiff neck, and blurred vision. He is presumed to have *N. meningitidis*. Which of the following is a characteristic physiological trait of this organism?

a. It causes spontaneous abortion and has tropism for placental tissue due to the presence of erythritol in allantoic and amniotic fluid
b. It has a capsule of polyglutamic acid, which is toxic when injected into rabbits
c. It possesses N-acetylneuraminic acid capsule and adheres to specific tissues by pili found on the bacterial cell surface
d. It secretes two toxins, A and B, in the large bowel during antibiotic therapy
e. It synthesizes protein toxin as a result of colonization of vaginal tampons

285. A 45-year-old cattle-farm worker goes to the public health clinic after experiencing 6 weeks of undulating fever, chills, sweating, headache, fatigue, muscle pain, and weight loss. History reveals that he enjoys drinking fresh unpasteurized milk with his other coworkers during the midmorning breaks. A blood sample is sent to the state laboratory for serologic testing because the physician assistant suspects *Brucella* infection. Which of the following best characterizes this organism?

a. It causes spontaneous abortion and has tropism for placental tissue due to the presence of erythritol in allantoic and amniotic fluid
b. It has a capsule of polyglutamic acid, which is toxic when injected into rabbits
c. It has 82 polysaccharide capsular types; capsule is antiphagocytic; type 3 capsule (β-D-glucuronic acid polymer) most commonly seen in infected adults
d. It secretes two toxins, A and B, in the large bowel during antibiotic therapy
e. It synthesizes protein toxin as a result of colonization of vaginal tampons

286. An 18-year-old male patient presents to the emergency room with a 3-day history of fever, dry cough, difficulty in breathing, and muscle aches and pains. His chest x-ray shows a diffuse left upper lobe infiltrate. *Mycoplasma pneumoniae* pneumonia (walking pneumonia) may be rapidly identified by which of the following procedures?

a. Cold agglutinin test
b. Culture of respiratory secretions in HeLa cells after centrifugation of the inoculated tubes
c. Culture of respiratory secretions on monkey kidney cells
d. Detection of specific antigen in urine
e. Electron microscopy of sputum

287. A 50-year-old male presents with severe bilateral pulmonary infiltrate, elevated temperature leucocytosis, elevated enzymes, and elevated creatine kinase. He recently visited his favorite restaurant that had a large water fountain, which was misty on the day of his visit. Which of the following procedures would most rapidly diagnose the suspected organism that is the etiologic agent of Legionnaires disease in this patient?

a. Cold agglutinin test
b. Culture of respiratory secretions on a charcoal-based nutrient agar
c. Detection of antigen in respiratory secretions
d. Detection of specific antigen in urine
e. Electron microscopy of sputum

288. A group of elementary school-age children meet for a birthday party, and in the next few days, about half of them experience a mild upper respiratory illness, with sore throat and runny nose. One family gets laboratory work done and finds that *Chlamydia pneumoniae* (TWAR) is involved. Which of the following procedures would be best if the laboratory wanted to isolate this bacterium?

a. Cold agglutinin test
b. Culture of respiratory secretions in HeLa cells after centrifugation of the inoculated tubes
c. Culture of respiratory secretions on monkey kidney cells
d. Detection of specific antigen in urine
e. Electron microscopy of sputum

289. A 70-year-old man with a history of diabetes presents with severe pain in his right ear. The patient was diagnosed with external otitis. Further tests suggested that the patient suffered bone and nerve damage. Clinical laboratory analysis showed that the isolated microorganism produced a distinct blue pigment as well as an ADP-ribosylating toxin. What is the most likely causative agent?

a. *Staphylococcus epidermidis*
b. *Staphylococcus aureus*
c. *Pseudomonas aeruginosa*
d. *Enterococcus faecalis*
e. *Candida albicans*

290. A 40-year-old woman has a history of several months of gastric pain that was temporarily relieved with antacid. Stomach biopsies revealed the presence of comma-shaped organisms. The patient responded very well to a combined treatment of proton pump inhibitors and amoxicillin. Which of the following factors produced by the etiologic agent is associated with the development of gastric cancer in persons with chronic infections?

a. CagA protein
b. Flagella
c. Mucinase
d. Urease
e. Vacuolating toxin

291. A 60-year-old man suffered from fever, watery diarrhea, abdominal pain, and nausea. Three weeks later, he was admitted to the hospital unable to speak but coherent and oriented. Neurological examination revealed bilateral muscle weakness in his legs. Within hours, the muscle weakness extended to his arms and chest. He was diagnosed with Guillain–Barré syndrome. With which organism was he most likely infected?

a. *Campylobacter jejuni*
b. *Clostridium tetani*
c. *Cytolmegalovirus*
d. *Salmonella enterica*
e. *Shigella sonnei*

292. An outbreak of gastroenteritis occurred in a youth group camp. Water at the camp, which was not chlorinated or filtered, was obtained from a spring on the premises. The farmland near the camp was grazed by cattle and sheep. Run-off from the pasture entered the camp spring. The isolated microorganism required an atmosphere containing reduced oxygen and increased carbon dioxide for its growth. In most cases, the gastroenteritis was self-limiting. Those requiring antibiotic treatment responded to erythromycin. Which is the most likely causative agent?

a. *Campylobacter jejuni*
b. Enteroinvasive *Escherichia coli* (EIEC)
c. *Enteropathogenic Escherichia coli* (EPEC)
d. *Vibrio cholerae*
e. *Vibrio parahaemolyticus*

293. A man who had been wading while fishing in the Gulf of Mexico developed painful swellings that evolved into vesicles and bullae (image). These lesions became necrotic and the man developed septicemia, severe sepsis, and multiorgan dysfunction syndrome. Which of the following is the most likely cause of this man's infection?

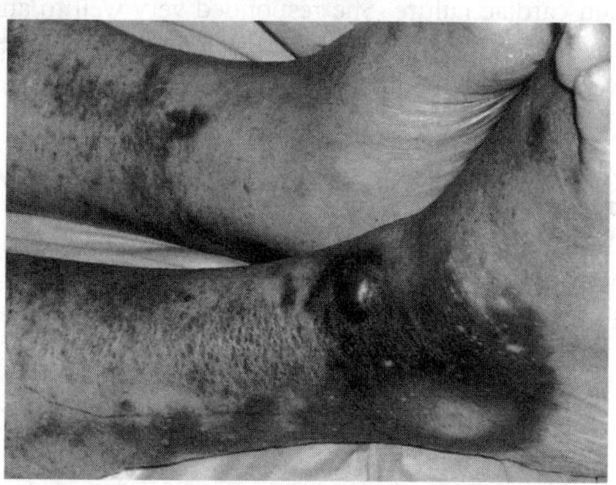

(Reproduced, with permission, from Goldsmith LA, Katz SI, Gilchrest BA, et al. Fitzpatrick's Dermatology in General Medicine. *8th ed. New York: McGraw-Hill Education; 2012. Fig. 183-4.)*

a. *Pseudomonas aeruginosa*
b. *Staphylococcus aureus*
c. *Streptococcus pyogenes*
d. *Vibrio parahaemolyticus*
e. *Vibrio vulnificus*

294. A 60-year-old male in the intensive care unit recovering from back surgery required intubation for respiratory support. Forty-eight hours after intubation, he developed ventilator-associated pneumonia. The microorganism isolated from tracheal secretions aspirated from the patient is a gram-negative, oxidase positive, obligate aerobe that produces a multitude of virulence factors including proteases, toxins, and rhamnolipid. The patient was treated with broad-spectrum antibiotics for several weeks, but the treatment was unsuccessful and he died. Which is the most likely causative agent of this patient's infection?

a. *Escherichia coli*
b. *Haemophilus influenzae*
c. *Klebsiella pneumoniae*
d. *Moraxella catarrhalis*
e. *Pseudomonas aeruginosa*

295. Four weeks after hurricane Rita, a 50-year-old man and his wife from southeastern Louisiana developed diarrhea. The man had mild diarrhea. However, his wife had severe watery diarrhea, fever, muscle cramps, and vomiting, which quickly progressed in to a loss of renal function and respiratory and cardiac failure. She responded very well to antibiotic and aggressive rehydration therapy. Stool samples from both patients contained gram-negative comma-shaped bacteria. Which is the most likely causative agent?

a. *Campylobacter jejuni*
b. *Salmonella enterica*
c. *Shigella flexneri*
d. *Vibrio cholerae*
e. *Vibrio vulnificus*

Bacteriology

Answers

180. The answer is a. (*Murray [2009], pp 277-285. Murray [2013], Ch 25; Ryan, Ch 27.*) *Mycoplasma hominis* and *Mycoplasma pneumoniae* are obviously incorrect because they do not possess a cell wall and would stain pink following the Gram stain. They also are not acid fast. That leaves the three *Mycobacterium* species as the possible correct answer. *Mycobacterium scrofulaceum* is incorrect because it is rarely pathogenic and is uncommon in the United States. *Mycobacterium tuberculosis* infections in AIDS patients are more common than *M. avium*-complex diseases in places like Asia and Africa where tuberculosis is more likely to occur. Recently, AIDS patients in the United States are more likely to be infected with *M. avium*-complex than *M. tuberculosis* due to the rarity of the disease tuberculosis in this country.

181. The answer is c. (*Murray [2009], pp 282-285. Murray [2013], Ch 25; Ryan, Ch 27.*) Lady Windermere syndrome is caused by *M. avium*-complex, usually in elderly female nonsmokers, resulting in a very serious lung infection with this organism. Scrofula is a term usually reserved for tuberculosis of the neck, but the disease is really a cervical lymphadenopathy caused by *Mycobacterium tuberculosis*. The woman obviously has leprosy due to the presence of acid-fast staining bacilli in the skin scrapings and the loss of feeling in her fingers and toes. This is caused by the bacterium infecting and destroying nervous tissue in these areas. Tuberculoid leprosy (also called paucibacillary Hansen disease) is the mild form of the disease with few organisms observed in skin scrapings. Lepromatous leprosy is the fulminant form of the disease with numerous bacilli seen in skin scrapings. Leprosy is also known as Hansen disease, after the discoverer of the causative organism of the disease, *Mycobacterium leprae*.

182. The answer is e. (*Murray [2009], pp 371-373. Murray [2013], Ch 35; Ryan, Ch 40.*) *Bacillus anthracis* causes anthrax and the man obviously does not have anthrax which is usually manifested as a cutaneous disease. *Brucella abortus* tends to produce a mild disease with rare pus forming complications. Therefore, the question becomes which of the stated *Bartonella* species causes

Trench fever and is spread by lice? *Bartonella bacilliformis* is spread by sand flies and causes Carrion disease, which is an acute febrile illness consisting of an anemia that is called Oroya fever. This is then followed by the cutaneous form of the disease called verruga peruana. The anemia is caused by the organism entering the red blood cells and altering them to the degree that they are cleared by the reticuloendothelial system. *Bartonella henselae* causes a medical problem called cat scratch disease (CSD). It is a chronic regional lymphadenopathy following the scratch of a cat. It is not spread by an insect vector. *Bartonella quintana* causes Trench fever, also known as 5-day fever because the fever reoccurs at 5-day intervals. This disease is characterized by severe headaches, pain in the long bones, and 5-day fever intervals. It is spread by the human body louse—*Pediculus humanus*. That is why this disease is often seen in the homeless who have a difficult time bathing regularly.

183. The answer is a. (*Murray, pp 365-369; Murray [2013], Ch 34; Ryan, Ch 34.*) Legionnaires' disease is a disease caused by infection with *Legionella pneumophila*. It is a disease caused by the organism growing in the air conditioning systems in buildings. Therefore, it is a disease that is most often seen in the summer. Legionnaires' disease is a disease primarily affecting the lungs. The organism will not grow on blood agar but will grow on buffered charcoal yeast extract as a Gram-negative rod. Because it produces a penicillinase, the antibiotic penicillin is ineffective against it. The mild form of Legionnaires' disease is called Pontiac fever because it was first observed in Pontiac, Michigan. Psittacosis, which is caused by *Chlamydophila psittaci*, is a lung infection, but the organism will not grow on buffered charcoal yeast extract agar. *Klebsiella pneumoniae* will cause a lobar lung infection and is a Gram-negative rod, but it will grow on blood agar media. *Streptococcus pneumoniae* will also cause a lobar pneumonia, but it is a Gram-positive coccus, and it will grow on blood agar media. Finally, tuberculosis, which is caused by *Mycobacterium tuberculosis,* is not a Gram-negative bacterium, and will not even stain with the Gram-stain due to the high concentration of lipid in its cell wall.

184. The answer is d. (*Murray [2009], pp 209-217; Murray [2013], Ch 18; Ryan, Ch 24.*) Staphylococcal food poisoning is caused by *Staphylococcus aureus* and not *Staphylococcus epidermidis*. It is a result of the ingestion of food contaminated with *S. aureus* that the bacterium has grown on and produced a heat-stable enterotoxin. This is a toxemia and not an infection and that is why no antibiotic intervention is necessary, as well as why it occurs so quickly (2-3 hours) following ingestion of the contaminated food. It also is self-limiting and usually resolves itself in 24 hours. *Bacillus cereus* also produces a rapid food poisoning (3-4 hours after the ingestion of contaminated food), but the usual food is rice because the organism is a spore former and the spores survive the heating of the rice. *Clostridium botulinum* also produces a food poisoning but it may take 36 hours to manifest itself and the end result is a flaccid paralysis and not vomiting and diarrhea. *Escherichia coli* is also a well-known cause of food poisoning but it takes at least 24 hours to manifest itself because the organism must grow in the gut and produce enough enterotoxin to cause the observed vomiting and diarrhea.

185. The answer is d. (*Murray [2009], pp 381-383; Murray [2013], Ch 36; Ryan, Ch 29.*) The boy met his unfortunate end for a variety of different reasons. The primary reason the boy died was because he had not recently received a tetanus booster. If he had told his parents about the nail puncture, they could have taken him to the doctor to get a tetanus shot. That shot would have saved his life. Now we will go to the microbiology of the question. The boy came down with tetanus because *Clostridium tetani* is a spore former, and because the spores can be found in the soil, they can also be found on rusty nails. The rust on the nail does not play a role in this question at all. The second important thing about *Clostridium tetani* is that it is a strict anaerobe. So the nail drives the spores into the boy's foot and causes tissue damage (necrosis), and where there is necrosis, there is no blood supply, and where there is no blood supply, there is no oxygen, and where there is no oxygen there are anaerobic conditions. Therefore, the *Clostridium tetani* spores can germinate (crack open) and allow the vegetative form of the organism to come out, and it is the vegetative form that produces the potent heat-labile neurotoxin. The *Clostridium tetani* neurotoxin blocks release of the neurotransmitters for inhibitory synapses, thus causing the involuntary muscle spasms and respiratory failure.

186. The answer is e. (*Murray [2009], pp 261-267. Murray [2013], Ch 23. Ryan, Ch 26.*) The disease that this child has is diphtheria, which is caused by *Corynebacterium diphtheriae*. *Bacillus anthracis* causes the disease anthrax and there is no leathery membrane structure produced in the pharynx in anthrax. None of the *Clostridium* species listed above (*botulinum*, *perfringens*, or *tetani*) produce a leathery membrane in the pharynx, and besides they are all strict anaerobes and would not grow in the oral cavity. *C. diphtheriae* does produce a leathery membrane in the oral cavity due to its production of the diphtheria toxin whose mechanism of action is inhibition of protein synthesis by inactivation of elongation factor 2, which is a mammalian protein that transfers the amino acid from the t-RNA to the growing polypeptide chain.

187. The answer is d. (*Brooks, pp 275-276. Levinson, pp 146, 496. Murray, pp 328-332. Ryan, pp 381-383. Toy, p 90.*) *Helicobacter pylori* was first recognized as a possible cause of gastritis and peptic ulcer by Marshall and Warren in 1984. This organism is readily isolated from gastric biopsies but not from stomach contents. It is similar to *Campylobacter* species and grows on chocolate agar at 98.6°F (37°C) in the same microaerophilic environment suitable for *C. jejuni* (Campy-Pak or anaerobic jar [Gas Pak] without the catalyst). *Helicobacter pylori*, however, grows more slowly than *C. jejuni*, requiring 5 to 7 days' incubation. *C. jejuni* grows optimally at 107.6°F (42°C), not 98.6°F (37°C), as does *H. pylori*.

DIAGNOSTIC TESTS FOR HELICOBACTER PYLORI

	Advantages	Disadvantages
Noninvasive		
Serum ELISA	Inexpensive	Not useful for follow-up
Urea breath test	Useful for follow-up	Expensive; may be falsely negative in patients on acid suppression therapy
Stool antigen test	Inexpensive; useful for follow-up	Inconvenient
Whole blood assay	Inexpensive; rapid	Less accurate than serum ELISA
Invasive (endoscopic)		
Histology	Visualization of pathology	May miss low-grade infection
Rapid urease	Rapid	May be falsely positive in bacterial overgrowth
Culture	Antibiotic susceptibility	Not maximally sensitive; not available routinely; requires 4-7 days

ELISA, enzyme-linked immunosorbent assay.

(*Reprinted, with permission, from Wilson WR, Sande MA.* Current Diagnosis and Treatment in Infectious Disease. *New York: McGraw-Hill; 2001:584.*)

188. The answer is a. (*Brooks, pp 280-282. Levinson, pp 152-153. Murray, pp 343-348. Ryan, pp 399-400.*) The major determinant of virulence in *H. influenzae* is the presence of a capsule. There is no demonstrable exotoxin, and the role of endotoxin is unclear. While one would expect that IgA protease would inhibit local immunity, the role of this enzyme in pathogenesis is as yet unclear. Flagella production is not considered a virulence factor. See the table accompanying the answer to question 190 for a comparison of gram-negative rods associated with the respiratory tract.

189. The answer is e. (*Brooks, pp 270-272. Levinson, pp 45, 143-145. Murray, pp 317-322. Ryan, pp 348, 375. Toy, p 102.*) The toxin of *V. cholerae* and LT enterotoxin from *E. coli* are similar. The B subunits of the toxins bind to ganglioside GM1 receptors on the host cell. The A subunits catalyze transfer of the ADP-ribose moiety of ADP to a regulatory protein known as G_s. This activated G_s stimulates adenyl cyclase. Cyclic AMP is increased, as is fluid and electrolyte release from the crypt cells into the lumen of the bowel. Watery, profuse diarrhea ensues. *Brucella abortus* disease starts in humans with an acute bacteremic phase followed by a chronic stage that may last for years. They are adapted to an intracellular habitat with complex nutritional requirements. *Brucella abortus* does not produce any product similar to the toxin of *V. cholerae*; *C. diphtheriae's* toxin causes an abrupt arrest of protein synthesis that results in the necrotizing and neurotoxic effects. Listeria enters the body through ingestion and infects cells of the CNS. No virulence factor similar to that of *V. cholerae* is produced by Listeria organisms. *Pseudomonas aeruginosa* is pathogenic only when introduced into areas where there are no normal defenses. It produces exotoxin A, which causes tissue necrosis and blocks protein synthesis similar to *C. diphtheriae*.

190. The answer is d. (*Brooks, pp 317, 751. Levinson, pp 25, 189, 503. Ryan, p 904.*) Microscopic examination can readily demonstrate clue cells (epithelial cells with *Gardnerella* bacteria attached) or pseudohyphae (*Candida*). A wet mount will be needed to demonstrate motile *Trichomonas* cells. *Candida*, *Trichomonas*, and bacterial vaginitis are seen most often. *Staphylococcus aureus* is involved much less frequently. While *E. coli* may be a common cause of genitourinary infection, clue cells are usually absent. See the below table for a comparison of these bacteria.

GRAM-NEGATIVE RODS ASSOCIATED WITH THE RESPIRATORY TRACT

Species	Major Diseases	Laboratory Diagnosis	Factors X and V Required for Growth	Vaccine Available	Prophylaxis for Contacts
Haemophilus influenzae	Meningitis[a]; otitis media, sinusitis, pneumonia, epiglottitis	Culture; capsular polysaccharide in serum or spinal fluid	+	+	Rifampin
Bordetella pertussis	Whooping cough (pertussis)	Fluorescent antibody on secretions; culture	–	+	Erythromycin
Legionella pneumophila	Pneumonia	Serology; urinary antigen; culture	–	–	None

[a]In countries where the *H. influenzae* b conjugate vaccine has been deployed, the vaccine has greatly reduced the incidence of meningitis caused by this organism.

(Reprinted, with permission, from Levinson W, Jawetz E. Medical Microbiology and Immunology. *7th ed. New York, NY: McGraw-Hill; 2002.)*

CLINICAL FEATURES OF VAGINITIS

	Normal	Vulvovaginal Candidiasis	Trichomoniasis	Bacterial Vaginosis
Symptoms	None	Pruritus Soreness Dyspareunia	Soreness Dyspareunia Often asymptomatic	Often asymptomatic Occasional abdominal pain
Discharge				
Amount	Variable	Scant/moderate	Profuse	Moderate
Color	Clear/white	White	Green-yellow	White/gray
Consistency	Nonhomogeneous floccular	Clumped, adherent	Homogeneous, frothy	Homogeneous adherent
Vaginal Fluid pH	4.0-4.5	4.0-4.5	5.0-6.0	>4.5
Amine test (fish odor)	None	None	Usually positive	Positive
Microscopy				
Saline	PMN:EC ratio < 1 Lactobacilli predominate	PMN:EC < 1 Pseudohyphae (~40%)	PMN:EC > 1 Motile trichomonads PMNs predominate	PMN:EC < 1 Clue cells Coccobacilli
10% KOH	Negative	Pseudohyphae (~70%)	Negative	Negative

PMN, polymorphonuclear leukocytes; EC, epithelial cells.

(Reprinted, with permission, from Wilson WR, Sande MA. Current Diagnosis and Treatment in Infectious Disease. *New York: McGraw-Hill; 2001:209.)*

191. The answer is d. (*Brooks, pp 224-230. Levinson, pp 106-110, 484. Murray, pp 209-220. Ryan, p 268.*) *Staphylococcus aureus* is a well-known pathogen that is very opportunistic and commonly causes abscess lesions. It routinely may resist phagocytosis by WBCs due to protein A. Osteomyelitis and arthritis, either hematogenous or traumatic, are commonly caused by *S. aureus*, especially in children. *Salmonella* are gram-negative. *Staphylococcus saprophyticus* is a common skin flora and is usually not pathogenic. *Streptococcus pneumoniae* is seldom or never involved in osteomyelitis infections, as is true for *L. monocytogenes*.

192. The answer is c. (*Brooks, p 293. Levinson, pp 160, 495. Murray, pp 344-350. Ryan, p 490.*) *Pasteurella* (gram-negative coccobacilli) are primarily animal pathogens, but they can cause a wide range of human diseases. They have a bipolar appearance on stained smears. *Pasteurella multocida* occurs worldwide in domestic and wild animals. It is the most common organism in human wounds inflicted by bites of cats and dogs. It is a common cause of hemorrhagic septicemia in a variety of animals. Wounds commonly present with an acute onset (within hours) of redness, swelling, and pain. The other organisms are routinely found in the environment and may be opportunistic pathogens. *Pasteurella multocida* is a gram-negative rod that usually responds to penicillin treatment. *Aeromonas, Campylobacter, Pseudomonas*, and *Yersinia* are also gram-negative rods.

193. The answer is a. (*Brooks, pp 320-326. Levinson, pp 161-165. Murray, pp 278-281. Ryan, pp 445-446.*) Most cases of tuberculosis are caused when patients inhale droplet nuclei containing infectious organisms. While the bacilli are deposited on the alveolar spaces, they do not clog up the alveoli but are engulfed by macrophages. Tissue injury is not a result of toxin secretion but of cell-mediated hypersensitivity; that is, "immunologic injury." Humoral (antibodies) immunity would not be responsible for tissue damage since CMI is reacting against the organism. Adhesion sites are not implicated as virulence factors and toxins apparently are not made by the organisms.

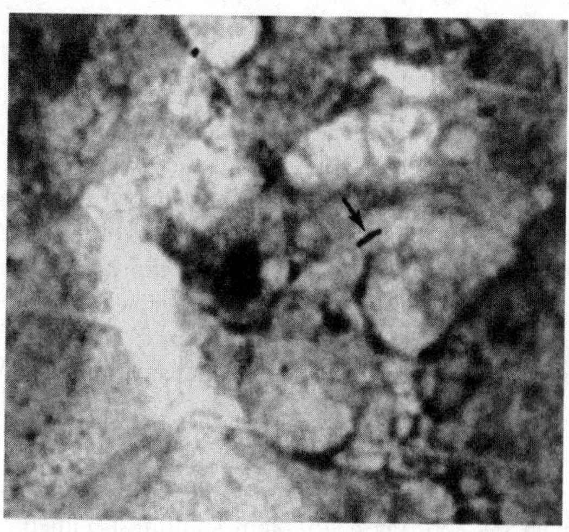

(Reproduced, with permission, from Brooks GF, et al. Jawetz's Medical Microbiology. *24th ed. New York: McGraw-Hill; 2007:322.)*

194. The answer is c. (*Brooks, p 190. Levinson, pp 70, 78-79. Murray, pp 207, 816-817. Ryan, p 33.*) A new class of antibiotics, the quinolones, has one member, nalidixic acid, that has been available for years. The new representatives are much more active biologically and are effective against virtually all gram-negative bacteria and most gram-positive bacteria. They include norfloxacin, ofloxacin, ciprofloxacin, enoxacin, and the fluorinated quinolones such as lomefloxacin. These antibiotics kill bacteria by inhibition of synthesis of nucleic acid, more specifically, DNA gyrase. Resistance to quinolones has been observed and appears to be a class-specific phenomenon. An exception is when an organism is resistant to nalidixic acid, elevated minimal inhibitory concentrations (MICs) will generally apply to other quinolones, although these MICs will still be within the range of susceptibility. Penicillin-binding proteins (PBPs) and β-lactamase involve penicillins, not quinolones, as does the glycine cross-linking. Inhibition of reverse transcriptase (RNA-dependent DNA polymerase) would not be involved in this clinical situation since RT inhibition would indicate HIV or HBV involvement.

195. The answer is c. (*Brooks, pp 225, 229. Levinson, pp 106-110. Murray, pp 211-220. Ryan, pp 269-270.*) VISA was first recognized in Japan.

Emergence in the United States soon followed. It is likely that the human VISA isolates have resulted from increased use of vancomycin for patients with MRSA or perhaps an increased pool of VISA in the environment selected out by the use of glycopeptides such as avoparcin, a growth promoter used in food-producing animals. In patients with VISA, the Centers for Disease Control and Prevention (CDC) strongly recommend compliance with isolation procedures and other infection control practices geared to control of VISA. Staphylococci are susceptible to vancomycin if the MIC is equal to or less than 2 μg/mL and of intermediate susceptibility if the MIC is 4 to 8 μg/mL. Vancomycin resistance in *S. aureus* is of major concern worldwide and surveillance should be maintained. VISA strains are usually nafcillin-resistant.

196. The answer is a. (*Brooks, pp 198, 280. Levinson, pp 62-64. Murray, p 808. Ryan, pp 854-855. Toy, p 90.*) Many sputum specimens are cultured unnecessarily. Sputum is often contaminated with saliva or is almost totally made up of saliva. These specimens rarely reveal the cause of the patient's respiratory problem and may provide laboratory information that is harmful. The sputum in the question appears to be a good specimen because there are few epithelial cells. The pleomorphic, gram-negative rods are suggestive of *Haemophilus*, but culture of the secretions is necessary. Normal flora from a healthy oral cavity consists of gram-positive cocci and rods, with few or no PMNs. Pneumococci are gram-positive diplococci. Vincent disease is an oral infection, which involves oral tissue only. The presence of PMNs indicates an inflammatory response.

197. The answer is b. (*Brooks, pp 306-309. Levinson, pp 150-151, 497. Murray, pp 400-403. Ryan, pp 324-325.*) *Bacteroides fragilis* is a constituent of normal intestinal flora and readily causes wound infections often mixed with aerobic isolates. These anaerobic, gram-negative rods are uniformly resistant to aminoglycosides and usually to penicillin as well. Reliable laboratory identification may require multiple analytical techniques. Generally, wound exudates smell bad owing to production of organic acids by such anaerobes as *B. fragilis*. Black exudates or a black pigment (heme) in the isolated colony is usually a characteristic of *Bacteroides* (*Porphyromonas*) *melaninogenicus*, not *B. fragilis*. Potent neurotoxins are synthesized by the gram-positive anaerobes such as *C. tetani* and *C. botulinum*.

198. The answer is b. (*Brooks, pp 296-301. Levinson, pp 119-123. Murray, pp 292-298. Ryan, p 336.*) Typical *Neisseria* are gram-negative diplococci. *Neisseria gonorrhoeae* contain pili, hairlike appendages that may be several micrometers long. They enhance attachment of the organism to mucous membranes, helping to make the organism more resistant to phagocytosis by WBCs. Gonococci isolated from clinical specimens produce small colonies containing piliated bacteria. Capsules appear to be less important in gonococcal infection than *N. meningitidis* infections. Flagella, peptidoglycan, LPS, and F pili do not significantly relate to pathogenesis, other than that LPS (endotoxin) release may become significant later in infection.

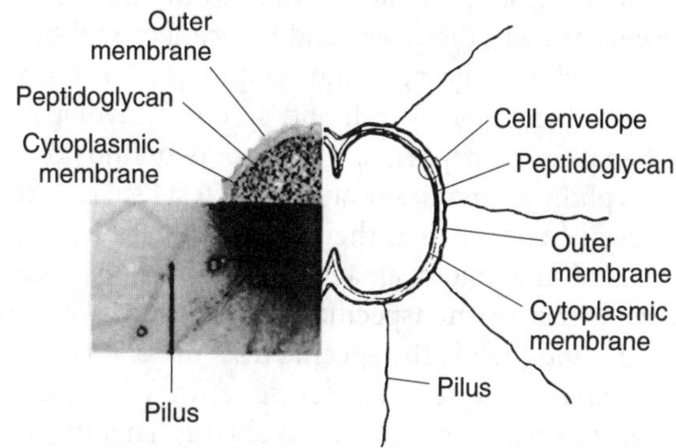

Collage and drawing of *N. gonorrhoeae* showing pili and the three layers of the cell envelope. *(Reproduced, with permission, from Brooks GF, et al.* Jawetz's Medical Microbiology. *22nd ed. New York: McGraw-Hill; 2001:256.)*

199. The answer is d. (*Brooks, pp 218-219. Levinson, pp 131-132. Murray, pp 255-258. Ryan, pp 302-304. Toy, p 102.*) *Listeria* multiplies both extracellularly and intracellularly, but under most circumstances, a competent immune system eliminates *Listeria.* As expected, listeriosis is seen in the very young and the very old, and in people with compromised immune systems. Reports of *Listeria* food outbreaks have implicated such foods as coleslaw and milk products, especially if not pasteurized. Early-onset-syndrome listeriosis is the result of infection in utero and characterized by sepsis and lesions in multiple organs. None of the other options (*Corynebacterium*, *Escherichia*, streptococci type B, or *S. pneumoniae*) would be likely to cause an in utero infection.

200 to 203. The answers are 200-d, 201-a, 202-c, and 203-d. (*Brooks, pp 332-335. Levinson, pp 8, 173, 501. Murray, pp 405-411. Ryan, pp 424-430. Toy, p 164.*) This patient appears to have primary syphilis, as evidenced by a penile chancre that was not tender. One of the differences between syphilis and herpes simplex virus (HSV) is that an HSV lesion is excruciatingly painful. The herpes lesion is vesicular in appearance whereas the classic syphilis chancre has an eroded appearance. Treponemal organisms may be seen microscopically in the lesion if the lesion is scraped. The syphilis lesion will resolve with antibiotic therapy. Acyclovir prescription at this time would be premature. If not treated, the chancre will disappear and the patient will be asymptomatic until he/she exhibits the signs and symptoms of secondary syphilis, which include a disseminated rash and systemic involvement such as meningitis, hepatitis, or nephritis. There are two kinds of tests for the detection of syphilis antibodies: nonspecific tests such as the RPR and VDRL, and specific tests such as the FTA, *T. pallidum* hemagglutination test (TPHA), and the microhemagglutination—*T. pallidum* (MHTP). The difference is that the nonspecific tests use a cross-reactive antigen known as cardiolipin, while the specific tests use a *T. pallidum* antigen. Although the nonspecific tests are sensitive, they lack specificity and often cross-react in patients who have diabetes, hepatitis, or infectious mononucleosis, or who are pregnant. Some patients, especially those with autoimmune diseases, will have both nonspecific (RPR) and specific tests (FTA) positive even if they do not have syphilis. Resolution of such a situation can be done by molecular methods for *T. pallidum*, such as PCR, or by the immobilization test using live spirochetes and the patient's serum. In the TPI test, the spirochetes will die in the presence of specific antibody.

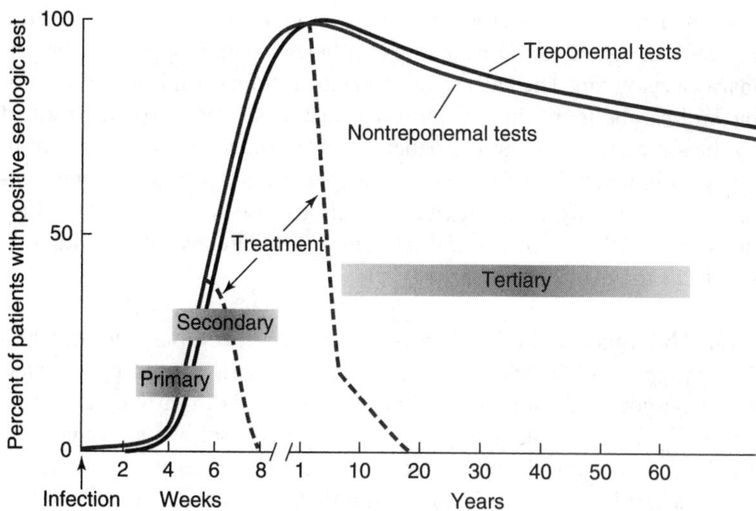

Treponemal and nontreponemal tests in syphilis. The time course of treated and untreated syphilis in relation to serologic tests is shown. The nontreponemal tests (VDRL, RPR) rise during primary syphilis and reach their peak in secondary syphilis. They slowly decline with advancing age. With treatment they revert to normal over a few weeks. The treponemal tests (FTA-Abs, MHTP) follow the same course but remain elevated even following successful treatment. *(Reprinted, with permission, from Ryan KJ, et al.* Sherris Medical Microbiology. *4th ed. New York: McGraw-Hill; 2001:429.)*

204. The answer is b. (*Brooks, p 211. Levinson, pp 129, 492-493. Murray, pp 378-387. Ryan, pp 322-324.*) Patients treated with antibiotics develop diarrhea that, in most cases, is self-limiting. However, in some instances, particularly in those patients treated with ampicillin or clindamycin, a severe, life-threatening pseudomembranous enterocolitis develops. This disease has characteristic histopathology, and membranous plaques can be seen in the colon by endoscopy. Pseudomembranous enterocolitis and antibiotic-associated diarrhea are caused by an anaerobic gram-positive rod, *C. difficile*. It has been recently shown that *C. difficile* produces a protein toxin with a molecular weight of about 250,000. The "toxin" is, in fact, two toxins, toxin A and toxin B. Both toxins are always present in fecal samples, but there is approximately 1000 times more toxin B than toxin A. Toxin A has enterotoxic activity—that is, it elicits a positive fluid response in ligated rabbit ileal loops—whereas toxin B appears to be primarily a cytotoxin. The bacteroides and clostridium organisms are anaerobic and can be found in the intestinal tract. Also, these would be killed by the antibiotics given to the patient. *Staphylococcus aureus* is resistant to many antimicrobials and can cause gastroenteritis if it becomes predominant, but it usually does not cause as serious disease as pseudomembranous enterocolitis. Commercial laboratory tests are available to identify *C. difficile* toxin and enterotoxin.

205. The answer is a. (*Brooks, pp 280-282. Levinson, pp 152-155. Murray, pp 343-349. Ryan, pp 397-401.*) Meningitis caused by *H. influenzae* cannot be distinguished on clinical grounds from that caused by pneumococci or meningococci. The symptoms described are typical for all three organisms. *H. influenzae* is a small, gram-negative rod with a polysaccharide capsule. It is able to grow on laboratory media if two factors are added. Heme (factor X) and NAD (factor V) provide for energy production. Use of the conjugate vaccine (type b polysaccharide) reduces the disease incidence more than 90%. Pneumococci are gram-positive diplococci, and meningococci are gram-negative diplococci, which grow on blood agar and chocolate agar with no X and V factors needed, respectively. Salt-mannitol agar is used to distinguish *S. aureus* from other oral flora. Streptococci do not produce catalase while many other organisms do. Coagulase production is another test to identify *S. aureus*. Commercial kits are available for immunologic detection of *H. influenzae* antigens in spinal fluids, but currently none are available to measure specific antibody in CSF.

206. The answer is a. (*Brooks, p 220. Levinson, pp 169-170, 500-501. Murray, pp 391-393. Ryan, pp 458-459.*) The patient presented with typical symptoms of actinomycosis. *Actinomyces israelii* is normal flora in the mouth. However, it causes a chronic draining infection, often around the maxilla or the mandible, with osteomyelitic changes. Treatment is high-dose penicillin for 4 to 6 weeks. The diagnosis of actinomycosis is often complicated by the failure of *A. israelii* to grow from the clinical specimen. It is an obligate anaerobe. FA reagents are available for direct staining of *A. israelii*. A rapid diagnosis can be made from the pus. FA conjugates are also available for *A. viscosus* and *A. odontolyticus*, anaerobic actinomycetes that are rarely involved in actinomycotic abscesses. *Corynebacterium diphtheriae* is a gram-positive rod, as is *P. acnes*, and *S. aureus* would be a large gram-positive cocci.

207. The answer is b. (*Brooks, pp 238-240. Levinson, pp 112-113, 485. Murray, pp 233-236. Ryan, pp 286-287.*) GBS can be reduced by intrapartum administration of penicillin. While GBS is relatively more resistant to penicillin than group A streptococci, the great majority of GBS isolates are still penicillin-susceptible. An aminoglycoside such as gentamicin may be added to GBS treatment regimens due to the relative reduced susceptibility of some strains. Experimentally, GBS polysaccharide vaccines have also been used. Screening pregnant females early in pregnancy probably offers little advantage because of the possible acquisition of GBS late in the pregnancy. Identification of possible high-risk births would be part of the physician's care of the pregnant patient and is too general for this question. Screening for GBS at the first office visit is premature since this is a first-time pregnancy with no history of GBS complications. Screening of GBS in the last trimester would probably not be done unless some indication of problems was identified. GBS is part of the normal vaginal flora and would be identified as such on culturing. No polysaccharide vaccine for GBS is currently available.

208. The answer is b. (*Brooks, pp 238-240. Levinson, pp 112-113, 485. Murray, pp 233-236. Ryan, pp 286-287.*) There has been speculation concerning the pathogenesis of GBS. This includes failure to activate complement pathways and immobilization of polymorphonuclear leukocytes due to the inactivation of complement C5a, a potent chemoattractant.

209. The answer is a. (*Brooks, pp 332-335. Levinson, pp 173-175. Murray, pp 405-411. Ryan, pp 424-429.*) In men, the appearance of a hard chancre on the penis characteristically indicates syphilis. Even though the chancre does not appear until the infection is 2 or more weeks old, the VDRL test for syphilis still can be negative despite the presence of a chancre (the VDRL test may not become positive for 2 or 3 weeks after initial infection). However, a lesion suspected of being a primary syphilitic ulcer should be examined by dark-field microscopy, which can reveal motile treponemes. Sending the patient home untreated would never occur, especially in light of the lesion being present. Since syphilis was suspected, the spirochete would not grow on T-M medium, and no pus discharge (suspect gonorrhea) was reported to justify culture for *N. gonorrhoeae*.

210. The answer is a. (*Brooks, pp 285-286. Levinson, pp 157, 491-492. Murray, pp 358, 361-363. Ryan, pp 483-484.*) *Brucella* are small, aerobic, gram-negative coccobacilli. Of the four well-characterized species of *Brucella*, only one—*B. melitensis*—characteristically infects both goats and humans. Brucellosis may be associated with GI and neurologic symptoms, lymphadenopathy, splenomegaly, hepatitis, and osteomyelitis. Susceptibility to dyes (thionin and basic fuchsin) can help in differentiation of the species. None of the remaining options (*C. jejuni, S. enteritidis*, and *S. marcescens*) are known to routinely be passed from animals to humans. *Francisella tularensis* is known to be so (see the table), but usually in connection with hunting and cleaning game animals. See the table below for a listing of gram-negative rods associated with animal sources.

GRAM-NEGATIVE RODS ASSOCIATED WITH ANIMAL SOURCES

Species	Disease	Source of Human Infection	Mode of Human Transmission from Animal to Human	Diagnosis
Brucella species	Brucellosis	Pigs, cattle, goats, sheep	Dairy products; contact with animal tissues	Serology or culture
Francisella tularensis	Tularemia	Rabbits, deer, ticks	Contact with animal tissues; ticks	Serology
Yersinia pestis	Plague	Rodents	Flea bite	Immunofluorescence or culture
Pasteurella multocida	Cellulitis	Cats, dogs	Cat or dog bite	Wound culture

(Reprinted, with permission, from Levinson W, Jawetz E. Medical Microbiology and Immunology. *7th ed. New York: McGraw-Hill; 2002:139.)*

SPIROCHETES OF MEDICAL IMPORTANCE

Species	Disease	Mode of Transmission	Diagnosis	Morphology	Growth in Bacteriologic Media	Treatment
Treponema pallidum	Syphilis	Intimate (sexual) contact; across the placenta	Microscopy; serologic tests	Thin, tight, spirals, seen by dark-field illumination, silver impregnation, or immunofluorescent stain	–	Penicillin G
Borrelia burgdorferi	Lyme disease	Tick bite	Clinical observations; microscopy	Large, loosely coiled; stain with Giemsa stain	+	Tetracycline or amoxicillin for acute; penicillin G for chronic
Borrelia recurrentis	Relapsing fever	Louse bite	Clinical observations; microscopy	Large, loosely coiled; stain with Giemsa stain	+	Tetracycline
Leptospira interrogans	Leptospirosis	Food or drink contaminated by urine of infected animals (rats, dogs, pigs, and cows)	Serologic tests	Thin, tight spirals, seen by dark-field illumination	+	Penicillin G

(Reprinted, with permission, from Levinson W, Jawetz E. Medical Microbiology and Immunology. *7th ed. New York: McGraw-Hill; 2002: 154.)*

211. The answer is a. (*Brooks, pp 270-272. Levinson, pp 143-145. Murray, pp 317-320. Ryan, pp 376-377.*) Cholera is a toxicosis. The mode of action of cholera toxin is to stimulate the activity of adenyl cyclase, an enzyme that converts ATP to cyclic AMP. Cyclic AMP stimulates the secretion of chloride ion, and affected patients lose copious amounts of fluid. A drug that inhibits adenyl cyclase thus might block the effect of cholera toxin. Water and electrolyte replacement are primary management mechanisms, while oral tetracycline may help reduce stool output. Many antimicrobial agents are effective against *V. cholerae*, notably oral tetracycline. A sensitivity test would be needed for choosing the best drug to kill the bacteria. Fluid secretion would be lessened if adenyl cyclase was inhibited. Our patient would not die with the described medical treatment, but be helped to overcome the infection. Reduction of bacterial motility has no association with bacterial virulence.

212. The answer is d. (*Brooks, pp 226-228. Levinson, pp 106-110. Murray, pp 210-223. Ryan, pp 263-264.*) Certain strains of staphylococci elaborate an enterotoxin that is frequently responsible for food poisoning. Typically, the toxin is produced when staphylococci grow on foods rich in carbohydrates and is present in the food when it is consumed. The resulting gastroenteritis is dependent only on the ingestion of toxin and not on bacterial multiplication in the GI tract. Characteristic symptoms are nausea, vomiting, abdominal cramps, and explosive diarrhea. The illness rarely lasts more than 24 hours. *Campylobacter perfringens* toxin contributes to a form of food poisoning, but the organism is ingested and grows in the patient, then releasing the toxin. *Campylobacter perfringens* also have toxins that can damage various tissues (gas gangrene). *Staphylococcus aureus* produces coagulase that clots plasma and does not contribute to *S. aureus* food poisoning. Penicillinase (β-lactamase) does not contribute to food poisoning symptoms. Leukocidin inactivates WBCs in the laboratory, but clinical significance is uncertain.

213. The answer is e. (*Brooks, pp 224-229. Levinson, pp 106-110. Murray, p 222, Ryan, pp 269-270.*) Staphylococci are gram-positive, nonspore-forming cocci. Clinically, their antibiotic resistance poses major problems. Many strains produce β-lactamase (penicillinase), an enzyme that destroys penicillin by opening the lactam ring. Drug resistance, mediated by plasmids, may be transferred by transduction. No known allergic reactions occur by release of staphylococcal proteins. Even if the penicillin penetrates the *S. aureus* membrane, external penicillinase would probably have broken the β-lactam ring, inactivating the drug. *S. aureus* most likely contains penicillin-binding proteins (PBPs) but nothing happens if the penicillin is inactivated. Acetyl is CH_3CO. The acetylase would break this bond, but it is uncertain whether this inactivates penicillin like β-lactamase does.

214. The answer is c. (*Brooks, p 207. Levinson, pp 127-128, 492. Murray, pp 383-386. Ryan, pp 320-322.*) *Campylobacter botulinum* growing in food produces a potent neurotoxin that causes diplopia, dysphagia, respiratory paralysis, and speech difficulties when ingested by humans. The toxin is thought to act by blocking the action of acetylcholine at neuromuscular junctions. Botulism is associated with high mortality; fortunately, *C. botulinum* infection in humans is rare. Activation of cyclic AMP is important in cholera disease, not botulism. Clostridia are gram-positive and have no endotoxin. Ingestion of the botulism toxin initiates the disease. The actual organism may or may not be alive when ingested. An enterotoxin, by definition, would affect the intestinal tract.

215. The answer is a. (*Brooks, pp 296-303. Levinson, pp 119-123. Murray, pp 73-78, 291-299. Ryan, p 327.*) Several *Neisseria* species make up part of the normal (nonpathogenic) flora of the human upper respiratory tract. While commensal organisms seldom cause disease, they may occasionally be opportunistic. These organisms are also "foreign" to the immune system and cause immune responses to occur, especially humoral (antibody). The pathogens (*N. gonorrhea* and *N. meningitidis*) produce factors that ensure successful colonization of tissue in spite of local immune defense mechanisms. *Neisseria* organisms are gram-negative and have endotoxin but not lipoteichoic acid residues. These are part of gram-positive cell walls. Since even nonpathogenic neisseria are foreign to the immune system, any antibody response would be specific to the bacterial strain.

216. The answer is d. (*Brooks, pp 273-275. Levinson, pp 145-146. Murray, pp 325-328. Ryan, pp 379-380.*) Until recently, both erythromycin and ciprofloxacin were the drugs of choice for *C. jejuni* enterocolitis. Recently, resistance to the quinolones (ciprofloxacin) has been observed. Ampicillin is ineffective against this gram-negative, curved rod. While Pepto-Bismol may be adequate for a related ulcer-causing bacterium, *Helicobacter*, it is not used for *C. jejuni*. While the pathogenesis of *C. jejuni* suggests an enterotoxin, an antitoxin is not available.

217. The answer is b. (*Brooks, pp 280-282. Levinson, pp 152-153. Murray, pp 344-348. Ryan, pp 397-401. Toy, p 96.*) *Haemophilus influenzae* is a gram-negative bacillus. In young children, it can cause pneumonitis, sinusitis, otitis, and meningitis. Occasionally, it produces a fulminative laryngotracheitis with such severe swelling of the epiglottis that tracheostomy becomes necessary. Clinical infections with this organism after the age of 3 years are less frequent, especially since approval of the type b vaccine. *Haemophilus haemolyticus* is a hemolytic variant of *H. influenzae* which that only occasionally causes disease. *Klebsiella pneumoniae* is present in about 5% of individuals and causes about 1% of pneumonias. *Treponema pneumoniae* is a prominent cause of pneumonia in persons 5 to 20 years old. *Neisseria meningitidis* can be part of the oral flora but is significant in disease when it enters the bloodstream and CNS.

218. The answer is a. (*Brooks, pp 240-243. Levinson, pp 27, 140, 537. Murray, pp 243-246. Ryan, pp 294-295. Toy, p 70.*) Enterococci cause a wide variety of infections ranging from less serious—for example, UTIs—to very serious, such as septicemia. A gram-positive coccus resistant to penicillin must be assumed to be enterococcus until other, more definitive biochemical testing places the isolate in one of the more esoteric groups of gram-positive cocci. Group A streptococci can cause a wide variety of diseases, including RF. Certain antigens of the Group A streptococci cross react with human heart antigens, causing damage to heart muscles and valves. GBS are part of the normal vaginal flora, are β-hemolytic, and test positive to the cAMP test. Gram-negative *Neisseria* species are seldom involved in heart disease, even as opportunists. *Streptococcus pneumoniae* can cause upper respiratory disease, bacteremia, and meningitis.

219. The answer is d. (*Brooks, p 243. Levinson, pp 111, 489-490. Murray, pp 243-246. Ryan, pp 294-295.*) *Enterococcus faecalis* causes 85% to 90% of enterococcal infections, while *E. faecium* causes 5% to 10%. The enterococci are among the most frequent causes of nosocomial infections, especially in intensive care units. *Streptococcus bovis* is a nonenterococcal Group D streptococcus. *Streptococcus pyogenes* is a Group A streptococcus, responsible for 95% of streptococci infections. *Streptococcus pneumoniae* are sensitive to many antimicrobials. Once isolated, there are a variety of tests to speciate enterococci. However, penicillin-resistant, non-β-lactamase-producing, vancomycin-resistant, gram-positive cocci are most likely *E. faecium* or *E. faecalis*.

220. The answer is e. (*Brooks, pp 240-243. Levinson, pp 77, 112. Murray, pp 243-246. Ryan, pp 294-295.*) There are a variety of mechanisms for vancomycin resistance in *E. faecium*, and they have been termed Van A, B, or C. These isolates have become one of the most feared nosocomial pathogens in the hospital environment. Unfortunately, no approved antibiotics can successfully treat vancomycin-resistant enterococci (VRE)—only some experimental antibiotics such as Synercid. Enterococci are highly resistant to cephalosporins, β-lactamase-resistant penicillins, and monolactams. They have low-level resistance to aminoglycosides and intermediate resistance to fluoroquinolones. They are inhibited by β-lactams (ampicillin) but not killed by them.

221. The answer is c. (*Brooks, pp 224-229. Levinson, pp 107-109, 484. Murray, pp 211-220. Ryan, p 824.*) *Staphylococcus aureus* is implicated in the majority of cases of acute osteomyelitis, which affects children most often. A superficial staphylococcal lesion frequently precedes the development of bone infection. In the preantibiotic era, *Streptococcus pneumoniae* was a common cause of acute osteomyelitis. *M. tuberculosis* and gram-negative organisms are implicated less frequently in this infection.

222. The answer is d. (*Brooks, pp 213-216. Levinson, pp 130-131, 481. Murray, pp 261-265. Ryan, p 170. Toy, p 64.*) All toxigenic strains of *C. diphtheriae* are lysogenic for β-phage carrying the *Tox* gene, which codes for the toxin molecule. The expression of this gene is controlled by the metabolism of the host bacteria. The greatest amount of toxin is produced by bacteria grown on media containing very low amounts of iron. Fragment B of the toxin is required for cell entry, while Fragment A stops protein production by inhibiting elongation factor 2 (EF-2). *Corynebacterium* diphtheriae does not possess a capsule, which is normally used to impede phagocytosis by WBCs. Glucose and/or sucrose fermentation is not a virulence factor. Endotoxin comes from gram-negative bacteria while corynebacteria are gram positive.

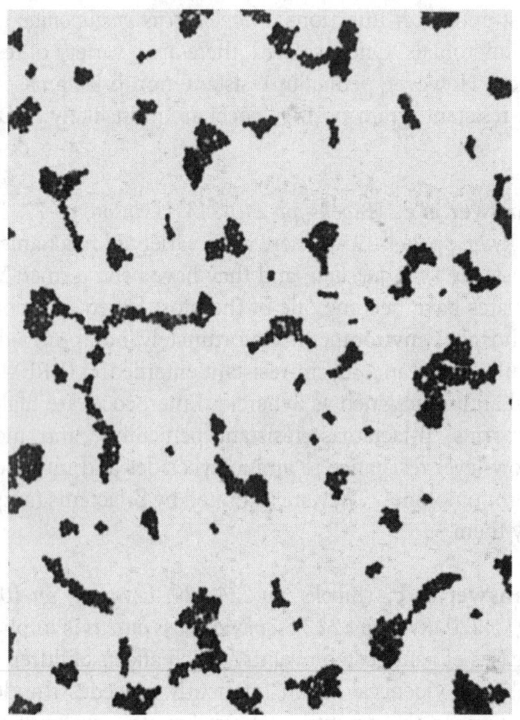

(Reproduced, with permission, from Brooks GF, et al. Jawetz's Medical Microbiology. *24th ed. New York: McGraw-Hill; 2007: 225.)*

223 to 225. The answers are 223-e, 224-e, and 225-b. (*Brooks, pp 226-228. Levinson, pp 40-44, 107-108. Murray, pp 211-220. Ryan, pp 264-266. Toy, p 156.*) TSS is a febrile illness seen predominantly, but not exclusively, in menstruating women. Clinical criteria for TSS include fever greater than 102°F (38.9°C), rash, hypotension, and abnormalities of the mucous membranes and the GI, hepatic, muscular, cardiovascular systems, or CNS. Usually three or more systems are involved. Treatment is supportive, including the aggressive use of antistaphylococcal antibiotics. Certain types of tampons may play a role in TSS by trapping O_2 and depleting magnesium. Most people have protective antibodies to the toxic shock syndrome toxin (TSST-1). Chicken pox (VZV) or varicella presents with a typical vesicular rash. Guillain–Barré syndrome is a demyelinating condition of the peripheral nerves. Scalded skin syndrome is caused by *S. aureus* exfoliative toxin that produces epidermal skin layer sloughing. Food poisoning is caused by *S. aureus* enterotoxins, which are produced in contaminated food and symptoms appear after ingestion.

TSS is caused by a toxin-producing strain of *S. aureus* (TSST-1). In this case, no actual organisms would likely be isolated since TSS is caused by an excreted toxin, not the actual organism. Blood culture would also most likely be negative. While there have been reports that *S. epidermidis* produces TSS, they have largely been discounted. Vaginal colonization with *S. aureus* is a necessary adjunct to the disease. *Staphylococcus aureus* is isolated from the vaginal secretions, conjunctiva, nose, throat, cervix, and feces in 45% to 98% of cases. The organism has infrequently been isolated from the blood. *Clostridium difficile* and *C. perfringens* produce pseudomembranous colitis and gas gangrene, respectively. *Gardnerella vaginalis* can be found in the normal vaginal flora and in vaginosis, where inflammatory cells are not present. "Clue cells" are vaginal epithelial cells covered with many gram-variable bacteria, including *G. vaginalis*.

Epidemiologic investigations suggest strongly that TSS is related to use of tampons, in particular, use of the highly absorbent ones that can be left in for extended periods of time. An increased growth of intravaginal *S. aureus* and enhanced production of TSST-1 have been associated with the prolonged intravaginal use of these hyperabsorbent tampons and with the capacity of the materials used in them to bind magnesium. The most severe cases of TSS have been seen in association with gram-negative infection. TSST-1 may enhance endotoxin activity. Recently, group A streptococci have been reported to cause TSS. Purchased fast-food ingestion, heavy menstrual flow, rubella exposure, and travel to Vermont would have no relevance to this clinical situation.

226 and 227. The answers are 226-c and 227-d. (*http://en.wikipedia.org/wiki/Bayesian_statistics.*) Bayesian statistics are often used to determine sensitivity, specificity, and predictive values of new diagnostic tests. A square is set up and the experimental numbers inserted: a = true positive, b = false positive, c = false negative, and d = true negative. The formulas for sensitivity, specificity, and predictive values are also given (see the below table.)

It is necessary to note that the incidence of the disease in the population affects predictive values but not sensitivity or specificity. At a given level of sensitivity and specificity, as the incidence of the disease in the population increases, the predictive value of a positive (PVP) increases, and the predictive value of a negative (PVN) decreases. For this reason, predictive values are difficult to interpret unless true disease incidence is known.

	CULTURE	
LA Test	Positive	Negative
Pos	(*a*) 25	(*b*) 5
NEG	(*c*) 5	(*d*) 95

$$\text{Sensitivity} = \frac{a}{a+c} = \frac{25}{25+5} = 85\%$$

$$\text{Specificity} = \frac{d}{d+b} = \frac{95}{95+5} = 95\%$$

$$\text{PVP} = \frac{a}{a+b} = \frac{25}{25+5} = 85\%$$

$$\text{PVN} = \frac{d}{d+c} = \frac{95}{95+5} = 95\%$$

228. The answer is d. (*Brooks, pp 263-265. Levinson, pp 149-150. Murray, pp 333-337. Ryan, pp 387-388.*) Pseudomonads occur widely in soil, water, plants, and animals. They are gram-negative, motile, aerobic rods that produce water-soluble pigments (blue and green). They are very opportunistic when abnormal host defenses are encountered. While motile, they do not "swarm" over the surface of an agar plate, as *Proteus* does. Being gram-negative, as many enteric and environmental organisms are, their cell walls contain endotoxin (LPS). Many of the pseudomonads are resistant to a wide range of antimicrobials, enhancing their opportunistic characteristics.

229. The answer is c. (*Brooks, pp 203-211. Levinson, pp 127-129. Murray, pp 377-389, 247-251. Ryan, pp 308, 314-317.*) *Clostridium* and *Bacillus* organisms exist widely in nature. While many *Clostridium* are pathogenic due to exotoxin production (*C. tetani, C. botulism*), and anthrax has multiple virulence factors (capsule, LF, EF, and PA), *C. perfringens* and *B. cereus* are found routinely in gastroenteritis outbreaks. Since both are spore formers, the usual epidemiological investigation finds that heating foods kills vegetative bacteria but not spores. If food is inappropriately stored (>40-140°F), spores may germinate into vegetative bacteria and be ingested, causing the disease. Most episodes are self-limited. Both produce enterotoxins that account for similar disease presentations.

230. The answer is e. (*Brooks, pp 224-229. Levinson, pp 48, 107-109. Murray, pp 211-220. Ryan, pp 269-270.*) The incidence of oxacillin and MRSA has been rapidly increasing. MRSA and methicillin-sensitive *S. aureus* (MSSA) coexist in heterologous populations. Treatment of a patient harboring this heterologous population may provide a selective environment for the MRSA. Prior to changing therapy, the susceptibility of the isolate should be determined. Vancomycin has often been used effectively for MRSA, but it is expensive and nephrotoxic. There is no evidence that MRSA is any more virulent or invasive than susceptible strains. See the table below for a listing of medically important staphylococci.

STAPHYLOCOCCI OF MEDICAL IMPORTANCE

Species	Coagulase Production	Typical Hemolysis	Important Features[a]	Typical Disease
Staphylococcus aureus	+	Beta	Protein A on surface	Abscess, food poisoning, TSS
Staphylococcus epidermidis	–	None	Sensitive to novobiocin	Infection of prosthetic heart valves and hips; common member of skin flora
Staphylococcus saprophyticus	–	None	Resistant to novobiocin	Urinary tract infection

[a]All staphylococci are catalase-positive.

(*Reprinted, with permission, from Levinson W, Jawetz E.* Medical Microbiology and Immunology. *7th ed. New York: McGraw-Hill; 2002:92.*)

231. The answer is c. (*Brooks, pp 253-255. Levinson, pp 136-140, 492. Murray, pp 303-307. Ryan, pp 355-357. Toy, p 76.*) Food poisoning with *E. coli* 0157/H7 causes hemorrhagic colitis; it is often seen in people who have eaten beef hamburgers. The same organism also causes a hemorrhagic uremic syndrome. The toxin, called *Shiga-like toxin*, can be demonstrated in Vero cells, but the cytotoxicity must be neutralized with specific antiserum. With the exception of sorbitol fermentation, there is nothing biochemically distinctive about these organisms.

232. The answer is b. (*Brooks, pp 253-255. Levinson, pp 136-140, 492. Murray, pp 303-307. Ryan, pp 355-357.*) ETEC is an important cause of traveler's diarrhea, producing a heat-labile exotoxin (LT) and a heat-stable enterotoxin (ST). To cause diarrhea, *E. coli* must produce not only LT and ST toxins but also adhere to the lining of the small intestine. Fimbrial antigens are involved in adherence. O657/H7 stain is called EHEC, while EPEC is also an important cause of diarrhea in infants. EIEC produces a shigellosis-type disease.

233. The answer is d. (*Brooks, pp 291-292. Levinson, pp 159-160. Murray, pp 311-313. Ryan, pp 484-488.*) Bubonic plague and pneumonic plague differ clinically. Bubonic plague, characterized by swollen lymph nodes and fever, is usually transmitted through a flea bite. Pneumonic plague, which is characterized by sepsis and pneumonia, is transmitted by the droplet route, usually after contact with an infected human or animal. Age of the patient, geographic location and/or health of the animal vector, and season of the year would all be insignificant in considering epidemiological differences between the clinical presentations of the two plagues.

234. The answer is a. (*Brooks, pp 315, 316. Levinson, pp 32, 186-187. Murray, p 372. Ryan, p 479.*) While the essential information (ie, the evidence that the child in question was scratched by a cat) is missing, the clinical presentation points to a number of diseases, including cat scratch disease (CSD). Until recently, the etiologic agent of CSD was unknown. Evidence indicated that it was a pleomorphic, rod-shaped bacterium that had been named *Afipia*. It was best demonstrated in the affected lymph node by a silver impregnation stain. However, it now appears that *Afipia* causes relatively few cases of CSD and that the small, pleomorphic, gram-negative rods present mainly in the walls of capillaries primarily responsible are *Rochalimaea henselae*, which has recently been renamed *B. henselae*. *Brucella*, *Mycobacterium*, and *Yersinia* species have not been shown to have any association with CSD.

235. The answer is c. (*Brooks, pp 233-239. Levinson, pp 110-115. Murray, pp 225-233. Ryan, p 273.*) There has been a marked increase in fatal streptococcal infections, including those that are described as "necrotizing fasciitis." The strains of group A streptococci isolated have a pyrogenic exotoxin with properties not unlike those of the toxic shock toxin of *S. aureus*. Mortality is high (30%) in spite of aggressive antibiotic therapy.

236. The answer is b. (*Brooks, pp 275-276. Levinson, pp 146-147, 496. Murray, pp 328-332. Ryan, pp 383-384.*) *Helicobacter pylori* antigen tests from a stool sample using an ELISA format and a monoclonal antibody to *H. pylori* are as sensitive as culture of the control portion of the stomach. Urea breath tests are also widely used. *Helicobacter pylori* has an active enzyme (urease) that breaks down radioactive urea. The patient releases radioactive CO_2 if *H. pylori* are present. *Helicobacter pylori* antibody tests, IgG and IgA, indicate the presence of *H. pylori* and usually decline after effective treatment. Culture of stomach contents is insensitive and not appropriate as a diagnostic procedure for *H. pylori*. Direct tests, such as antigen or culture of gastric mucosa, are preferred because they are the most sensitive indication of a cure.

237. The answer is e. (*Brooks, pp 337-338, Levinson, pp 24, 176-177. Murray, pp 411-415. Ryan, pp 434-437. Toy, p 40.*) At present, Lyme disease may be diagnosed clinically and serologically. Patients who are from endemic areas such as eastern Pennsylvania and report joint pain and swelling months subsequent to exposure to ticks must be evaluated for Lyme disease and treated if the test is positive. Patients may also report a variety of neurologic problems such as tingling of the extremities, Bell palsy, and headache. IgM antibody appears soon after the tick bite (10 days-3 weeks) and persists for 2 months; IgG appears later in the disease but remains elevated for 1 to 2 years, especially in untreated patients. A significant IgG titer is at least 1:320. Most investigators feel that IgM titers of 1:100 are significant; some investigators say that any IgM titer is significant. Management of this patient would best be done by immediately starting treatment with tetracycline, effective against *B. burgdorferi*.

238. The answer is c. (*Brooks, pp 320-327. Levinson, pp 161-168. Murray, pp 282-285, 289. Ryan, p 613.*) There are some interesting characteristics of *M. avium* from AIDS patients. According to data from the National Jewish Hospital and Research Center in Denver and the CDC, 75% of the isolates were serovar 4, and 76% produced a deep-yellow pigment. Yellow pigment is not a characteristic of most isolates of *M. avium*. The significance of these findings is unknown. Most *M. avium* isolates are resistant to isoniazid and streptomycin but susceptible to clofazimine and ansamycin. In vitro susceptibility testing, however, may not be reliable for *M. avium*. A blood culture is often the most reliable way to diagnose the disease. Finally, all isolates of *M. avium* are acid-fast, by definition.

239. The answer is b. (*Brooks, pp 142, 170, 238. Levinson, pp 115, 470. Murray, pp 231, 233. Ryan, p 279.*) Rheumatic fever (RF) is a disease that causes polyarthritis, carditis, chorea, and erythema marginatum. The mechanism of damage appears to be autoimmune; that is, antibodies are synthesized to a closely related streptococcal antigen such as M-protein, but these same antibodies cross react with certain cardiac antigens such as myosin. Until recently, RF was very rare in the United States. In 1986, there were at least 135 cases of RF in Utah. Subsequently, scattered cases of RF have occurred in other states. Epidemiologists do not have a reason for this increase in RF. Some evidence suggests that there may be a genetic predisposition to the disease. Intramuscular injection of benzathine penicillin is effective treatment for and prophylaxis against group A streptococcal infection. While it appears that certain strains of streptococci contain cell membrane antigens that are identical to human heart tissue antigens, the strains can infect skin and cause pharyngitis. The first attack of RF (rheumatic fever) usually produces only slight cardiac damage. It is important to protect such patients from recurrent *S. pyogenes* infections by prophylactic penicillin use to prevent increased damage from multiple future bacterial attacks. Answer option (e) refers to a staphylococcal antigen as similar, but the correct comparison would be with streptococcal antigen and cardiac antigen.

240. The answer is d. (*Brooks, pp 198, 240. Levinson, pp 27, 112. Murray, pp 73-78. Ryan, pp 293-294.*) In the healthy oral cavity, gram-positive, α-hemolytic streptococci make up the predominant flora. Any dental manipulation causes bleeding, allowing the oral flora to get into the blood (bacteremia). Phagocytic activity by WBCs usually clears this in a few minutes. However, these same organisms are quite efficient at attaching to and colonizing heart valve defects. *Streptococcus viridans* is a typical member of this α-hemolytic group and is commonly found in SBE. *Staphylococcus aureus* and *S. epidermidis* are present in the oral flora in very small numbers, as is *S. pneumoniae*. If *E. faecalis* gets into the bloodstream from the GI tract, it could potentially also cause heart valve problems. The α-hemolytic viridans streptococci are reported as being isolated from SBE most often.

241. The answer is e. (*Brooks, pp 241-242. Levinson, pp 11, 66, 153. Murray, p 241. Ryan, p 291.*) The quellung test determines the presence of bacterial capsules. Specific antibody is mixed with the bacterial suspension or with clinical material. The polysaccharide capsule–antibody complex is visible microscopically. The test is also termed *capsular swelling*. The capsules of *S. pneumoniae* as well as *N. meningitidis, H. influenzae*, and *K. pneumoniae* play a role in the pathogenicity of the organisms. These surface structures inhibit phagocytosis, perhaps by preventing attachment of the leukocyte pseudopod. *Corynebacterium diphtheriae, Enterobacter*, and *H. parainfluenzae* are nonencapsulated.

242. The answer is b. (*Brooks, pp 218, 280. Levinson, pp 112, 114, 136, 139. Murray, pp 255-258. Ryan, pp 302-305. Toy, p 102.*) No vaccine is available for *Listeria*. Except during a meningococcal epidemic, *H. influenzae* is the most common cause of bacterial meningitis in children. The organism is occasionally found to be associated with respiratory tract infections or otitis media. *Haemophilus influenzae, N. meningitidis, S. pneumoniae*, and *Listeria* account for 80% to 90% of all cases of bacterial meningitis. A purified polysaccharide vaccine conjugated to protein for *H. influenzae* type B is available. A tetravalent vaccine is available for *N. meningitidis* and a 23-serotype vaccine for *S. pneumoniae.*

243. The answer is e. (*Brooks, p 149. Levinson, pp 30-37. Murray, pp 73-76.*) Organisms may be transmitted in a number of ways, such as by air, food, hands, sexual contact, and infected needles. However, for each disease or disease category, there is usually a portal of entry not always unique to the organism. The skin is a tough integument and, in fact, is resistant to most infectious organisms except those that may breakdown human skin. Breaches of the skin as by wounds, burns, and the like predispose patients to a variety of infections such as tetanus caused by wound contamination with spores of *C. tetani*, or direct infection by *Staphylococcus*, *Streptococcus*, or gram-negative rods (such as *Serratia* or *Pseudomonas*).

244 to 246. The answers are 244-d, 245-a, and 246-b. (*Brooks, pp 148-151. Levinson, pp 30-37. Murray, pp 73-76.*) The respiratory tract is a common portal of entry to such airborne organisms as *M. tuberculosis*. This is why respiratory precautions must be taken when patients are harboring viable *M. tuberculosis*. The GI tract is usually infected from ingestion of contaminated food or water (*Shigella*, *Salmonella*, and *Campylobacter*) or by an alteration of the normal microbial flora such as with *C. difficile* disease. The genital tract may become infected either by sexual contact or by alteration of the genital environment, as often occurs with yeast infections. Several bacteria such as *N. gonorrhoeae*, *Chlamydia*, and *T. pallidum* are transmitted by direct sexual contact with infected partners.

247. The answer is d. (*Brooks, pp 268, 296, 303-304. Levinson, pp 190, 504. Murray, pp 334, 338-340. Ryan, pp 390-391.*) While admittedly rare in human medicine, the bacteria referred to should be appreciated for their role in human disease. *Branhamella* is a gram-negative diplococcus. It has recently been renamed *Moraxella catarrhalis*. While it is a member of the normal flora, it may cause severe upper and lower respiratory tract infection, particularly in the immunosuppressed patient. Most isolates produce β-lactamase and are resistant to penicillin. *M. catarrhalis* is not a gram-negative rod that causes endocarditis, nor a gram-negative, fusiformed (pointed ends) rod associated with periodontal disease or sepsis. It is not the cause of rat-bite fever or the causative agent of trench fever.

248. The answer is b. (*Brooks, pp 220, 267. Levinson, p 187. Murray, pp 372, 374. Ryan, pp 390-391.*) *Capnocytophaga* grows best in a carbon dioxide atmosphere, as the name implies. It is isolated frequently from patients with periodontal disease but may also cause septicemia in susceptible patients. Rat-bite fever is caused by *Spirillum*, and the agent of CSD is *B. henselae*.

249. The answer is b. (*Brooks, pp 350-354. Levinson, pp 183, 503. Murray, pp 436-440. Ryan, pp 477-478.*) *Coxiella burnetii* is a rickettsial organism that causes upper respiratory infections in humans. These can range from subclinical infection to influenza-like disease and pneumonia. Transmission to humans occurs from inhalation of dust contaminated with rickettsiae from placenta, dried feces, urine, or milk, or from aerosols in slaughterhouses. *Campylobacter burnetii* can also be found in ticks, which can transmit the agent to sheep, goats, and cattle. No skin rash occurs in these infections. Treatment includes tetracycline and chloramphenicol. *Coxiella burnetii* is not transmitted by flea or tick vectors. Since Q fever involves the upper respiratory tract, liver, or CNS, there is no transmission by urethral discharge.

250 to 252. The answers are 250-a, 251-d, and 252-b. (*Brooks, pp 243, 219-221. Levinson, pp 69-84. Murray, pp 199-208. Ryan, pp 294, 457-459, 870-871.*) These questions demonstrate commonly occurring clinical infectious diseases and microbiologic problems. Enterococci may be resistant to ampicillin and gentamicin. Vancomycin would be the drug of choice. However, laboratory results do not always correlate well with clinical response. The National Committee on Clinical Laboratory Standards recommends testing enterococci only for ampicillin and vancomycin. Some symptomatic patients may have 10 leukocytes per milliliter of urine but relatively few bacteria. The patient is likely infected and the organisms, particularly if in pure culture, should be further processed.

The patient in Question 252 probably has actinomycosis. These laboratory data are not uncommon. There is no reason to work up all the contaminating bacteria. A fluorescent microscopy test for *A. israelii* is available. If positive, the FA provides a rapid diagnosis. In any event, it may be impossible to recover *A. israelii* from such a specimen. High-dose penicillin has been used to treat actinomycosis. One of the options suggests no further clinical work-up on the patients be done. Clearly, laboratory results may help the clinician make patient management decisions but each of these three cases show that physicians need to have a good understanding that laboratory tests may give conflicting information for the patient being treated. The physician must help the laboratory to understand how to use the data produced to give the patient the best possible medical care. Antibiotic sensitivity tests today are mostly automated and reliable. If a repeat is needed, a new blood sample should be drawn for the new test.

253 to 257. The answers are 253-c, 254-d, 255-b, 256-d, and 257-e. (*Brooks, pp 170-172. Levinson, pp 69-84. Murray, pp 199-208. Ryan, p 195. Toy, p 40.*) There are few bacteria for which antimicrobial susceptibility is highly predictable. However, some agents are the drug of choice because of their relative effectiveness. Among the three antibiotics that have been shown to treat legionellosis effectively (erythromycin, rifampin, and minocycline), erythromycin is clearly superior, even though in vitro studies show the organism to be susceptible to other antibiotics.

Penicillin remains the drug of choice for *S. pneumoniae* and the group A streptococci, although a few isolates of penicillin-resistant pneumococci have been observed. Resistance among the pneumococci is either chromosomally mediated, in which case the minimal inhibitory concentrations (MICs) are relatively low, or plasmid-mediated, which results in highly resistant bacteria. The same is generally true for *H. influenzae*. Until the mid-1970s, virtually all isolates of *H. influenzae* were susceptible to ampicillin. There has been a rapidly increasing incidence of ampicillin-resistant isolates—almost 35% to 40% in some areas of the United States. Resistance is ordinarily mediated by β-lactamase, although ampicillin-resistant, β-lactamase-negative isolates have been seen. No resistance to penicillin has been seen in group A streptococci.

Lyme disease, caused by *B. burgdorferi*, has been treated with penicillin, erythromycin, and tetracycline. Treatment failures have been observed. Ceftriaxone has become the drug of choice, particularly in the advanced stages of Lyme disease.

The most common infection due to β-hemolytic *S. pyogenes* (GAS) is strep sore throat or pharyngitis. From here, the infection is able to spread to all parts of the body. Significant symptoms, as described, are often experienced, with only 20% of infections being asymptomatic. The organisms grow fairly well in the laboratory and easily identified. All *S. pyogenes* strains are susceptible to penicillin G, and most are susceptible to erythromycin. Antimicrobial drugs have no effect on established glomerulonephritis and RF. In acute infections, efforts must be made to eradicate streptococci from the patient quickly to eliminate the antigenic stimulus.

Campylobacter difficile causes toxin-mediated pseudomembranous enterocolitis as well as antibiotic-associated diarrhea. Pseudomembranous enterocolitis is normally seen during or after administration of antibiotics. One of the few agents effective against *C. difficile* is vancomycin. Alternatively, bacitracin can be used.

258 to 261. The answers are 258-a, 259-d, 260-b, and 261-c. *(Brooks, pp 270-276. Levinson, pp 133-146. Murray, pp 325-328. Ryan,* *pp 373-378. Toy, p 172.*) Some organisms originally thought to be vibrios, such as *C. jejuni*, have been reclassified. *Campylobacter jejuni*, which grows best at 107.6°F (42°C), has its reservoir in birds and mammals and causes gastroenteritis in humans.

Vibrio cholerae causes cholera, which is worldwide in distribution. Vibrios are the most common bacteria in surface waters worldwide. They are curved rods with a polar flagellum. *Vibrio cholerae* subgroups O1 and O139 (older serotype designations: Ogawa [AB], Inaba [AC], Jolpka [ABC]) cause cholera in humans. A person with normal gastric acidity may have to ingest 10^{10} or more *V. cholerae* to become infected when the vehicle is water because the organisms are susceptible to acid. When ingested with food, as few as 10^2 to 10^4 may be able to produce disease. The organisms do not reach the bloodstream but remain in the intestinal tract.

Vibrio parahaemolyticus is a halophilic marine vibrio that causes gastroenteritis in humans, primarily from ingestion of cooked seafood. It is lactose-negative and sucrose-negative.

Vibrio vulnificus is also halophilic. It has been suggested that these halophilic vibrios do not belong to the genus *Vibrio* but in the genus *Beneckea*. *Vibrio vulnificus* is lactose-positive and produces heat-labile, extracellular toxin. Organisms that, unlike *V. cholerae*, do not agglutinate in 0 to 1 antiserum were once called nonagglutinable (NAG), or noncholera (NC), vibrios. Such a classification can be confusing because *V. vulnificus*, which is an NCV, nevertheless causes severe cholera-like disease. In addition, *V. vulnificus* can produce wound infections, septicemia, meningitis, pneumonia, and keratitis.

262 to 265. The answers are 262-b, 263-d, 264-a, and 265-e. (*Brooks, pp 280-287. Levinson, pp 152-156. Murray, pp 311-313, 358-363. Ryan, pp 401-402, 481-488.*) All the organisms described in the questions are short, ovoid, gram-negative rods. For the most part, they are nutritionally fastidious and require blood or blood products for growth. These and related organisms are unique among bacteria in that, though they have an animal reservoir, they can be transmitted to humans. Humans become infected by a variety of routes, including ingestion of contaminated animal products (*B. abortus* in cattle), direct contact with contaminated animal material or with infected animals themselves (*Y. enterocolitica* and *B. bronchiseptica* in dogs), and animal bites (*P. multocida* in many different animals). The laboratory differentiation of these microbes may be difficult and must rely on a number of parameters, including biochemical and serologic reactions, development of specific antibody response in affected persons, and epidemiologic evidence of infection.

Yersinia enterocolitica are motile at 77°C (25°C) and nonmotile at 98.6°F (37°C). They are found in the intestinal tract of animals and cause a variety of clinical syndromes in humans. Transmission to humans probably occurs via animal fecal contamination of food, drink, or fomites.

The brucellae are obligate parasites of animals and humans and are located intracellularly. *Brucella abortus* is typically found in cattle. Brucellosis (undulant fever) has an acute bacteremic phase followed by a chronic stage that may last years and involve many tissues. *Brucella abortus* requires CO_2 for growth and is most often isolated from blood and bone marrow. Species differentiation is due to dye (thionine) sensitivity.

Bordetella bronchiseptica causes diseases in animals (kennel cough in dogs) and occasionally respiratory disease and bacteremia in humans. *Bordetella* requires enriched medium (Bordet-Gengou) and is strongly urease-positive.

Pasteurella multocida occurs worldwide in the respiratory and GI tracts of many domestic and wild animals. It is the most common organism in human wounds inflicted by cat and dog bites. It is one of the common causes of hemorrhagic septicemia in rabbits, rats, horses, sheep, fowl, cats, and swine. It can affect many systems in humans, as well as bite wounds.

266 to 268. The answers are 266-d, 267-e, and 268-b. (*Brooks, pp 63-71. Levinson, pp 62-68. Murray, pp 189-198. Ryan, pp 339, 373, 449. Toy, p 122.*) The medium of choice for the isolation of pathogenic *Neisseriae* is TMTM agar. TM agar is both a selective and an enriched medium; it contains hemoglobin, the supplement Isovitalex, and the antibiotics vancomycin, colistin, nystatin, and trimethoprim. *Vibrio cholerae* as well as other vibrios, including *V. parahaemolyticus* and *V. alginolyticus*, are isolated best on thiosulfate citrate bile salts sucrose medium, although media such as mannitol salt agar also support the growth of vibrios. Maximal growth occurs at a pH of 8.5 to 9.5 and at 98.6°F (37°C) incubation. Löwenstein–Jensen slants or plates, which are composed of a nutrient base and egg yolk, are used routinely for the initial isolation of mycobacteria. Small inocula of *M. tuberculosis* can also be grown in oleic acid albumin media; large inocula can be cultured on simple synthetic media.

Loeffler medium is an enriched nonselective medium used for the cultivation of corynebacteria, especially *C. diphtheriae*. Horse serum and egg coagulate during sterilization and provide nutrients. This medium enhances the production of metachromatic granules (observed with methylene blue stain). Columbia agar with 5% sheep blood is a general-purpose medium for isolation of a variety of organisms, including fastidious organisms. Along with nutrition, blood agar allows the observation of alpha (incomplete) and beta (complete lysis) hemolysis caused by bacteria.

269. The answer is b. (*Brooks, pp 206-207. Levinson, pp 127-128. Murray, pp 383-386. Ryan, pp 320-322.*) Botulism is a disease brought about by ingesting a preformed toxin. Anaerobic bacteria have grown in food, deposited the botulism toxin, and died. The toxin affects the CNS by inhibiting the release of acetylcholine at the neuronal synapse. This results in a flaccid paralysis and death by respiratory failure. At no stage of the disease will any antibiotic be able to modify or arrest the disease. Antitoxins (A, B, and E) must be promptly administered, and ventilation assisted mechanically. In all other choices, antibiotics will provide a mechanism to kill or inhibit the microorganisms, bringing the infection under control.

270. The answer is d. (*Brooks, pp 339-340. Levinson, pp 67, 174-177, 541. Murray, pp 416-418. Ryan, pp 430-431.*) Leptospirosis is a zoonosis of worldwide distribution. Human infection results from ingestion of water or food contaminated with leptospirae. Rats, mice, wild rodents, dogs, swine, and cattle excrete the organisms in urine and feces during active illness and during an asymptomatic carrier state. Drinking, swimming, bathing, or food consumption may lead to human infection. Children acquire the disease from dogs more often than do adults. Treatment can include doxycycline, ampicillin, or amoxicillin. Symptoms in humans range from fever and rash to jaundice through aseptic meningitis.

Leptospirae are tightly coiled, thin, flexible spirochetes 5 to 15 μm long, with one end bent into a hook. It stains best where silver can be impregnated into the organism. The gram stain would not be useful. The organisms derive energy from oxidation of fatty acids, so EMB or TM agar would be inadequate. Agglutination testing and CIE is complicated by the fact that all *Leptospirae* strains exhibit cross-reactivity in serologic tests.

271 to 274. The answers are 271-e, 272-a, 273-b, and 274-d. (*Brooks, pp 196-201. Levinson, pp 25-30. Murray, pp 73-78. Ryan, p 143.*) An understanding of normal, or indigenous, microflora is essential in order to appreciate the abnormal. Usually, anatomic sites contiguous to mucous membranes are not sterile and have characteristic normal flora.

The skin flora differs as a function of location. Skin adjacent to mucous membranes may share some of the normal flora of the GI system. Overall, the predominant bacteria on the skin surface are *S. epidermidis* and *Propionibacterium*, an anaerobic diphtheroid.

The mouth is part of the GI tract, but its indigenous flora shows some distinct differences. While anaerobes are present in large numbers, particularly in the gingival crevice, the eruption of teeth at 6 to 9 months of age leads to colonization by organisms such as *S. mutans* and *Streptococcus sanguis*, both α-hemolytic streptococci. An edentulous person loses β-hemolytic streptococci as normal flora.

The GI tract is sterile at birth and soon develops characteristic flora as a function of diet. In the adult, anaerobes such as *B. fragilis* and *Bifidobacterium* may outnumber coliforms and enterococci by a ratio of 1000:1. The colon contains 10^{11} to 10^{12} bacteria per gram of feces.

Soon after birth, the vagina becomes colonized by lactobacilli. As the female matures, lactobacilli may still be predominant, but anaerobic cocci, diphtheroids, and anaerobic, gram-negative rods also are found as part of the indigenous flora. Changes in the chemical or microbiologic ecology of the vagina can have marked effects on normal flora and may promote infection such as vaginitis or vaginosis.

Escherichia coli are among the most common group of gram-negative rods isolated in the laboratory. It is fairly easily identified in the laboratory. It ferments mannitol and is lactose positive. The organism is part of normal body flora, but is a very efficient opportunist. Urinary tract infections are commonly caused with this organism.

275 to 278. The answers are 275-c, 276-d, 277-a, and 278-e. (*Brooks, pp 196-201. Levinson, pp 25-30. Murray, pp 73-78. Ryan, pp 274-275, 457-459.*) *Streptococcus salivarius, S. mutans, A. israelii*, and *A. viscosis* are all part of the normal microbiota of the human mouth. Both genera are common causes of bacterial endocarditis. *Streptococcus mutans* is highly cariogenic (ie, capable of producing dental caries), in large part because of its unique ability to synthesize a dextran bioadhesive that sticks to teeth.

S. salivarius settles onto the mucosal epithelial surfaces of the human mouth soon after birth and is often found in the saliva. Streptococcus pyogenes (group A streptococcus) is responsible for about 95% of human infections caused by streptococci and is the cause of RF. Members of the genus *Actinomyces* that are clinically significant and can be differentiated by specific FA microscopy as well as a battery of physiologic tests, such as those assessing requirements for oxygen. *Actinomyces* organisms are opportunistic members of the normal oral microbiota. Both *A. israelii* and *A. viscosis* are pathogenic and can cause osteomyelitis in the cervicofacial region. Of the two species, *A. israelii*, which is anaerobic, is the more common causative agent of actinomycosis. *A viscosis*, a facultative anaerobe, appears to be cariogenic. Group A streptococci (GAS) are β-hemolytic and produces cellulitis as a typical lesion. Cellulitis is recognized as a diffuse, rapidly spreading lesion in the body tissues.

279 to 285. The answers are 279-b, 280-a, 281-e, 282-d, 283-c, 284-c, and 285-a. (*Brooks, pp 213-216, 283-287, 253-255. Levinson, pp 130-131, 138, 153-155, 158-159. Murray [2009], pp 261-265, 303-307, 351-361. Toy, p 122.*) Diphtheria, a disease caused by *C diphtheriae*, usually begins as pharyngitis associated with pseudomembrane formation and lymphadenopathy. Growing organisms lysogenic for a prophage produce a potent exotoxin that is absorbed in mucous membranes and causes remote damage to the liver, kidneys, and heart; the polypeptide toxin inhibits protein synthesis of the host cell. Although *C. diphtheriae* may infect the skin, it rarely invades the bloodstream and never actively invades deep tissue. Diphtheria toxin (DT) kills sensitive cells by blocking protein synthesis. DT is converted to an enzyme that inactivates EF-2, which is responsible for the translocation of polypeptidyl-tRNA from the acceptor to the donor site on the eukaryotic ribosome. The reaction is as follows:

$$\text{NAD} + \text{EF-2} = \text{ADP-ribosyl} - \text{EF-2} + \text{nicotinamide} + \text{H}^+$$

Bordetella pertussis and *B. parapertussis* are similar and may be isolated together from a clinical specimen. However, *B. parapertussis* does not produce pertussis toxin. Pertussis toxin, like many bacterial toxins, has two subunits: A and B. Subunit A is an active enzyme, and B promotes binding of the toxin to host cells. Pertussis toxin has ADP-ribosylating activity, with an A/B structure and mechanism of action similar to that of cholera toxin (cAMP).

Francisella tularensis is a short, gram-negative organism that is markedly pleomorphic; it is nonmotile and cannot form spores. It has a rigid growth requirement for cysteine. Human tularemia usually is acquired from direct contact with tissues of infected rabbits but also can be transmitted by the bites of flies and ticks. *Francisella tularensis* causes a variety of clinical syndromes, including ulceroglandular, oculoglandular, pneumonic, and typhoidal forms of tularemia.

The pathogenesis of infection with *E. coli* is a complex interrelation of many events and properties. *Escherichia coli* may serve as a model for other members of the Enterobacteriaceae. Some strains of *E. coli* are EIEC, some ETEC, some EHEC, and others EPEC. At present, there is little clinical significance in routinely discriminating the various types, with the possible exceptions of the ETEC and the *E. coli* 0157/H7 that are hemorrhagic. *Escherichia coli* 0157/H7 secretes a toxin called *verotoxin*. The toxin is very active in a Vero cell line. More correctly, the toxin(s) should be called *Shiga-like*.

Streptococcal infection usually is accompanied by an elevated titer of antibody to some of the enzymes produced by the organism. Among the antigenic substances elaborated by group A β-hemolytic streptococci are erythrogenic toxin, streptodornase (streptococcal DNase), hyaluronidase, and streptolysin O (a hemolysin). Streptolysin S is a nonantigenic hemolysin. Specifically, erythrogenic toxin causes the characteristic rash of scarlet fever.

Many factors play a role in the pathogenesis of *N. meningitidis*. A capsule containing *N*-acetylneuraminic acid is peculiar to *Neisseria* and *E. coli* K1. Fresh isolates carry pili on their surfaces, which function in adhesion. *Neisseria* has a variety of membrane proteins, and their role in pathogenesis can only be speculated upon at this time. The LPS of *Neisseria*, more correctly called lipooligosaccharide (LOS), is the endotoxic component of the cell.

There are no known toxins, hemolysins, or cell-wall constituents known to play a role in the pathogenesis of disease by *Brucella*. Rather, the ability of the organisms to survive within the host phagocyte and to inhibit neutrophil degranulation is a major disease-causing factor. Brucella has a predilection for tissues and organs rich in erythritol such as the uterus and placenta. Tropism to theses tissues results in abortion in cattle.

286 to 288. The answers are 286-a, 287-c, and 288-b. (*Ryan, pp 851-855. Toy, pp 90, 96.*) "Atypical pneumonia" is an old classification used for respiratory disease that is not lobar and is not "typical." That is, it does not include pneumonia caused by pneumococcus, *Klebsiella, Haemophilus*, or β-hemolytic streptococci that results in a typical lobular infiltrate. In recent years, the atypical pneumonias have become much more frequent than pneumococcal pneumonia. They are characterized by a slower onset with headache, joint pain, fever, and signs of an acute upper respiratory infection. There are usually no signs of acute respiratory distress, but patients report malaise and fatigue. The most common cause of atypical pneumonia is *M. pneumoniae*. A quick test for *M. pneumoniae* infection is cold agglutinins. The test may lack both sensitivity and specificity, but it is rapid and readily available compared with culture of *M. pneumoniae* or specific antibody formation.

In certain age groups (men over 55 years old), Legionnaires disease must be ruled out. While direct microscopy, culture, and serology are available, the detection of *Legionella* antigen in respiratory secretions is the most sensitive test available.

Campylobacter pneumoniae may also cause respiratory infection particularly in, but not limited to, children. Diagnosis is best made by growing these energy-defective bacteria in tissue culture such as HeLa cells. Serology is usually not helpful.

During the winter months, *Bordetella* infection may be quite prevalent, particularly in those patients whose immunizations are not updated. Adult *Bordetella* infection may not present with typical whooping cough symptoms and must be differentiated from other forms of acute bronchitis by culture on specific media or direct fluorescent microscopy.

Direct microscopy of sputum is an important preliminary test for sputum and other exudate specimens. One needs to be aware that the information obtained is limited in interpretation. No specific identity of a microorganism can be determined by gram staining and even mixtures of bacteria can be inferred. On the other hand, examination of gram stains may provide enough information for the physician to make immediate decisions on treatment and other management that may be modified by future laboratory results. Fluorescent Ab detection of an organism in sputum is more specific than gram staining. Here specific known Abs (single or in a mixture) are used to identify organisms present.

289. The answer is c. (*Murray: Medical Microbiology [2013], Ch 18, 20, 30, and 66.*) External otitis or swimmer's ear is an inflammation of the outer ear and the ear canal. In the virulent form of the disease—malignant external otitis, which occurs in people with diabetes, damage to the cranial nerves and bone may occur. External otitis is caused by either bacterial or fungal pathogens. Bacterial pathogens include *Pseudomonas aeruginosa, Staphylococcus aureus*, *Staphylococcus epidermidis*, and *Enterococcus faecalis*. Fungal pathogens include *Candida albicans* and *Aspergillus* spp. The majority of bacterial external otitis is caused by *P. aeruginosa*. *P. aeruginosa* produces pyocyanin, which is a blue pigment that catalyzes the production of superoxide and hydrogen peroxide. Pyocyanin also stimulates the release of IL-8 (CXCL8 in humans). *P. aeruginosa* also produces exotoxin A, which ADP-ribosylates EF-2 in the eukaryotic cell leading to the cessation of protein synthesis and cell death. Neither pyocyanin nor exotoxin A is produced by the other pathogens listed (*S. aureus, S. epidermidis, E. faecalis*, and *C. albicans*).

290. The answer is a. (*Murray: Medical Microbiology [2013], Ch 29; Ryan: Sherris Medical Microbiology [2010], Ch* 32.) The virulence factors produced by *Helicobacter pylori* are urease, flagella, mucinase, vacuolating toxin, and the Cag protein. Urease neutralizes gastric acid by hydrolyzing urea produced by gastric cells to produce ammonia and CO_2. Urease also stimulates the production of inflammatory cytokines. Mucinase degrades gastric mucus and reduces mucus viscosity to facilitate bacterial movement. *H. pylori* carry 4-7 polar flagella which provide the bacterium with motility that is essential to penetrate gastric mucus. *H. pylori* is sensitive to the acidic lumen of the stomach. Therefore, the highly motile *H. pylori* quickly penetrate the lumen and colonize the mucus layer that covers gastric mucosa where the pH is slightly alkaline. The vacuolating cytotoxin, which produces large cytoplasmic vacuoles, causes apoptosis in epithelial cells. The CagA protein, which is injected into cells via the type III secretion system, triggers reorganization of the actin skeleton within the intoxicated cells. It also stimulates neutrophil migration to the gastric mucosa. While the specific mechanism of *H. pylori* carcinogenesis is unknown, the CagA protein is the leading candidate for the oncogenic protein involved.

291. The answer is a. (*Murray: Medical Microbiology [2003], Ch 23, 29, 36.*) Guillain–Barré syndrome is an autoimmune disorder affecting the peripheral nervous system. The syndrome is an uncommon complication of infection with *Campylobacter jejuni* (the leading infectious cause in the United States). The ascending paralysis is characterized by weakening that begins in the feet and hands and migrates toward the trunk. The symptoms occur within few days and the recovery is slow. The likely cause of the disease is antigenic cross-reactivity between oligosaccharides of *C. jejuni* and glycosphingolipids on the surface of neuronal tissues. Antibodies to certain strains of *C. jejuni* (primarily serotype O:19) may also damage the myelin of the peripheral nervous system leading to muscle paralysis. Cytomegalovirus is the second most common infectious agent associated with GBS, but it does not cause the clinical symptoms described for this patient. *Clostridium tetani* produces a heat labile neurotoxin (tetanospasmin) which causes either localized or generalized muscle spasms; diarrhea is not a clinical syndrome caused by *C. tetani*. *Salmonella* and *Shigella* are associated with the autoimmune condition. Reiter syndrome, a form of reactive arthritis, characterized by conjunctivitis plus arthritis and, when caused by *Chlamydia trachomatis* and other genitourinary pathogens, urethritis. *Campylobacter jejuni* can also cause Reiter syndrome.

292. The answer is a. (*Murray: Medical Microbiology [2013], Ch 27, 28, 29.*) *Campylobacter jejuni* may be part of the normal flora of different domesticated animals including poultry, sheep, and cattle. Surface waters and soil where animal graze may be contaminated with *C. jejuni*. Therefore, *C. jejuni* outbreaks, which are zoonotics, may result from the ingestion of contaminated water that has not been treated. The main symptoms of *C. jejuni* infection are gastroenteritis, abdominal pain, fever, and malaise. The symptoms often peak at 24 to 48 hours after onset or may last for 7 to 10 days. The disease is generally self-limited. Due to the susceptibility of *Campylobacter* to different antibiotics including macrolides, erythromycin is the drug of choice to treat severe enteritis caused by *C. jejuni*. Optimum growth of *Campylobacter* occurs under reduced oxygen and increased carbon dioxide (5%-10%). Infection with *V. cholerae* results in a massive watery diarrhea that progresses to severe dehydration and hypovolemic shock. Infection with *V. parahaemolyticus* is associated with explosive watery diarrhea, abdominal pain, and fever. The gastroenteritis is self-limited. *V. parahaemolyticus* is usually found in an estuarine and marine environment and is associated with ingestion of contaminated shellfish. Enteropathogenic and enteroinvasive *E. coli* strains are major causes of diarrhea in underdeveloped countries. Both cause watery diarrhea and vomiting. *E. coli* grows rapidly under aerobic conditions.

293. The answer is e. (*Murray: Medical Microbiology [2013], Ch 18, 19, 28, 30.*) *Vibrio vulnificus* is a gram-negative rod that produces a number of virulence factors including capsule, cytolysin, collagenase, and protease. The bacteria may enter the body while one is swimming or wading in contaminated seawater. It also enters the body through open wounds. Initial features of *V. vulnificus*–infected wounds are swelling, erythema, and pain. This is usually followed by the development of vesicles or bullae, eventual tissue necrosis, and septicemia. *V. vulnificus*, which may produce large disfiguring ulcers, is commonly found in the Gulf of Mexico. In severely burned patients, *Pseudomonas aeruginosa* causes wound infection followed by localized tissue necrosis and bacteremia. Immersion in *P. aeruginosa*–contaminated hot tubs or swimming pools may result in localized infection of hair follicles (folliculitis), but not usually the development of bullae. Staphylococcus aureus may infect traumatic or surgical wounds. Infected areas are characterized by erythema, edema, pain, and the accumulation of purulent discharge. The infection is usually treated by opening the wound and draining the purulent discharge. *Streptococcus pyogenes* (Group *A Streptococcus*) causes various suppurative infections including pyoderma, a localized skin infection characterized by vesicles that progress to pustules; erysipelas, a localized skin infection characterized by inflammation and lymphadenopathy; and necrotizing fasciitis, which involves extensive destruction of muscles and fat. *V. parahaemolyticus* causes gastroenteritis and wound infection. However, *V. parahaemolyticus* wounds do not have the special features of *V. vulnificus*–infected wounds.

294. The answer is e. (*Murray: Medical Microbiology [2013], Ch 27, 30.*) *Pseudomonas aeruginosa* is a major cause of nosocomial pneumonia in health-care related settings. A major portion of the *P. aeruginosa*-associated nosocomial pneumonia occurs in immunocompromised patients in intensive care units who have undergone intubation (ventilator-associated pneumonia). Among the conditions that predispose immunocompromised patients to *P. aeruginosa* infection is the utilization of contaminated respiratory equipment during intubation. *P. aeruginosa* is a gram-negative, oxidase-positive, obligate aerobe that produces numerous extracellular virulence factors including exotoxins, proteases, and rhamnolipid. All of the microbes can cause pneumonia. However, none of the other microorganisms listed produce rhamnolipids. *Escherichia coli* and *Klebsiella pneumoniae* are members of the Enterobacteriaceae, which are oxidase negative. *Moraxella catarrhalis* is a gram-negative diplococcus that is also oxidase positive, but it does not produce toxins and is more fastidious in its growth than *P. aeruginosa*. *Haemophilus influenzae* is a fastidious, facultative anaerobe that requires hemin and NAD for growth.

295. The answer is d. (*Murray: Medical Microbiology [2013], Ch 27, 28, 29.*) *Vibrio cholerae* causes cholera, which is acquired by drinking water that has been contaminated with human feces. *V. cholerae* can also be acquired by eating food that has been washed with contaminated water. Cholera outbreaks usually occur in communities with poor sanitary systems. Even in developed countries, a breakdown in the sanitary systems by natural disasters such as floods or hurricanes may produce cholera outbreak. Infection with *V. cholerae* may result in simple colonization, mild gastroenteritis, or a severe often fatal watery diarrhea. Cholera is characterized by abrupt onset of watery diarrhea and vomiting. As the disease progresses, the stool becomes colorless and speckled with mucus (rice stool). Continuous fluid loss results in severe dehydration, metabolic acidosis, and hypovolemic shock (loss of potassium). This leads to a cardiac arrhythmia and renal failure. To avoid the hypovolemic shock, cholera patients must be immediately treated with electrolytes and fluid replacements. In untreated patients, the mortality rate may reach 60% but is reduced to 1% with the immediate treatment with electrolytes and fluid replacements. *Salmonella enterica* infection causes gastroenteritis, nausea, and vomiting. *Salmonella enterica* may also cause bacteremia. *Shigella flexneri* invades the colonic mucosa. Therefore, shigellosis is characterized by abdominal cramps, fever, and diarrhea with blood in stool. *Campylobacter jejuni* infection results in diarrhea, fever, and abdominal pain. Most infections are self-limited. *Vibrio vulnificus* causes wound infections characterized by tissue necrosis and accompanied by septicemia. *V. vulnificus* infection has a high mortality rate.

Rickettsiae, Chlamydiae, and Mycoplasma

Questions

296. Mycoplasmas have been cultivated from human mucous membranes and tissues, especially from the genital, urinary, and respiratory tracts. Chlamydia can be isolated from many of these sources as well. Both cause respiratory and genital tract infections. Adults may present with asymptomatic respiratory infection to serious pneumonitis, and identification of the etiologic agent usually determines the best antimicrobial treatment. Which of the following best describes the difference between mycoplasmas and chlamydiae?

a. Able to cause disease in humans
b. Able to cause urinary tract infection
c. Able to grow on artificial cell-free media
d. Being able to stain well with Gram stain
e. Susceptible to penicillin

297. A 39-year-old man presents with sudden, influenza-like symptoms. He states that he works in a slaughterhouse, and several of his coworkers have similar symptoms. Early stages of pneumonia are detected. Which of the following is the most likely etiologic organism?

a. *Coxiella burnetii*
b. *Rickettsia rickettsiae*
c. *Taenia solium*
d. *Taenia saginata*

298. Many survivors of military or natural disasters are at risk of infection due to loss of public health services. Rickettsial infections—except Q fever and the ehrlichiosis—typically are manifested by fever, rashes, and vasculitis. Which of the following best characterizes rickettsiae, which include the spotted fevers, Q fever, typhus, and scrub typhus?

a. Easily stained (gram-negative) with a Gram stain
b. Maintained in nature, with humans as the mammalian reservoir
c. Obligate intracellular parasites
d. Stable outside the host cell
e. The cause of infections in which a rash is always present

299. A man with chills, fever, and headache is thought to have "atypical" pneumonia. History reveals that he raises chickens, and that approximately 2 weeks ago he lost a large number of them to an undiagnosed disease. Which of the following is the most likely diagnosis of this man's condition?

a. Anthrax
b. Leptospirosis
c. Ornithosis
d. Relapsing fever
e. Q fever

300. An ill patient denies being bitten by insects. However, he spent some time in a milking barn and indicates that it was dusty. Of the following rickettsial diseases, which one has he most likely contracted?

a. Brill–Zinsser disease
b. Q fever
c. Rickettsial pox
d. Rocky Mountain spotted fever (RMSF)
e. Scrub typhus

301. A 23-year-old college senior presents to the student health clinic with symptoms of a suspected sexually transmitted disease (STD). Neisseria and chlamydia agents are ruled out. Which of the following organisms is the most likely cause of his nongonococcal urethritis (NGU)?

a. *Mycoplasma fermentans*
b. *Mycoplasma hominis*
c. *Mycoplasma mycoides*
d. *Mycoplasma pneumoniae*
e. *Ureaplasma urealyticum*

302. A young man, home on leave from the military, went camping in the woods to detect deer movement for future hunting. Ten days later, he developed fever, malaise, and myalgia. Leukopenia and thrombocytopenia were observed, as well as several tick bites. Which of the following statements best describes human monocytic ehrlichiosis (HME)?

a. Clinical diagnosis is based on the presence of erythema migrans (EM)
b. Diagnosis is usually made serologically but morulae may be seen in the cytoplasm of monocytes
c. It is a fatal disease transmitted by the bite of a dog
d. Symptoms include vomiting and paralysis
e. The HME agent grows on artificial media

303. A couple, who did not know each other very well, dated and had sexual contact. Several weeks later, the man noticed a small, painless vesicle on his penis, which ruptured and then healed. Soon, his inguinal lymph nodes enlarged and discharged pus through multiple sinus tracts. Lymphogranuloma venereum (LGV) is a venereal disease caused by serotype L1, L2, or L3 of *Chlamydia trachomatis*. The differential diagnosis should include which of the following?

a. Babesiosis
b. Chancroid
c. Mononucleosis
d. Psittacosis
e. Shingles

304. A forest worker experiences a sudden onset of fever, headache, myalgias, and prostration. A macular rash develops several days later, with it appearing first on the hands and feet before moving onto his trunk. Which of the following treatments is most appropriate?

a. Amphotericin B
b. Cephalosporin
c. Erythromycin
d. Sulfonamides
e. Tetracycline

305. Chlamydiae are true bacteria with an unusual three-stage cycle of development. These characteristics are important to understand to be able to distinguish them from other bacteria and viruses that can cause similar disease presentations and choice of treatments. For the growth of *Chlamydia*, which of the following is the correct sequence of these events?

a. Development of an initial body, synthesis of elementary body progeny, penetration of the host cell
b. Penetration of the host cell, development of an initial body, synthesis of elementary body progeny
c. Penetration of the host cell, synthesis of elementary body progeny, development of an initial body
d. Synthesis of elementary body progeny, development of an initial body, penetration of the host cell
e. Synthesis of elementary body progeny, penetration of the host cell, development of an initial body

306. Young children in a small Egyptian village have eye infections that present with lacrimation, discharge, and conjunctival hyperemia. Scarring of the conjunctiva and noticeable loss of vision occur in some. Which of the following statements best describes the etiologic agent that caused these infections and relative treatment?

a. The organisms are gram-positive and treatable with penicillin
b. The organisms have no cell wall and will only respond to tetracycline
c. The organisms are gram-negative, and prophylactic use of tetracyclines can prevent infections
d. Gram stains of conjunctival scrapings are useful diagnostic tests to justify treatment with sulfonamides
e. The organisms are isolated on blood agar plates and respond to cell wall-inhibiting antibiotics

307. The ehrlichia group organisms are obligate intracellular bacteria that are taxonomically grouped with the rickettsiae and have tick vectors. Human granulocytic ehrlichiosis (HGE) is a disease transmitted to humans by the bite of a tick, *Ixodes scapularis.* Three ehrlichia species are present in different parts of the United States and produce inclusions in circulating WBCs. Which of the following statements about HGE is correct?

a. Clinical diagnosis is based on the presence of EM
b. HGE is caused by *Ehrlichia chaffeensis*
c. HGE is a self-limiting disease
d. HGE is characterized by an acute onset of fever, severe headache, and influenza-like symptoms
e. The causative organism can be grown on ordinary laboratory media

308. The "spotted fever" group of rickettsial diseases is caused by a variety of rickettsial species. While not critical for treatment of disease, the speciation of these organisms is essential for epidemiologic studies. Which of the following rickettsiae is found in the United States and is a member of the spotted fever group?

a. *Rickettsia akari*
b. *Rickettsia australis*
c. *Rickettsia conorii*
d. *Rickettsia prowazekii*
e. *Rickettsia sibirica*

309. A 36-year-old man presents to his primary care physician's office complaining of fever and headache. On examination, he has leucopenia, increased liver enzymes, and inclusion bodies are seen in his monocytes. History reveals that he is outdoorsman and that he remembers removing a tick from his leg. Which of the following is the most likely diagnosis?

a. Ehrlichiosis
b. Lyme disease
c. Q fever
d. Rocky Mountain spotted fever
e. Tularemia

310. Rickettsial organisms infect humans worldwide, although geographic locations may be limited for some species and possibly produce some challenges in medical diagnosis. All are obligate intracellular parasites, except *C. burnetii*, and transmitted by an insect vector. Typhus, spotted fever, and scrub typhus share which of the following manifestations of disease?

a. Arthritis
b. Common vector
c. Fever and rash
d. Short incubation period (<48 hours)
e. Similar geographic distribution

311. Humans are the natural hosts for *C. trachomatis*, which is widespread in the population and a well-known cause of STD. The organism is a well-documented cause of NGU in men and urethritis, cervicitis, and pelvic inflammatory disease in women. This organism is also implicated in which of the following?

a. Blindness
b. Middle ear infection in young children
c. Perinatal retinitis
d. Sexually transmitted cardiac disease in adults
e. Urinary tract infection in children

312. A homosexual male presents to his physician with bilateral inguinal buboes (lymph nodes), one of which seems ready to rupture. He recalls having two small, painless genital lesions that healed rapidly. The etiologic agent is isolated using McCoy cells. Which of the following statements best characterizes LGV?

a. It is most common in temperate regions
b. In the United States, it is more common among women
c. The causative agent is *C. trachomatis*
d. LGV does not become chronic
e. Penicillin is effective in early treatment

313. Dozens of political refugees fleeing from active warfare and living in a dense forest environment with crowded, unsanitary conditions experienced nonspecific symptoms, followed by high fever, severe headache, chills, myalgia, and arthralgia. All had body lice. Improved living conditions in a refugee camp and treatment with tetracycline brought resolution to most individuals. Which of the following statements describes the etiological agent responsible for their infection?

a. The disease was caused by an organism with no cell walls
b. The disease was caused by a viral agent
c. The disease was derived from rodents living in the forest area
d. Reoccurrence of milder disease may occur in later years
e. The disease was caused by a tick vector

314. An 18-year-old student develops symptoms consistent with primary atypical pneumonia (PAP). This is generally a mild disease, ranging from subclinical infection to serious pneumonitis; the latter characterized by onset of fever, headache, sore throat, and cough but requires laboratory tests to determine which organism is involved and a basis for antimicrobial choices. Which of the following organisms causes this disease in humans?

a. *Mycoplasma fermentans*
b. *Mycoplasma hominis*
c. *Mycoplasma pneumoniae*
d. *Mycoplasma orale*
e. *Ureaplasma urealyticum*

315. NGU is the most common STD in men. Within 2 weeks, the symptoms usually include painful urination and a urethral discharge. Because of the similarity of NGU symptoms with *Neisseria gonococcus* infection, diagnosis depends on culture of the discharge. While the majority of NGU are caused by *C. trachomatis*, which of the following organisms is very significant in causing additional cases in humans?

a. *Mycoplasma fermentans*
b. *Mycoplasma hominis*
c. *Mycoplasma pneumoniae*
d. *Mycoplasma orale*
e. *Ureaplasma urealyticum*

316. A healthy oral cavity has a microbial population consisting of gram-positive streptococci and diphtheroids. Anaerobic rods and spirochetes are present in low numbers and may be opportunistic for disease. Which of the following organisms also normally inhabits the healthy human oral cavity?

a. *Mycoplasma fermentans*
b. *Mycoplasma hominis*
c. *Mycoplasma pneumoniae*
d. *Mycoplasma orale*
e. *Ureaplasma urealyticum*

317. At least 15 species of *Mycoplasma* are of human origin, and five are of primary importance. Which of the following organisms normally inhabits the female genital tract and is strongly associated with salpingitis and ovarian abscesses?

a. *Mycoplasma fermentans*
b. *Mycoplasma hominis*
c. *Mycoplasma pneumoniae*
d. *Mycoplasma orale*
e. *Ureaplasma urealyticum*

318. Suppurative inguinal adenitis usually starts by the appearance of small, painless lesions on the external genitalia that heal spontaneously. Then regional lymph nodes enlarge and become painful and often discharge pus through multiple sinus tracts. Which organism listed below is responsible for this STD?

a. *Bartonella (Rochalimaea) henselae*
b. *Chlamydia trachomatis*
c. *Coxiella burnetii*
d. *Ehrlichia chaffeensis*
e. *Rickettsia rickettsii*

319. Which of the following is transmitted by the bite of a hard *Ixodes* tick, where circulating leukocytes are infected and morulae (clusters of microorganisms) form, which can be treated with tetracyclines and rifamycins?

a. *Bartonella (Rochalimaea) henselae*
b. *Chlamydia trachomatis*
c. *Coxiella burnetii*
d. *Ehrlichia chaffeensis*
e. *Rickettsia rickettsii*

320. Six laboratory technicians at the state health laboratory were working on a study using rabbits. The experiments involved an outbreak of acute febrile illnesses in workers from a slaughterhouse. The organism of interest was a gram-negative bacterium with tropism for mononuclear cells. A dysfunction of the animal cage air safety system allowed contaminated air to escape into the animal care facility and research laboratories. Four of the six technicians now suffer from a flu-like illness and pneumonitis. Which organism listed below is most likely the cause of this outbreak?

a. *Bartonella (Rochalimaea) henselae*
b. *Chlamydia trachomatis*
c. *Coxiella burnetii*
d. *Ehrlichia chaffeensis*
e. *Rickettsia rickettsii*

321. A 56-year-old woman in Uganda presents to an emergency clinic. The woman is homeless and extremely dirty. She is also very dehydrated and the duty nurse notices lice in her hair and clothing. The patient reported high fever, severe headaches, and muscle pain. A petechial rash was observed all over her body. After 72 hours in the hospital, the woman died. A Gram-stain of the organism showed a weakly staining Gram-negative bacterium that could not be grown in vitro. What organism was the most likely cause of her infection?

a. *Chlamydia trachomatis*
b. *Coxiella burnetii*
c. *Rickettsia prowazekii*
d. *Rickettsia rickettsii*
e. *Rickettsia typhi*

322. A 25-year-old male patient presents to the emergency room in July in Texas. He complains of shortness of breath and a low-grade fever. The emergency room physician suspects tracheobronchitis. The patient also complains of a dry, nonproductive cough. A patchy bronchopneumonia was observed on x-ray. Cold agglutinins were observed in the patient's serum. The physician suspects a *Mycoplasma pneumoniae* infection. Which of the following antibiotics does the physician know that he cannot or should not administer in this situation?

a. Clindamycin
b. Erythromycin
c. Kanamycin
d. Penicillin
e. Tetracycline

323. A 45-year-old man living in Uganda presents to the emergency clinic. He complains that he has a "groin swelling." He says that this "groin swelling" has broken open and a thick, white fluid has leaked out. This patient stated that he had been sexually active for 30 years and that he observed a "sore" on his penis about a month ago. The patient also complained of recent headaches, fever, and muscle pain. A bacterium was isolated from this thick white fluid, but it would not grow in vitro. It would only grow in tissue culture. The organism was a Gram-negative rod. Which of the following bacteria was the cause of this man's infection?

a. *Chlamydophila psittaci*
b. *Chlamydophila pneumoniae*
c. *Chlamydia trachomatis*
d. *Neisseria gonorrheae*
e. *Treponema pallidum*

324. A week after returning from a July camping trip to the Blue Ridge Mountains in North Carolina, a 10-year-old boy is brought to the emergency room with a severe headache, fever, and muscle pain. He also has a maculopapular rash on his arms and legs. Although the rash began on his arms and legs, it has now spread to his trunk. He remembers removing several ticks from around his ankles on the camping trip. What is the organism most likely to the cause of this young man's infection?

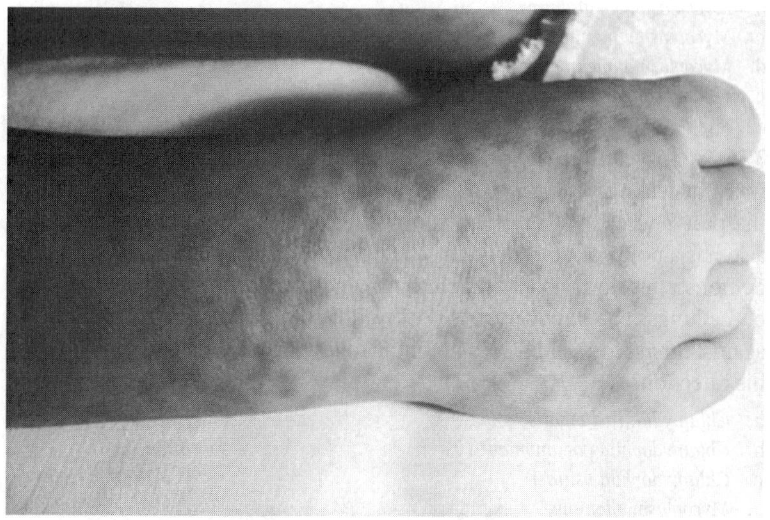

(From Public Health Image Library. Content provider: Center for Disease Control.)

a. *Coxiella burnetii*
b. Group A streptococci (*Streptococcus pyogenes*)
c. *Rickettsia prowazekii*
d. *Rickettsia ricketsii*
e. *Salmonella typhi*

325. A 19-year-old college student presents to the university infirmary with what the doctor thought was NGU. The physician had a very hard time isolating a causative organism from the young man. The clinical lab finally got the organism to grow in vitro and they reported that the offending organism produced extremely small colonies and would only grow in the presence of urea. The organism often died rapidly after the initial isolation. The organism causing this student's NGU was which of the following?

a. *Coxiella burnetii*
b. *Mycoplasma genitalium*
c. *Mycoplasma hominis*
d. *Mycoplasma pneumoniae*
e. *Ureaplasma urealyticum*

326. A 15-year-old boy presents to his family doctor and reports that he was not feeling very good. He says that he has been feeling "lousy" for the past 2 weeks with a fever, runny nose, headaches, and no energy. He also has a nonproductive cough. The doctor orders a pulmonary x-ray that demonstrates no consolidation and only patchy opacity in the lower lobes of the lungs. The boy's serum is positive for cold agglutinins and antibodies against *Streptococcus* MG. Which of the following bacteria is responsible for his infection?

a. *Chlamydia trachomatis*
b. *Chlamydophila pneumoniae*
c. *Chlamydophila psittaci*
d. *Mycoplasma hominis*
e. *Mycoplasma pneumoniae*

327. A 40-year-old man develops a cough that is nonproductive and goes to see his family doctor. He says that he has been feeling "lousy" and has bronchitis, sinusitis, and a sore throat. The doctor orders an x-ray that does not show consolidation, but rather a patchy infiltrate in his upper right lung. The man denies taking any new pets or animals recently into his house. A Gram-stain of the sputum specimen shows a few Gram-negative rods that do not stain very well. Samples sent to the clinical laboratory do not grow on normal laboratory media (eg, blood agar), but do grow in monolayer cells in tissue culture. What bacterium is most likely to be the cause of this man's infection?

a. *Chlamydia trachomatis*
b. *Chlamydophila psittaci*
c. *Chlamydophila pneumoniae*
d. *Mycoplasma pneumoniae*
e. *Streptococcus pneumoniae*

328. A 35-year-old woman living in Minnesota goes to her family physician. She complains that for the past 8 days she has experienced a flu-like illness. The illness consisted of muscle pain, lethargy, headaches, and a high fever (almost 41°C). She states that she had removed several ticks from around her ankles about 14 days ago. The physician gives her a shot of penicillin, but when she returns to see him about a week later, she reports no improvement. The physician then draws her blood and submits it to a clinical laboratory for identification. No bacteria grew out on blood agar, but a Giemsa stain of the blood culture showed coccobacillary organisms inside polymorphonuclear neutrophils. Which of the following bacteria was most likely to be the cause of her illness?

a. *Anaplasma phagocytophilum*
b. *Coxiella burnetii*
c. *Chlamydophila pneumoniae*
d. *Chlamydophila psittaci*
e. *Rickettsia rickettsii*

329. A 27-year-old man presents to his family doctor because he has been having a mucopurulent discharge from his penis. He had recently visited a prostitute and he had unprotected sex with her. He was afraid that he had caught the "clap". He did not have a fever and he said he experienced no pain upon urination. The doctor noted a white urethral discharge from the man's penis. This discharge was then sent to the clinical laboratory. Because the physician suspected *Neisseria gonorrheae* infection, the lab stained the specimen and tried to grow it on blood agar. The causative organism did not grow on blood agar, but would only grow in certain cells lines. What was the organism that caused this man's infection?

a. *Chlamydophila pneumoniae*
b. *Chlamydophila psittaci*
c. *Chlamydia trachomatis*
d. *Neisseria gonorrheae*
e. *Treponema pallidum*

330. A physician was asked to come to an Indian reservation in South Dakota because of an outbreak of a serious eye infection. The infection was believed to have spread from person to person by infected towels at the gymnasium. Patients reported conjunctivitis with widespread inflammation. In some cases, the patient's conjunctiva became so damaged, that the eyelids turned inward, thus scratching the eyeball every time they blinked. In some patients, there was corneal scarring and invasion of blood vessels into the cornea. Fortunately, the physician recognized what the disease was, its cause, and how to treat it. He administered azithromycin in one dose and the infections resolved. What organism was causing the described symptoms?

a. *Chlamydia trachomatis*
b. *Chlamydophila pneumoniae*
c. *Chlamydophila psittaci*
d. *Rickettsia prowazekii*
e. *Rickettsia rickettsii*

331. A 45-year-old man reported to the emergency room in respiratory distress. His symptoms included muscle pain, congestion, a dry cough, and difficulty breathing. He also was experiencing fever and chills. A chest x-ray showed consolidation of the left lower lobe, and a patchy infiltrate of his right upper lobe. He was given a shot of penicillin and hospitalized. He did not improve on this antibiotic so he was given doxycycline, which allowed for his improvement. It was decided to give doxycycline after his attending physician learned he was a bird enthusiast and had recently received an African parrot that had arrived sick and had died. What was the name of the organism with which the man was infected?

a. *Chlamydophila pneumoniae*
b. *Chlamydophila psittaci*
c. *Chlamydia trachomatis*
d. *Rickettsia prowazekii*
e. *Rickettsia rickettsii*

332. A 50-year-old man presented to his family doctor complaining of flu-like symptoms. The doctor gave him a shot of penicillin and sent him home. The man came back a week later and in fact, felt worse. The man was a rancher and raised a lot of cattle. He told the doctor that he had congenital heart disease and an attack of rheumatic fever when he was young. The man now complained of fever, night sweats, continual coughing, weight loss, and lethargy. The doctor had the man hospitalized because he now suspected subacute bacterial endocarditis (SBE). A culture of his blood did not show any bacterial growth, but a serum analysis for antibodies against a certain bacterium was positive. As a result of finding antibodies to this organism, treatment with doxycycline was begun and the patient improved and was released from the hospital. What was the name of the organism with which the man was infected?

a. *Chlamydophila psittaci*
b. *Chlamydophila pneumoniae*
c. *Chlamydia trachomatis*
d. *Coxiella burnetii*
e. Viridans streptococci

333. In July of 1987 in Texas, a man went to his family doctor complaining of flu-like symptoms, high fever, lethargy, muscle pain, and a headache. He complained that he just felt "lousy". When the doctor took the patient's history, he learned that the man was an avid hiker and camper. In fact, the man just came back from a recent camping trip to South Carolina. The man remembered removing a blood-filled tick from his leg on that trip. He had killed the tick and thought nothing more of it. Now, he felt it might be relevant. The doctor also felt this information was relevant and asked for a Giemsa stain of the man's blood by the clinical lab. The results came back stating that there were morulae inside the monocytes in the man's blood. The doctor, based on these results, immediately started the man on doxycycline because he felt the man was infected with which organism?

a. *Amblyomma americanum*
b. *Anaplasma phagocytophilum*
c. *Ehrlichia canis*
d. *Ehrlichia ewingii*
e. *Ehrlichia chaffeensis*

334. A United States businessman presented to the emergency room in New York City. He complained of severe headaches, muscle pain, and fever. He had a maculopapular rash on his trunk that was moving to his arms and legs. The emergency room doctors were stumped as to what might be causing this disease state. When they took his history, he told them that he had just come back from a business trip to Japan where he had spent a few days camping in the mountains and had been bitten by some insects. He stated that he never saw the insects, so he did not know what kind they were. He said he knew what fleas and ticks looked like and he was sure that he was not bitten by either of those. In fact, he could show the doctors the eschars of the insect bites. When asked how long ago this was, he replied "about 11 days". Because of this information gathered by taking the patient's history, the emergency room doctors felt confident they knew what had caused the patient's symptoms. They gave the patient doxycycline and told him to see his family doctor for a follow-up after 1 week. When this man went to his family doctor, he was greatly improved. What organism did the New York businessman have that had caused his infection?

a. *Dermacentor andersoni*
b. *Orientia tsutsugamushi*
c. *Rickettsia prowazekii*
d. *Rickettsia rickettsii*
e. *Rickettsia typhi*

Rickettsiae, Chlamydiae, and Mycoplasma

Answers

296. The answer is c. (*Brooks, pp 344-345. Levinson, pp 171-172. Murray, pp 421-426. Ryan, pp 409, 463. Toy, p 116.*) Unlike chlamydiae, mycoplasmas can replicate in cell-free media. They lack a rigid cell wall and are bound by a triple-layer unit membrane. For this reason, they are completely resistant to the action of penicillins.

297. The answer is a. (*Brooks, pp 353-354. Levinson, pp 182-184. Murray, pp 438-439. Ryan, p 477.*) Q fever is an acute, flu-like illness caused by *C. burnetii.* It is one rickettsial disease not transmitted by the bite of a tick. *C. burnetii* is found in high concentrations in the urine, feces, and placental tissue/amniotic fluid of cattle, goats, and sheep. Transmission to humans is by aerosol inhalation of those specimens. *Rickettsia* is present in the United States and South America, but is transmitted by ticks that feed on rodents or dogs. The parasitic *Taenia* species are transmitted by ingestion of undercooked meat.

298. The answer is c. (*Brooks, pp 350-354. Levinson, pp 182-184. Murray, pp 427-436. Ryan, pp 472-473.*) Rickettsiae are obligate intracellular parasites that depend on host cells for their phosphorylated energy compounds. The significant rickettsial diseases in North America include RMSF (*R. rickettsii*), Q fever (*C. burnetii*), and typhus (*R. prowazekii, R. typhi*). Laboratory diagnosis of rickettsial disease is based on serologic analysis rather than isolation of the organism.

299. The answer is c. (*Brooks, pp 364-365. Levinson, pp 179-181. Murray, pp 441-450. Ryan, p 469.*) Ornithosis (psittacosis) is caused by *C. psittaci.* Humans usually contract the disease from infected birds kept as pets or from infected poultry, including poultry in dressing plants. Although ornithosis may be asymptomatic in humans, severe pneumonia can develop. Fortunately, the disease is cured easily with tetracycline. *Bacillus anthracis* is a spore-forming, gram-positive bacillus that has a protective capsule made of glutamic acid (amino acid) residues. Humans are infected accidentally by contact with infected animals or their products. Skin lesions, seen most often, are known as woolsorter's disease. *Leptospira* organisms are tightly coiled spirochetes. Human contact is often in water, where the organism enters breaks in the skin. They produce hemorrhage and necrosis in the liver and kidneys and often present as aseptic meningitis. Relapsing fever is caused by *Borrelia recurrentis* and is transmitted by the body louse or *Ornithodoros* ticks. An unusual feature of this disease is the selection of new antigenic forms of the organism after host antibody formation. Q fever is caused by a rickettsial organism, *C. burnetii*.

300. The answer is b. (*Brooks, pp 350-354. Levinson, pp 182-184. Murray, pp 427-436. Ryan, p 477.*) Most rickettsial diseases are transmitted to humans by way of arthropod vectors. The only exception is Q fever, which is caused by *C. burnetii*. This organism is transmitted by inhalation of contaminated dust and aerosols or by ingestion of contaminated milk. Brill–Zinsser disease is a recurrence of epidemic typhus (louse borne). Rickettsial pox is transmitted by a mite from the mouse reservoir. RMSF is caused by *R. rickettsii* and is transmitted by ticks from the rodent or dog reservoirs. Scrub typhus is an Asian/Pacific area disease with a mite transferring the organism from a rodent reservoir.

301. The answer is e. (*Brooks, p 347. Levinson, pp 171-172. Murray, pp 421-426. Ryan, p 413.*) *Ureaplasma urealyticum* has been associated with NGU as well as infertility. *Mycoplasma pneumoniae* is the etiologic agent of PAP. *Mycoplasma hominis*, although isolated from up to 30% of patients with NGU, has yet to be implicated as a cause of that disease. *Mycoplasma fermentans* has, on rare occasions, been isolated from the oropharynx and genital tract. *Mycoplasma mycoides* causes bovine pleuropneumonia.

302. The answer is b. (*Brooks, p 355. Levinson, pp 182-184. Murray, pp 435-437. Ryan, p 478.*) HME, caused by the bite of the tick *Amblyomma americanum* infected with *E. chaffeensis*, causes an illness not unlike RMSF, except a rash usually does not occur. Diagnosis is usually made serologically, and treatment of choice is tetracycline. Symptoms include high fever, severe headache, and myalgias. EM is the characteristic skin lesion seen in Lyme disease. HME is transmitted by a tick vector, as mentioned previously, and not by a dog bite. Vomiting and paralysis are not usual symptoms seen in HME cases. Cultures can be isolated using tissue culture cell lines, but not artificial media (agar, broth, etc).

303. The answer is b. (*Brooks, p 362. Levinson, pp 179-181. Murray, pp 441-450. Ryan, pp 466-467.*) The differential diagnosis of LGV includes syphilis, genital herpes, and chancroid. Several clinical tests can be used to rule out syphilis and genital herpes. These include a negative (negative to rule out; positive to rule in) dark-field examination as well as positive serologic findings for syphilis and the demonstration of herpes simplex virus by cytology or culture. *Haemophilus ducreyi* can usually be isolated from the ulcer in chancroid. Babesiosis is an RBC-infecting tick-borne disease, usually derived from dogs or Texas cattle. Most cases are asymptomatic, but clindamycin or azithromycin are effective treatments. Mononucleosis is seen most often in infectious mononucleosis caused by EBV. Psittacosis is caused by inhaling aerosols or direct contact with birds infected with *C. psittaci* and is usually a mild upper respiratory illness. Shingles would be evidenced by masses of painful herpetic lesions caused by reactivation of VZV (chicken pox).

304. The answer is e. (*Brooks, pp 350-354. Levinson, pp 182-184. Murray, pp 427-436. Ryan, p 475.*) Tetracyclines and chloramphenicol are effective, provided that treatment is started early for rickettsial diseases, including RMSF, as in this case. Those should be given orally daily and continued for several days after the rash subsides. Intravenous dosage can be used in severely ill patients. Sulfonamides enhance the disease and are contraindicated. The other antibiotics are ineffective. Antibiotics only suppress the bacteria's growth, and the patient's immune system must eradicate them.

305. The answer is b. (*Brooks, p 359. Levinson, pp 179-181. Murray, pp 441-450, Ryan, p 465. Toy, p 52.*) The developmental cycle of *Chlamydia* begins with the elementary body attaching to and then penetrating the host cell. The elementary body, now in a vacuole bounded by host-cell membrane, becomes an initial body. Within about 12 hours, the initial body has divided to form many small elementary particles encased within an inclusion body in the cytoplasm; these progeny are liberated by host-cell rupture.

306. The answer is c. (*Brooks, pp 360-361. Levinson, pp 179-181. Murray, pp 441-450. Ryan, pp 464-466.*) *Chlamydia trachomatis* serovars A, B, Ba, and C are responsible for endemic trachoma. While diagnosis is usually dependent upon observation of intracellular inclusions with a glycogen matrix in which elementary bodies are embedded, Gram stain preparations are not useful diagnostic tools. The cell wall most closely resembles a high lipid content and may stain gram-negative or variable. A single monthly dose of doxycycline can result in significant clinical improvement and be preventative. Cell wall inhibitors (penicillins, cephalosporins) result in cell-wall defective forms but are not effective in clinical diseases treatment. Inhibitors of protein synthesis (tetracyclines, erythromycin) are effective in most clinical infections.

307. The answer is d. (*Brooks, p 355. Levinson, pp 182-184. Murray, pp 435-437. Ryan, p 478.*) HGE is caused by the bite of *I. scapularis* infected with either *E. phagocytophila* or *E. ewingii* or *Ehrlichia equi.* A rash rarely occurs and EM does not occur, but the symptoms (fever, chills, headache, myalgia, nausea, vomiting, anorexia, and weight loss) are similar to those seen in RMSF. Serological tests show that subclinical ehrlichiosis occurs frequently. *Ehrlichia chaffeensis* causes human monocyte ehrlichiosis and may cause severe or fatal illness. Seroprevalence studies suggest that subclinical ehrlichiosis occurs frequently. The organisms can be isolated using cell culture procedures.

308. The answer is a. (*Brooks, pp 350-354. Levinson, pp 182-184. Murray, pp 427-436. Ryan, p 473.*) The primary cause of RMSF is *R. rickettsii*, although rickettsial pox is caused by *R. akari*, the only other member of the spotted fever group that resides in the United States. *Rickettsia sibirica* is responsible for tick typhus in China; *R. australis* causes typhus in Australia, as the name signifies; and *R. conorii* causes European and African rickettsioses. *Rickettsia prowazekii* is not a member of the spotted fever group; it causes epidemic typhus.

309. The answer is a. (*Brooks, p 355. Levinson, pp 182-184. Murray, pp 435-437. Ryan, p 478.*) All the listed diseases except Q fever are tick-borne. Two human forms of ehrlichiosis can occur: HME, caused by *E. chaffeensis*, and HGE, caused by *E. ewingii*. Ehrlichiosis was previously recognized only as a veterinary pathogen. HME infection is transmitted by the brown dog tick and *A. americanum.* HGE infection is transmitted by *I. scapularis*, the same tick that transmits Lyme disease. Both infections cause fever and leukopenia. A rash rarely occurs. *E. chaffeensis* infects monocytes, and HGE infects granulocytes; both organisms produce inclusion bodies called *morulae*. *Francisella tularensis* is a small, gram-negative, nonmotile coccobacillus. Humans most commonly acquire the organism after contact with the tissues or body fluid of an infected mammal or the bite of an infected tick. The Rickettsia *C. burnetii* causes Q fever, and humans are usually infected by aerosol of a sporelike form shed in milk, urine, feces, or placenta of infected sheep, cattle, or goats. Lyme disease is caused by a spirochete, *B. burgdorferi*, and produces the characteristic lesion erythema chronicum migrans (ECM). The etiologic agent of RMSF is *R. rickettsii.* It usually produces a rash that begins in the extremities and then involves the trunk.

310. The answer is c. (*Brooks, pp 350-354. Levinson, pp 182-184. Murray, pp 427-436. Ryan, pp 473-475.*) Typhus, spotted fever, and scrub typhus are all caused by rickettsiae (*R. prowazekii, R. rickettsii*, and *R. tsutsugamushi*, respectively). Clinically, the diseases have several similarities. Each has an incubation period of 1 to 2 weeks, followed by a febrile period, which usually includes a rash. During the febrile period, rickettsiae can be found in the patient's blood, and there is disseminated focal vasculitis of small blood vessels. The geographic area associated with these diseases is usually different. Scrub typhus is usually found in Japan, Southeast Asia, and the Pacific, while spotted fever is usually found in the western hemisphere. Typhus has a worldwide incidence. (Typhus is caused by lice and fleas, spotted fever is caused by ticks and mites, and scrubs are caused by mites.)

311. The answer is a. (*Brooks, p 360. Levinson, pp 179-181. Murray, pp 441-450. Ryan, p 464. Toy, p 52.*) Trachoma has been the greatest single cause of blindness in the world. *Chlamydia trachomatis* is the most common cause of STD in the United States and is also responsible for the majority of cases of infant conjunctivitis and infant pneumonia. Middle ear infection in children is most often caused by bacteria normally found in the oral cavity or upper respiratory system. Gram-positive cocci, *Pseudomonas* species, and a host of other normal flora can be involved. Trachoma involves the keratoconjunctiva area of the eye, not the retina. Sexually transmitted cardiac in adults and children's urinary tract infections are not reported to be caused by *C. trachomatis.*

312. The answer is c. (*Brooks, p 362. Levinson, p 179. Murray, pp 441-450. Ryan, pp 466-468.*) LGV is an STD caused by *C. trachomatis* of immunotypes L1, L2, and L3. It is more commonly found in tropical climates. In the United States, the sex ratio is reported to be 3.4 males to 1 female. Tetracycline has been successful in treating this disease in the early stages; however, late stages usually require surgery. Unless effective antimicrobial drug treatment is given promptly, chronic inflammatory processes can lead to fibrosis, lymphatic obstruction, and rectal strictures.

313. The answer is d. (*Brooks, pp 350-354. Levinson, pp 182-184. Murray, pp 427-436. Ryan, pp 475-476.*) The disease described is epidemic typhus or louse-borne typhus. It is caused by *R. prowazekii* and is spread by the human body louse, *Pediculus humanus*. Lice obviously occur most readily in unsanitary conditions brought on by war or natural disasters, where normal healthy living conditions are unavailable. Rickettsial diseases respond to tetracycline treatment and vector control. The organisms replicate in endothelial cells, resulting in vasculitis. Recrudescent disease (recurrence in later years) has been demonstrated in people exposed to epidemic typhus during World War II. This form of disease is generally milder, and convalescence is shorter. Rickettsiae are pleomorphic coccobacilli with cell walls that do not stain well in Gram stain procedures. No viruses were involved in this problem because tetracycline was able to kill the infecting organisms. Humans are the main reservoir of the causative agent.

314 to 317. The answers are 314-c, 315-e, 316-d, and 317-b. (*Brooks, pp 344-347. Levinson, pp 171-172. Murray, pp 421-426. Ryan, pp 409-412. Toy, p 116.*) Members of the mycoplasma group that are pathogenic for humans include *M. pneumoniae* and *U. urealyticum*. *Mycoplasma pneumoniae* is best known as the causative agent of PAP, which may be confused clinically with influenza or legionellosis. It also is associated with arthritis, pericarditis, aseptic meningitis, and the Guillain–Barré syndrome. *M. pneumoniae* can be cultivated on special media and identified by immunofluorescence staining and "fried egg" colonies on agar.

Ureaplasma urealyticum (once called *tiny*, or *T. strain*) has been implicated in cases of NGU. As the name implies, this organism is able to split urea, a fact of diagnostic significance. *Ureaplasma urealyticum* is part of the normal flora of the genitourinary tract, particularly in women.

Both *M. orale* and *M. salivarium* are inhabitants of the normal human oral cavity. These species are commensals and do not play a role in disease.

The only other species of *Mycoplasma* associated with human disease is *M. hominis*. A normal inhabitant of the genital tract of women, this organism has been demonstrated to produce an acute respiratory illness that is associated with sore throat and tonsillar exudate, but not with fever. *M. hominis* can cause disease outside the urinary tract in immunosuppressed patients or immunocompetent patients after trauma of the genitourinary tract. Other opportunistic infections known to be caused by *M. hominis* include wound infections, osteomyelitis, brain abscess, pneumonia, and peritonitis. It has been associated with neonatal pneumonia and sepsis. *Mycoplasma fermentans* is an animal isolate.

318. The answer is b. (*Brooks, pp 360-361. Levinson, pp 179-181. Murray, pp 441-450. Ryan, pp 463-470, 471-479. Toy, p 52.*) Chlamydiae are gram-negative bacteria that are obligate, intracellular parasites. They are divided into three species: *C. trachomatis*, *C. pneumoniae*, and *C. psittaci*. Chlamydiae have a unique developmental cycle. The infectious particle is the elementary body. Once inside the cell, the elementary body undergoes reorganization to form a reticulate body. After several replications, the reticulate bodies differentiate into elementary bodies, are released from the host cell, and become available to infect other cells. Three of the 15 serovars of *C. trachomatis* (L1, L2, and L3) are known to cause LGV, an STD. *C. trachomatis* is a leading cause of STD in the United States. It is insidious because so many early infections are asymptomatic, particularly in women. The painless papule or vesicle develops on any part of the external genitalia, anus, rectum, or elsewhere. This lesion may ulcerate and heal without notice. Lymph nodes enlarge and discharge pus through sinuses. Unless effective antibiotics (tetracycline, erythromycin) are given promptly, a chronic inflammatory process may lead to fibrosis and lymphatic obstruction.

319. The answer is d. (*Brooks, p 355. Levinson, pp 182-184. Murray, pp 435-437. Ryan, pp 463-470, 471-479.*) *Ehrlichia* is an obligate, intracellular parasite that resembles *Rickettsia*. *Ehrlichia chaffeensis* has been linked to human ehrlichiosis, although this infection is primarily seen in animals. The majority of patients with this disease report exposure to ticks. It is thought that *I. scapularis* carries *Ehrlichia*, although the Lone Star tick, *A. americanum*, may also transmit the disease. These gram-negative bacteria infect circulating leukocytes where they multiply within phagocytic vacuoles, forming clusters with inclusion-like appearance. These clusters of ehrlichiae are called morulae (mulberry-like). Diagnosis is confirmed by observing these morulae in white blood cells.

320. The answer is c. (*Brooks, pp 350-351. Levinson, pp 182-184. Murray, pp 438-439. Ryan, pp 463-470, 471-479.*) *Coxiella* is transmitted through the respiratory tract rather than through the skin, and *B. henselae* from animal scratches. *Coxiella* may cause chronic endocarditis that is not very responsive to either antimicrobial therapy or valve replacement. About 50% of Q-fever cases in humans are asymptomatic. Symptomatic cases usually present with an acute febrile illness (flu-like disease, fever, pneumonitis, and possibly hepatitis). Diagnosis depends on a history with contact with newborn or infected adult animals (sheep, cattle, cats, rabbits, and dogs). About 2% to 10% of Q-fever patients progress to a chronic infection with endocarditis, which occurs in about 60% to 70% of those cases. No vaccine exists and doxycycline is effective when symptoms appear.

321. The answer is c. (*Murray [2009], pp 427-433. Murray [2013], Ch 41; Ryan, Ch 40.*) The source of the woman's infection is *Rickettsia prowazekii*. Her disease is louse-borne typhus. Louse-borne typhus is a disease with a mortality of approximately 30%. *Chlamydia trachomatis* is obviously incorrect because the woman does not have trachoma, which is primarily a disease of the eye or genital tract. *Coxiella burnetii* is incorrect because this organism causes Q fever, which is primarily a disease presenting with nonspecific flu-like symptoms. *Rickettsia rickettsii* causes Rocky Mountain spotted fever, which is the most common *Rickettsia* disease in the United States, but is spread by ticks. *Rickettsia typhi* causes endemic typhus or murine typhus and is spread by fleas. Therefore, it is important to know the arthropod vectors that spread *Rickettsia* diseases to be able to tell them apart.

322. The answer is d. (*Murray [2009], pp 199-208. Murray [2013], Ch 40; Ryan, Ch 38.*) Penicillin causes disruption of the cell wall of bacteria. The *Mycoplasma* are unique among bacteria (along with the *Ureaplasma*) because they do not possess a cell wall. Their cell membranes contain a high concentration of sterols, which strengthen them by allowing the organism to resist the difference between the internal and external osmotic pressure. The other four antibiotics (clindamycin, erythromycin, kanamycin, and tetracycline) are all protein synthesis inhibitors and would be expected to have some activity against *M. pneumoniae*. Erythromycin, the fluoroquinolones, and the tetracyclines have been used to treat infections by this organism. The fluoroquinolones and the tetracyclines are more commonly used in adults.

323. The answer is c. (*Murray [2009], pp 441-449. Murray [2013], Ch 43; Ryan, Ch 39.*) This man has LGV, which is a STD caused by the L serotypes of *Chlamydia trachomatis*. While *C. trachomatis* can cause diseases such as ocular infections and infant pneumonia, it can also cause the very serious STD of LGV. Different serotypes (in this case the L serotypes) of *C. trachomatis* are responsible for the different diseases. *Chlamydophila psittaci* causes human respiratory infections in man. *Chlamydophila pneumoniae* can also cause respiratory infections in man that range from asymptomatic to serious atypical pneumonias. *Neisseria gonorrheae* is a Gram-negative coccus that can cause STD, and *Treponema pallidum* is a Gram-negative spirochete that can also cause STDs.

324. The answer is d. (*Murray [2009], pp 427-433. Murray, Ch 41; Ryan, Ch 40.*) The disease that this young man has is Rocky Mountain spotted fever (RMSF). RMSF is the most common *Rickettsia* disease in the United States and is spread by ticks. This disease causes a maculopapular rash on the arms and legs that spreads to the trunk. The skin disease most often associated with the group A streptococci is erysipelas. *Coxiella burnetii* causes Q-fever, which is primarily a disease presenting with nonspecific flu-like symptoms. Typhoid fever, which is caused by *Salmonella typhi*, is a febrile illness with severe gastrointestinal distress. *Rickettsia prowazekii* causes the disease typhus, which is a disease with a 30% fatality rate and a maculopapular rash that is spread by lice and is rare in the United States.

325. The answer is e. (*Murray [2009], pp 421-425. Murray [2013], Ch 40; Ryan, Ch 38.*) *Ureaplasma urealyticum* can cause NGU and it produces colonies even smaller than the colonies of the *Mycoplasma*. The *Ureaplasma* species require the presence of urea in order to grow and it is thought that they use urea to generate energy. They also often die rapidly after their initial isolation. *Coxiella burnetii* does not cause NGU and does not require urea to grow. The three *Mycoplasma* species (*genitalium, hominis*, and *pneumoniae*) do not require urea to grow and are therefore incorrect.

326. The answer is e. (*Murray [2009], pp 421-425. Murray, Ch 40; Ryan, Ch 38.*) *Mycoplasma pneumoniae* produces an atypical pneumonia that shows up as a patchy opacity on chest x-ray. The most common clinical presentation with this organism is tracheobronchitis. The atypical pneumonia produced by *M. pneumoniae* is often referred to as "walking pneumonia". Cold agglutinins are antibodies that agglutinate type O red blood cells at 4°C. *Streptococcus* MG is a clinical strain of bacteria that rarely causes disease. These antibodies are often found in the serum of persons infected with *M. pneumoniae*. Antibodies to these organisms and cold agglutinins are not found in the serum of patients infected with *Chlamydia trachomatis, Chlamydophila pneumoniae, Chlamydophila psittaci*, or *Mycoplasma hominis*.

327. The answer is c. (*Murray [2009], pp 441-449. Murray [2013], Ch 43; Ryan, Ch 39.*) *Chlamydophila pneumoniae* produces pharyngitis, bronchitis, sinusitis, and pneumonia in humans. The lungs will show a patchy infiltrate upon x-ray. It is a Gram-negative bacterium that does not stain well upon Gram-stain. It will not grow in vitro (eg, on blood agar), but will grow in tissue culture cells because it is a strict intracellular bacterial pathogen. *Streptococcus pneumoniae* and *Mycoplasma pneumoniae* will both cause pneumonia, but they will both grow in vitro and are not obligate intracellular bacterial pathogens. Both *C. trachomatis* and *C. psittaci* are obligate intracellular bacterial pathogens. *C. trachomatis* causes ocular and genital infections, so is therefore incorrect. *C. psittaci* can cause pneumonia, but is also incorrect because the man has not recently obtained any new birds into his household.

328. The answer is a. (*Murray [2009], pp 435-440. Murray [2013], Ch 42; Ryan, Ch 40.*) Human anaplasmosis is caused by *Anaplasma phagocytophilum.* The cells that are primarily infected by this organism are granulocytes, which include neutrophils, basophils, and eosinophils. Human anaplasmosis presents as flu-like symptoms, with muscle pain, lethargy, high fever, and headaches. The disease is observed following the bite of a tick about 7 to 21 days after the injury. Antibiotics such as penicillin, cephalosporin, and the aminoglycosides are not effective against human anaplasmosis. *Coxiella burnetii* causes Q-fever, which is primarily a respiratory disease.

Both *Chlamydophila psittaci* and *Chlamydophila pneumoniae* cause respiratory diseases, and *Rickettsia rickettsii* causes Rocky Mountain spotted fever, which is characterized by a rash, which this patient does not have.

329. The answer is c. (*Murray [2009], pp 441-449. Murray [2013], Ch 43; Ryan, Ch 39.*) *Chlamydia trachomatis* is the most common sexually transmitted organism in the United States, so it is not surprising that this man picked up this organism after an unprotected sexual encounter with a prostitute. Most *C. trachomatis* genital infections in men are symptomatic. However, in women as many as 80% of their genital tract infections with this organism are asymptomatic. Asymptomatic women are an important reservoir for the distribution of this organism. *C. trachomatis* will not grow on blood agar and is an obligate intracellular bacterial pathogen. Both the *Chlamydophila* (*pneumoniae* and *psittaci*) cause respiratory tract infections. The infecting organism did not grow on blood agar, so it was not *N. gonorrheae*. The infecting organism was not *T. pallidum* because the initial chancre is on the genitals, and the second phase of syphilis, which is a rash, did not occur in this man.

330. The answer is a. (*Murray [2009], pp 441-449. Murray [2003], Ch 43. Ryan, Ch 39.*) The described disease is trachoma, an ocular disease caused by the A, B, and C serotypes of *C. trachomatis*. Trachoma is the most important cause of preventable blindness in the world. This infection is spread from eye to eye by fomites like contaminated towels. The conjunctiva becomes scarred as the infection continues and blindness can be the end result. The infection can be cured by one dose of azithromycin or by a seven day course of doxycycline. The two *Chlamydophila* (*psittaci* and *pneumoniae*) cause respiratory tract infections, while the two *Rickettsia* (*prowazekii* and *rickettsii*) produce rashes and these patients had no rashes.

331. The answer is b. (*Murray [2009], pp 441-449. Murray [2013], Ch 43; Ryan, Ch 39.*) *Chlamydophila psittaci* is the cause of psittacosis, which can be transmitted to humans from infected birds. When birds are shipped long distances (eg, from Africa), if they are infected with *C. psittaci*, their immune system begins to wane. If they get sick, the disease is called shipping fever. So when the person who ordered the parrot gets the bird, they may become infected with *C. psittaci* by inhalation. The organism then moves by hematogenous spread to the spleen and liver where the bacteria multiply. The lungs are then infected from the blood stream which induces an inflammatory reaction in the alveoli. Mucous plugs can then be produced in the smaller airways causing difficulty in breathing. *Chlamydophila pneumoniae* is incorrect because this organism is not spread by birds, and birds also do not spread *Chlamydia trachomatis*. The two *Rickettsia* organisms (*prowazekii* and *rickettsii*) do not cause respiratory tract infections and are not spread by birds.

332. The answer is d. (*Murray [2009], pp 435-440. Murray [2013], Ch 42; Ryan, Ch 40.*) The man had Q-fever. This disease is caused by infection with *Coxiella burnetii*. This organism is extremely stable and can survive in milk and soil for a very long time. Infections in man occur when the organisms become airborne from a contaminated source such as soil or milk from a farm. Man can also become infected by drinking contaminated milk. That is why it is a good idea to drink only pasteurized milk. Most of the people exposed to *Coxiella burnetii* suffer an asymptomatic infection and most symptoms that people do experience are flu-like. Q-fever can occur a long time after the original exposure to the organism and this occurs primarily in people with congenital heart disease. In this case, SBE is most commonly seen. The two *Chlamydophila* organisms (*psittaci* and *pneumoniae*) are incorrect. The man got his infection working on his cattle ranch. The *Chlamydophila* are not extremely stable and do not survive in dust. *Chlamydia trachomatis* is incorrect because this organism is not extremely stable and does not survive in dust. While the viridans streptococci do cause SBE, they did not cause this man's infection because they are sensitive to penicillin and they would have grown out in his blood culture had they been present.

333. The answer is e. (*Murray [2009], pp 435-440. Murray [2013], Ch 42; Ryan, Ch 40.*) The man had HME. This disease is spread by ticks and is caused by *Ehrlichia chaffeensis*. This organism results in the infection of monocytes in the patient's blood. Giemsa staining of the patient's peripheral blood should be performed to examine the monocytes for morulae (structures inside the monocytes that contain the intracellular organisms), because this is diagnostic of this disease. Patients with HME should be treated with doxycycline. *Ehrlichia canis* is incorrect because this organism causes infections in dogs. *Ehrlichia ewingii* is incorrect because this organism causes primary granulocytic ehrlichiosis. *Amblyomma americanum* is the tick arthropod vector for *E. chafeensis* and therefore incorrect.

334. The answer is b. (*Murray [2009], pp 427-433. Murray [2013], Ch 41. Ryan, Ch 40.*) The New York businessman had scrub typhus, which is caused by *Orientia tsutsugamushi.* This disease is spread by the bite of mites carrying the organism. Mites are so small that most people that get bit by them never see them. Scrub typhus develops suddenly after about a 2-week incubation period. It occurs in eastern Asia, Japan, Australia, and other western Pacific islands. The businessman's trip to Japan explains his infection. The disease is characterized by myalgia, fever, and severe headaches. A rash develops about 50% of the time. It can be treated with doxycycline. The three *Rickettsia* organisms (*prowazekii, rickettsii*, and *typhi*) are incorrect because the businessman had no lice (*prowazekii*), no flea bites (*typhi*), and no tick bites (*rickettsii*). Doxycycline would have cured all these organisms if they had been present. *Dermacentor andersoni* is the name of the wood tick that spreads Rocky Mountain spotted fever, so that is obviously incorrect.

[illegible]

334. The answer is b. [illegible] York [illegible] which is caused by [illegible] *tsutsugamushi*, [illegible] carrying the [illegible] [illegible] Asia, [illegible] Australia and [illegible] islands. The [illegible] The disease is characterized by [illegible] headache. A rash develops about [illegible] [illegible] because the [illegible] bites [illegible] and tick [illegible] would have [illegible] [illegible] is obviously incorrect.

Mycology

Questions

335. About 90 days post-bone marrow transplant, a 55-year-old white woman began to complain of dry cough, shortness of breath, and chest pain. She was started on antibiotics and blood culture obtained at the time was negative and there was not improvement. A computed tomography (CT) scan of the lungs showed a halo of low attenuation around a nodular lesion. Analysis of lung biopsy was similar to methenamine silver-stained section below. The most likely diagnosis for this patient is

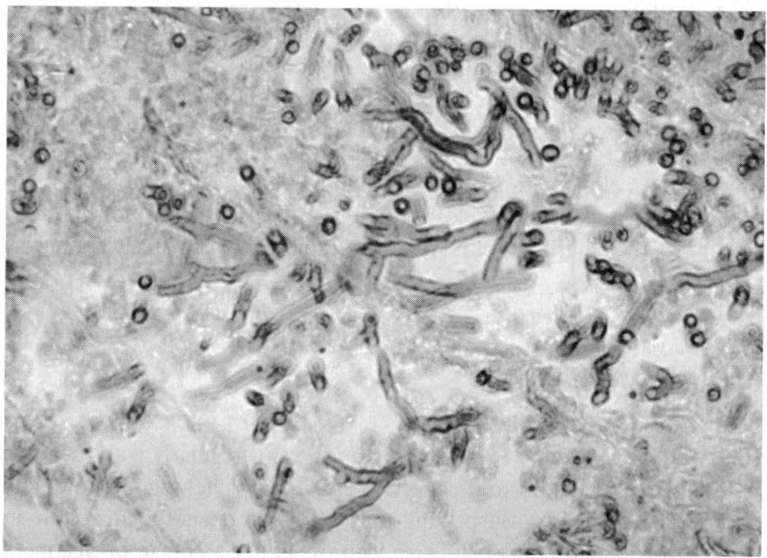

(Courtesy of Dr. William Kaplan; Public Health Image Library, Centers for Disease Control and Prevention; Atlanta, Georgia.)

a. Aspergillosis
b. Candidiasis
c. Histoplasmosis
d. Mucormycosis

336. A 65-year-old man was diagnosed with pseudomembranous candidiasis and given a prescription for oral fluconazole. This drug acts by:

a. Binding to membrane ergosterol
b. Incorporation into RNA leading to mistranslation and inhibits DNA synthesis
c. Inhibition of 1,3-β-glucan biosynthesis
d. Inhibition of mitosis
e. Inhibition of squalene 2,3-epoxidase
f. Inhibition P450-dependent sterol demethylase (lanosterol 14α-demethylase)

337. An AIDS patient with a CD4 count in the range 100 to 50 cells/mm^3 complains of headache and neck stiffness and appears disoriented. The possibility of fungal meningitis is considered and tests for the common fungal etiology of meningitis ordered. Tests included direct examination of spinal fluid for the organism and serology. The purpose of the serology test is detection of

a. Antibody to capsular polysaccharide
b. Antibody to cell wall mannoprotein
c. Capsular polysaccharide
d. Cell wall mannoprotein

338. A 6-year-old African American girl resident of a very large US city presents to a clinic with scaly patches and areas of alopecia on the scalp with hair shafts broken off close to the scalp. The hair did not fluoresce under Wood's light. If this child has tinea capitis, the most likely etiology is

a. *Epidermophyton floccosum*
b. *Microsporum audouinii*
c. *Microsporum canis*
d. *Trichophyton rubrum*
e. *Trichophyton tonsurans*

339. A 25-year-old male physical therapist trains regularly with the hope of qualifying for the Boston Marathon. He develops itching in interdigital spaces on his left foot. Suspecting tinea pedis he treats the area with an over-the-counter product. The area improves after a course of treatment but two months later reappears and again responded to the same treatment. However, there was reappearance 3 months later. If the self-diagnosis is correct, the normal habitat of the etiologic agent is most likely described as

a. Anthropophilic
b. Geophilic
c. Zoophilic

340. A patient receiving corticosteroid treatment for lupus developed headache and fever and when she began to display some memory loss she was brought to her physician by her spouse. Considered in the differential diagnosis was cryptococcal meningitis. Which of the following, if found upon examination of cerebrospinal fluid would support that diagnosis?

a. Encapsulated yeast cells
b. Hyphae
c. Intracellular yeast cells
d. Yeast cells with multiple buds
e. Yeast cells with a broad base between mother and daughter cells

341. A 35-year-old male, a legal resident in the USA, presented with a complaint of a lesion on the bottom of his foot that was smooth and shiny and somewhat discolored. He reported that it bothered him when wearing some shoes. He reported no chronic diseases or recent illnesses and he was a nonsmoker. Travel history determined that he frequently visited relatives in India. Histopathology of the biopsy specimen showed at 2.4-mm granule surrounded by neutrophils. Tissue staining suggested that the granule contained filaments >1 μm in width. The most likely diagnosis is

a. Actinomycetoma
b. Aspergillosis
c. Chromomycosis
d. Eumycetoma
e. Phaeohyphomycosis

342. A healthy 55-year-old man resident of Louisville, Kentucky, presented to his physician complaining of fever, headache, nonproductive cough, and chest pain of 10 days duration. As part of the history, the patient reported that he was still employed as a construction worker and for several weeks prior to becoming ill had been engaged in tearing down houses and structures as part of an urban renewal project. The most likely fungal infection considered in the differential diagnosis is

a. Blastomycosis
b. Coccidioidomycosis
c. Cryptococcosis
d. Histoplasmosis
e. Paracoccidioidomycosis
f. Sporotrichosis

343. A 40-year-old woman sees her primary care physician complaining of an ulcer on her finger. She reported that it started as a red bump. Knowing that her patient was a long-time avid gardener, the physician asked if that finger had been injured by a thorn. The patient responded that she did not remember about that particular finger but she certainly had received thorn punctures in past weeks. Based on this information, which of the following is the most likely fungal etiology?

a. *Fonsecaea pedrosoi*
b. *Malassezia furfur*
c. *Microsporum canis*
d. *Sporothrix schenckii*
e. *Stachybotrys chartarum*

344. Several young men from the local high school football team complain of a sudden onset of athlete's foot (tinea pedis). Which of the following observations in a skin scraping will support the diagnosis?

a. Hyaline hyphae and arthroconidia
b. Pigmented hyphae
c. Sclerotic bodies
d. Spherules
e. Yeast cells

345. A 57-year-old obese, white female with type 1 diabetes mellitus is diagnosed with strep throat and prescribed penicillin. A week later she returns complaining of a sore mouth and white patches on the tongue. Your examination confirms the white pseudomembranous lesions. Material from the lesion is obtained and prepared for microscopic examination. Your suspicion of the most likely clinical diagnosis will be confirmed by observation of buccal epithelial cells, leukocytes, and which of the following

a. Gram-positive bacteria
b. Gram-negative bacteria
c. Hyphae with septa and acute angle branching
d. Spherules containing endospores
e. Yeast cells, hyphae, and pseudohyphae

346. A small brownish irregular macule on the palm of a 13-year-old girl is examined by a dermatologist in her Louisiana home town. A skin scraping from the lesion is obtained for microscopic observation and culture. Microscopic examination of the specimen shows brownish filaments or hyphae and yeast cells. The most likely diagnosis is

a. Tinea capitis
b. Tinea corporis
c. Tinea manuum
d. Tinea nigra
e. Tinea pedis

347. You have been designated as a coordinator of construction of a bone marrow transplant unit (BMTU). There will be extensive removal of walls and floors in order to install the laminar flow rooms required for a BMTU. From the standpoint of frequency and lethality, which of the following fungi should be your biggest concern?

a. *Aspergillus* species
b. *Candida* species
c. *Cryptococcus* species
d. *Penicillium* species
e. *Pneumocystis jiroveci*

348. A 50-year-old man, newly employed by a commercial farm that supplies eggs and chickens to industry, develops a flu-like syndrome with fever, chills, myalgia, headache, and a nonproductive cough. He is diagnosed with histoplasmosis. A positive tissue biopsy would show the presence of

a. Arthrospores
b. Oval budding yeast cells inside macrophages
c. Spherules containing endospores
d. Tuberculate macroconidia
e. Yeast cells, hyphae, and pseudohyphae
f. Yeast cells with broad-based bud

349. A 65-year-old female patient with a long history of diabetes is brought the emergency room by her daughter with an immediate complaint of sudden swelling on the right side of the face and bleeding from the right nostril. Questioning of the patient and daughter suggests the possibility of ketoacidosis. The nasal bleeding is troublesome and a swab of the nares is rushed to the clinical laboratory for immediate attention along with blood to test for acidosis. The patient was admitted. The facial lesion became partially necrotic and there was slight protrusion of the right eye and facial paralysis. The patient died on the second day. If this patient died of a fungal infection, histopathologic examination of the lesions would most likely show…

a. Hyphae, some with arthroconidia
b. Septate dematiaceous hyphae
c. Septate hyphae with acute angle branching
d. Nonseptate hyphae
e. Narrow (<1 μm) Gram-positive filaments
f. Yeast cells

350. A normally healthy young man in Arizona was diagnosed with coccidioidomycosis. The most likely route of infection for the etiologic agent is

a. Aspiration
b. Cutaneous contact
c. Ingestion
d. Inhalation
e. Implantation

351. An immunocompromised patient is suspected of having aspergillosis due to *A. fumigatus*. Which of the following clinical conditions is most likely to occur?

a. Allergic bronchopulmonary response
b. Aspergilloma
c. Invasive pulmonary infection
d. Otomycosis
e. Wound infection

352. A 25-year-old pregnant woman, living in the San Joaquin Valley (California), experiences an influenza-like illness with fever and cough. She is diagnosed with *Coccidioides* infection. The most likely recommended treatment for the infection of this patient is

a. Amphotericin B or fluconazole
b. 5-fluorocytosine
c. None, the infection resolves without treatment
d. Supportive treatment only for symptoms
e. Terbinafine

353. Months after a kidney transplant, a 45-year-old woman who was receiving immunosuppressive therapy experienced a rapid onset of respiratory insufficiency and a dry cough. High-resolution computed tomographic scanning was ordered of the lungs. There were findings of interstitial disease. Bronchoalveolar lavage was performed and the material examined by Giemsa staining. The report stated that trophic forms and cysts were observed. The most likely infecting organism is

a. *Aspergillus fumigatus*
b. *Candida albicans*
c. *Pneumocystis jiroveci*
d. *Rhizopus arrhizus (oryzae)*

354. Bacteria and fungi share some common mechanisms of resistance to drugs used in treatment of bacterial or fungal infection. However, bacteria have a resistance mechanism not described in fungi. This mechanism is

a. Alteration in the drug target
b. Efflux of drug
c. Inactivation of drug
d. Influx of drug
e. Overexpression of drug target

355. An isolate of *Candida albicans* was found to be resistant to caspofungin due to mutation in the drug target which is

a. Cytosine permease
b. Ergosterol
c. P450 14-α-demethylase
d. Squalene 2,3-epoxidase
e. Subunit of β-1,3-glucan synthase

356. A 25-year-old man made a self-diagnosis of athlete's foot and purchased a product advertised to treat this condition that listed the active ingredient as tolnaftate. The mode of action of this drug is

a. Binding to membrane ergosterol
b. Incorporation into RNA leading to mistranslation and inhibition DNA synthesis
c. Inhibition of 1,3-β-glucan biosynthesis
d. Inhibition of mitosis
e. Inhibition of squalene 2,3-epoxidase
f. Inhibition P450-dependent sterol demethylase (lanosterol 14α-demethylase)

357. A 37-year-old HIV-positive male presented with fever, cough, facial papules, and pustules. Microscopic examination of a stained smear of material obtained from a pustule showed structures that could be described as those stained red or dark in the periodic acid Schiff stained tissue specimen below. These pustular lesions are most likely attributable to infection with

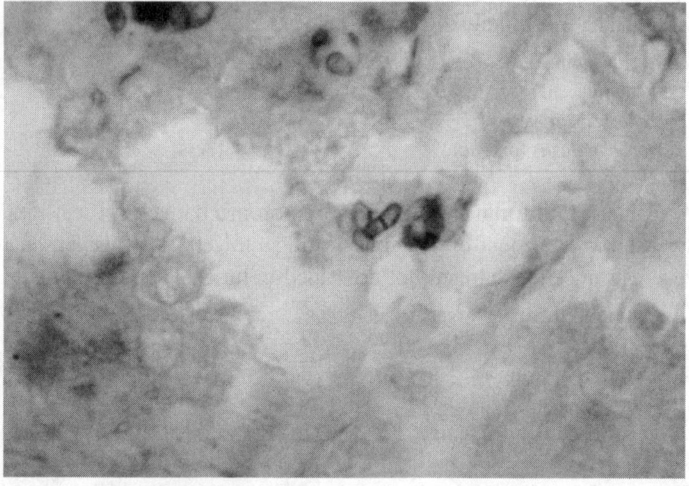

(Courtesy of Dr. Libero Ajello; Public Health Image Library, Centers for Disease Control and Prevention; Atlanta, Georgia.)

a. *Blastomyces dermatitidis*
b. *Candida albicans*
c. *Cryptococcus* spp.
d. *Histoplasma capsulatum*
e. *Penicillium marneffei*

358. An 18-year-old white male high-school student visits the family physician complaining of a diffuse, painful rash extending from his midthigh to his navel region. In recounting the history of the rash, he indicates that one of his football teammates gave him topical hydrocortisone to treat a minor groin rash. A KOH scraping of the lesion reveals hyaline hyphae and a portion of the scraping is submitted for culture. A schematic of the microscopic observation of the culture is shown below. The most likely etiology is

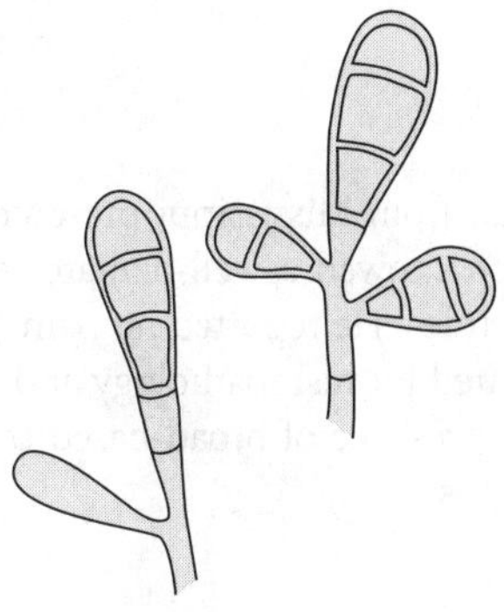

(Reproduced, with permission, from Brooks GF et al. Jawetz's Medical Microbiology. *22nd ed. New York: McGraw-Hill; 2001:536.)*

a. *Epidermophyton floccosum*
b. *Microsporum canis*
c. *Trichophyton rubrum*
d. *Trichophyton tonsurans*

359. A 37-year-old male presented with a lesion on the left leg. He reported receiving abrasions in the area 3 or 4 months earlier while on tour in Brazil. The lesion was a pink, smooth papular lesion, which he reported itched. The lesion was biopsied and the clinical pathology laboratory reported the presence of short, brownish hyphal fragments and sclerotic or Medlar bodies. The most likely diagnosis for this patient is

a. Blastomycosis
b. Chromoblastomycosis
c. Lacaziosis
d. Eumycetoma
e. Sporotrichosis

360. An 87-year-old man complained that his feet hurt when he put on shoes because of his toenails. Upon inspection several toenails on both feet showed yellowing and thickening. A scraping was obtained from one nail as well as subungual debris and prepared for culture and direct examination with potassium hydroxide and Calcofluor. Microscopic examination showed fluorescent hyphae. The most likely diagnosis is

a. Tinea capitis
b. Tinea corporis
c. Tinea manuum
d. Tinea pedis
e. Tinea unguium

361. A 55-year-old man from Mississippi presented with a lesion below his left eye. Examination showed a well-demarcated lesion with a raised border, scaling, and pustules. He reported no pain. Material from the edge of the lesion was submitted for histopathology and culture. The pathology laboratory reported the presence of broad-based budding yeast cells. The diagnosis for this patient is

a. Blastomycosis
b. Chromomycosis
c. Paracoccidioidomycosis
d. Penicilliosis
e. Sporotrichosis

362. A 47-year-old man from Cincinnati, Ohio, suspected to have community-acquired pneumonia was treated with antibiotics. When he failed to improve, histoplasmosis was considered. Among the tests ordered were serology, direct examination, and culture of induced sputum. In culture, the microscopic morphology most useful in identification of the etiologic agent is

a. Arthroconidia
b. Microconidia
c. Sclerotic bodies
d. Spherules
e. Tuberculate macroconidia

363. A 25-year-old female had surgery for a crush injury to the chest. She had a central venous catheter, was intubated, and was on a mechanical ventilator. Three days postsurgery she developed a fever and was treated empirically for bacterial infection but fever persisted. Fungemia was suspected and blood culture for fungi was ordered. Empiric antifungal therapy was initiated and the central venous catheter line was removed. Removal of the catheter is indicated because

a. Of the suspected presence of *Aspergillus fumigatus* biofilm
b. Of the suspected presence of *Candida albicans* biofilm
c. Of the suspected presence of *Cryptococcus neoformans* biofilm
d. Of the suspected presence of *Aspergillus fumigatus* planktonic organisms
e. Of the suspected presence of *Candida albicans* planktonic organisms
f. Of the suspected presence of *Cryptococcus neoformans* planktonic organisms

364. A 75-year-old African American male who had recently retired to the Tucson, Arizona area from Ohio, presented with history of cough, fever, and chills for 3 weeks. Because of the recent move and ethnicity, the patient was tested for coccidioidomycosis. This infection is initiated following inhalation of structures best described as

a. Arthroconidia
b. Blastoconidia
c. Endospores
d. Spherules
e. Sporangiospores

365. A 4-year-child develops tinea corporis (ringworm). The lesions clear using a preparation for treatment of athlete's foot obtained from local drug store. The lesions reappear on the child and a playmate in a few weeks. Internet research suggested to the mother that the family pet might be the source of infection and should be taken to a veterinarian. If this is the mode of transmission, the etiology is most likely

a. *Epidermophyton floccosum*
b. *Hortaea werneckii*
c. *Malassezia* spp.
d. *Microsporum canis*
e. *Trichosporon beigelii*

366. A patient from a small Mississippi town presented with a complaint of several weeks of productive cough, hemoptysis, weight loss, and chest pain. Radiologic findings were consistent with a pulmonary infiltrate. Among the possible diagnoses, blastomycosis was considered and culture for this organism was included in the orders for the clinical laboratory. The structure distinctive for identification in microscopic examination of a culture of the etiologic agent is

a. Arthroconidia
b. Broad-based budding yeast cells
c. Encapsulated yeast cells
d. Multiply budding yeast cells
e. Tuberculate macroconidia

367. *Candida albicans* is isolated in blood culture from a patient in a surgical intensive care unit. This most likely source of the infecting organism is

a. A health care worker
b. A visitor
c. Ambient air
d. The patient
e. The surgeon

368. A 30-year-old female of the US military was on assignment in a subtropical area. She reported to the physician with a complaint of patchy light-colored lesions on her chest and upper arms. She reported no other symptoms. Upon examination the lesions were irregular and well demarcated. Included in the differential diagnosis was pityriasis versicolor. A scraping on an affected area was obtained. If the diagnosis of pityriasis versicolor is correct, the best description of what will be observed in a positive specimen is

a. Hyaline hyphae
b. Hyaline hyphae and arthroconidia
c. Dematiaceous hyphae
d. Yeast cells with broad-based buds
e. Yeast cells and short hyphae

369. A 56-year-old man retired from the military to his hometown in Wisconsin. While in the military he had been stationed in several states and served in several parts of the world including South America, Africa, Southeast Asia, and most recently in Iraq and Afghanistan. He complained to his physician of a lesion inside his mouth on the left side. Histopathology of a biopsy specimen stained with methenamine silver was similar to that shown below. The most likely diagnosis is

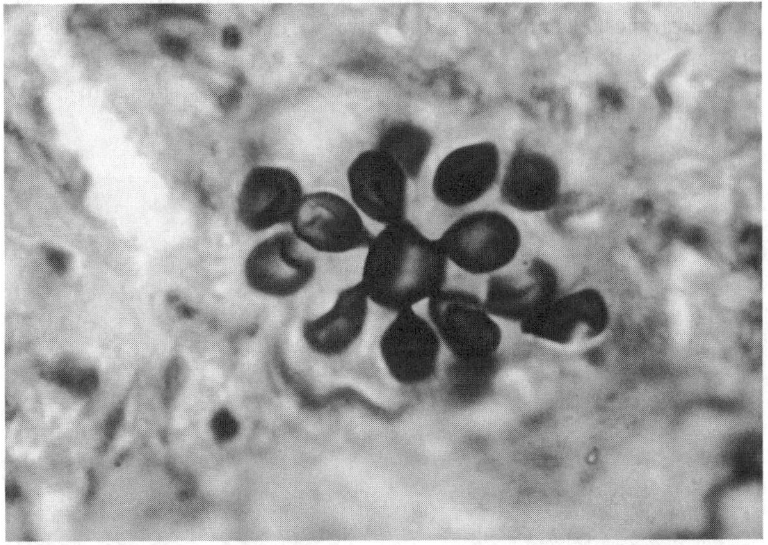

(Courtesy of the Public Health Image Library, Centers for Disease Control and Prevention; Atlanta, Georgia.)

a. Blastomycosis
b. Candidiasis
c. Histoplasmosis
d. Leishmaniasis
e. Paracoccidioidomycosis

370. The overexpression of drug efflux pumps in *Candida albicans* is an important mechanism in reduced susceptibility to

a. Azole class drugs
b. Echinocandin class drugs
c. Flucytosine
d. Polyene class drugs

371. A 28-year-old woman experienced vaginal and vulvar itching, a slightly watery discharge and pain with intercourse. Her gynecologist performed physical examination of the vulva, vagina, and cervix. The vaginal pH was estimated as 4.4. Microscopic examination was performed on some Gram-stained discharge material. The observation was similar to below. The most likely diagnosis is

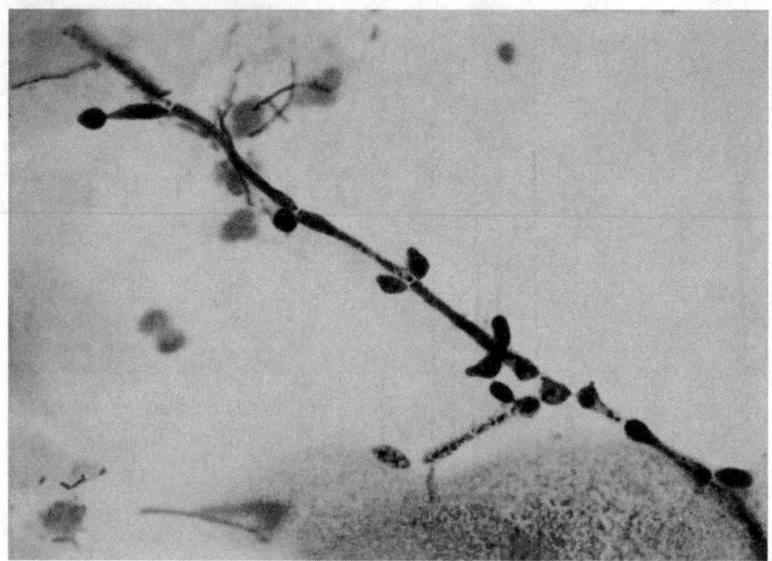

(Courtesy of Dr. Stuart Brow; Public Health Image Library, Centers for Disease Control and Prevention; Atlanta, Georgia.)

a. Bacterial vaginosis
b. Candidiasis
c. Chlamydial vaginitis
d. Trichomoniasis
e. Viral vaginitis

372. A 53-year-old white woman with end-stage renal disease received a kidney transplant and was maintained on an immunosuppressive regimen. Three months later she had a fever (38.3°C) and was found to have acute renal failure. Renal transplant biopsy was performed. Periodic acid-Schiff staining of a biopsy section showed yeast cells and hyphae. The most likely diagnosis for this patient is infection with

a. *Aspergillus fumigatus*
b. *Candida albicans*
c. *Candida glabrata*
d. *Cryptococcus neoformans*
e. *Rhizopus arrhizus (oryzae)*

373. Amphotericin B is noted for both its antifungal efficacy and side effects when administered to humans. The basis for the side effects is most likely

a. Binding of drug to cholesterol
b. Binding of drug to ergosterol
c. Binding of drug to phospholipids
d. Inhibition of cholesterol biosynthesis
e. Inhibition of ergosterol biosynthesis

374. A fungal teleomorph is

a. Asexual reproductive form
b. Infective form for humans
c. Sexually reproductive form
d. Dormant form

Mycology

Answers

335. The answer is a. (*Brooks, pp 646-647. Levinson, pp 351-352. Murray, Ch 73. Ryan, pp 723-733, 743-746.*) *Aspergillus* is widespread in nature and produces small conidia that are easily aerosolized. Atopic individuals often develop severe allergic reactions to the conidial antigens. In immunocompromised patients, the conidia may germinate to produce hyphae that invade the lungs and other tissues. Progress of disease can be rapid. A diagnosis of aspergillosis is supported by a tissue biopsy showing invasion by the organism and a positive culture from a normally sterile site. Aspergilli may be airborne in the environment and be laboratory culture contaminants or present in orally obtained samples from patients without apparent clinical illness and at low risk for invasive aspergillosis and such finding should be interpreted with caution. In tissue *Aspergillus* spp. (most commonly *A. fumigatus*) have septate hyphae 3 to 6 μm in width that are described as having acute angle branching. In bone marrow transplant patients infection may occur early after transplant or after several months as in this case. The other infections can occur in a compromised host but would differ from what is shown. Particularly, the septate hyphae and acute angle branching are not consistent with agents of mucormycosis that have wide nonseptate hyphae. *Histoplasma capsulatum*, which causes histoplasmosis in humans, grows in yeast form in the infected person. Normal healthy individuals may be infected; however, in the immunocompromised host the infection can be more severe.

336. The answer is f. (*Brooks, Ch 45. Levinson, Ch 47. Murray, Ch 69. Ryan, pp 707-710.*) Ergosterol is the major sterol component of the fungal cell membrane while cholesterol is found in mammalian membranes (see table on the next page). The difference is exploited by major antifungal drugs. Azole (imidazole and triazole) class drugs, for example miconazole, fluconazole, itraconazole, and voriconazole, inhibit a cytochrome P450-dependent demethylase (lanosterol 14-α-demethylase), which is in the latter part of the biosynthetic pathway for ergosterol. This pathway

SELECTED ANTIFUNGAL DRUGS, MODE OF ACTION AND MECHANISMS OF RESISTANCE

Antifungal Agent	Route	Mode of Action	Mechanism(s) of Resistance
Tolnaftate	Topical	Inhibition of squalene epoxidase (enzyme in the ergosterol biosynthesis pathway)	Resistant isolates very rare; likely mechanisms include efflux pumps, mutation, or overexpression target, nonspecific stress adaptation
Allylamines			
Naftifine	Topical		
Terbinafine	Oral, topical		
Flucytosine (5-flurocytosine)	Oral	Inhibition of DNA and RNA synthesis	Change in permease, cytosine deaminase, or uracil phosphoribosyl transferase activity
Echinocandins	IV	Inhibition of fungal cell wall glucan synthesis	Mutation in subunit β-1,3-glucan synthase
Anidalufungin			
Caspofungin			
Micafungin			
Azoles		Inhibits a cytochrome P450 enzyme 14-α-demethylase (enzyme in the ergosterol biosynthesis pathway)	Mutation or overexpression of 14-α-demethylase
Ketoconazole	Topical, oral		Overexpression of drug efflux pump(s)
Clotrimazole, bifonazole, econazole, miconazole, oxiconazole, sulconazole, terconazole, tioconazole	Topical		
Fluconaozle	Oral, IV		
Itraconazole	Oral, IV		
Posaconazole	Oral		
Voriconazole	Oral, IV		
Polyenes		Main mechanism binds to ergosterol creating channels resulting in metabolite leakage	Alteration or decrease in ergosterol content
Amphotericin	IV		
Natamycin	Topical (eye)		
Nystatin	Topical, oral	Oxidative pathways may enhance activity	
Griseofulvin	Oral	Acts on microtubules and interferes mitosis/cell division	Putative mechanism drug efflux

is also inhibited at an earlier stage prior to ring formation by allylamines (Terbinafine, naftifine) and tolnaftate. These drugs inhibit squalene-2,3-epoxidase. The inhibition of ergosterol production results in aberrant cell membrane. Polyene class drugs, for example amphotericin B, also exploit ergosterol by binding the sterol leading to channel formation in the membrane that allows leakage of intracellular constituents, for example potassium, and cell death. 5-Fluorocytosine (5FC, flucytosine) is a pyrimidine analog that after conversion to other compounds (5-fluorouracil, 5-fluorodeoxyuridylic acid, and 5-fluorouridine) leads to inhibition of DNA synthesis and RNA miscoding. Echinocandins, for example caspofungin, inhibit the synthesis of 1,3-β-glucan with inhibition of the glucan synthesis enzyme complex. Griseofulvin is thought to inhibit fungal growth by interaction with microtubules resulting in aberrant mitosis and cell division.

337. The answer is c. (*Brooks, Ch 45. Levinson, Ch 50. Murray, Ch 73. Ryan, pp 739-742.*) *Cryptococcus neoformans* is the most common cause of meningitis in AIDS patients. The frequency has declined in areas with robust antiretroviral treatment but can still occur in patients receiving treatment. Patients immunocompromised by other factors, for example maintained on corticosteroids, are also at risk. The organism is inhaled as a desiccated, minimally encapsulated organism or perhaps a basidiospore often after disturbance of soil rich in avian feces such as pigeon guano. The capsule can enlarge upon reaching the lung. Initial pulmonary infection may be asymptomatic and exposure may occur early in life. Symptomatic infection may mimic an influenza-like respiratory infection and resolve spontaneously. Particularly in immunocompromised patients the organism may multiply and disseminate with a predilection for the CNS causing meningoencephalitis. This is often the presenting complaint. The organism grows as encapsulated yeast that, in culture and cerebrospinal fluid, may be highlighted by mounting in India ink. Frequently, detection of capsular polysaccharide antigen is used as a diagnostic tool. There are commercial kits based on latex agglutination or enzyme immunoassay that can be used to detect antigen in serum or cerebrospinal fluid.

338. The answer is e. (*Brooks, Ch 45. Levinson, Ch 48. Murray, Ch 70. Ryan, pp 713-718.*) The large majority of fungal cutaneous skin infections are due to dermatophytes. These infections can occur from head to toe and

DERMATOPHYTE INFECTIONS

Manifestation	Lesion Location	Clinical Features	Dermatophytes Most Frequently Isolated
Tinea capitis	Scalp hair Endothrix: fungus inside hair shaft. Ectothrix: fungus on surface of hair	Scaling of scalp skin with variable inflammation and hair loss with short hair stubs or broken hair within hair follicles. Rare kerion formation with zoophilic ectothrix infection	Endothrix: *Trichophyton tonsurans* (dominant US); *T. mentagrophytes*,[a] *T. violaceum*, others Ectothrix: *Microsporum* canis, *M. audouinii*, others
	Favic pattern (tinea favus): fungus inside hair and empty spaces	Inflammatory crust or scutulum around hair shaft	Favic: *T. schoenleinii*
Tinea corporis (Classical ringworm)	Hairless, smooth skin	Classical: well-demarcated annular erythematous pruritic plaques with raised border and central clearing associated zoophilic and geophilic species; infection anthropophilic species may appear less inflammatory and annular or demarcated	*T. rubrum*; most common in North America; also *T. mentagrophytes*,[a] *Epidermophyton floccosum*; *M. canis*; others
Tinea cruris (jock itch)	Groin	Erythematous scaling lesion in intertriginous area. Pruritic	*T. rubrum*, *E. floccosum*, *T. mentagrophytes*[a]

(Continued)

DERMATOPHYTE INFECTIONS (CONTINUED)

Manifestation	Lesion Location	Clinical Features	Dermatophytes Most Frequently Isolated
Tinea faciei	Face	Similar to tinea corporis	*T. rubrum*, *T. mentagrophytes*,[a] *M. canis*
Tinea barbae	Neck and beard area	May be pustular with inflammation	Usually zoophilic spp., for example, *T. verrucosum*
Tinea manuum	Hand	Scaling, well-demarcated patches usually palmar surface, often one hand, may also have tinea pedis	*T. rubrum*
Tinea pedis (athlete's foot)	Foot soles and interdigital web spaces (associated with wearing shoes)	Erythema, scaling, cracks between toes most common	*T. rubrum*, *T. mentagrophytes*,[a] *E. floccosum*
Tinea unguium (onychomycosis caused by dermatophytes)	Nail	Nail thicken, discolored, crumbly, usually distally; usually occurs with adjacent skin infection and more often toenails	*T. rubrum*, *T. mentagrophytes*,[a] *E. floccosum*
Dermatophytid (id reaction)	Hands, any body site	Itchy, vesicular lesion	Usually sterile

[a]*T. mentagrophytes* has been reported with two variants, a zoophilic var. *mentagrophytes* and an anthropophilic var. *interdigitale*, and these are sometime listed as separate species *T. mentagrophytes* and *T. interdigitale*, respectively.

the infections are termed tinea followed by a description of the site (see table on the preceding page). These infections have been called ringworm, a misnomer from the misconception that the cause was a worm. However, that notion is perpetuated in the current terminology as tinea is from the Latin for a gnawing worm. The case is a classic description of tinea capitis that occurs primarily in children before puberty. There are two forms of childhood tinea capitis. One manifestation whose etiology is *M. audouinii* is sometimes called "gray patch". Over the past decades, this form has almost disappeared in the USA and been replaced by the second form. The second manifestation of childhood tinea capitis is caused by *T. tonsurans* and is sometimes called "black dot" because of the "dot" visible within the area of hair loss where a hair shaft broke off leaving a stump. Infections are primarily seen in children 3 to 9 years of age, although some adults may be asymptomatic carriers. If not resolved by treatment, the infection generally resolves with puberty. Among inner-city children the prevalence may be as high as 8%. Both *M. audouinii* and *T. tonsurans* are anthropophilic dermatophytes. Microscopic observation of infected hairs shows arthroconidia around the hair shaft (ectothrix) with *M. audouinii* infection and inside (endothrix) the hair shaft with *T. tonsurans* infection. Wood's light is a device that produces ultraviolet light rays. Hairs infected with *M. audouinii* fluoresce with a yellow-green color under Wood's light, while *T. tonsurans* does not. Other species may be more prevalent in other parts of the world as the cause of infection.

339. The answer is a. (*Brooks, Ch 45. Levinson, Ch 48. Murray, Ch 70. Ryan, pp 715-718.*) Tinea pedis (athlete's foot) is caused by dermatophytes. There are several etiologies of this infection (see table on the preceding page). Dermatophytes are adapted to one of three natural habitats: man (anthropophilic dermatophytes), animals other than man (zoophilic dermatophytes) and soil (geophilic dermatophytes). Infections with anthropophilic dermatophytes tend to be milder, recurrent or chronic, and less likely to completely resolve with topical treatment while those with the other two habitats tend to produce more inflammatory lesions that are not recurrent and respond well to treatment. The patient, in this instance has recurrent episodes, which is usually associated with anthropophilic species of which the most common is *Trichophyton rubrum*.

340. The answer is a. (*Brooks, Ch 45. Levinson, Ch 50. Murray, Ch 73. Ryan, pp 740-742.*) *Cryptococcus neoformans* occurs widely in nature, particularly in soil contaminated with bird droppings and is frequently associated with pigeon guano. The organism grows predominately in the yeast form as an encapsulated structure but as a basidiomycete may form hyphae and produce spores. Fungal structures may become dessicated in the environment and small enough to be inhaled into the lungs when material containing the organisms is disturbed. In the lung, the capsule can enlarge and encapsulated yeast cells are found in tissue. Lung infection is often asymptomatic, particularly in a normal host, but can result in pneumonia. Meningitis occurs through dissemination, particularly in immunosuppressed patients. India ink preparations of CSF reveal a budding yeast with a wide, unstained capsule in infected persons. A second species, *C. gattii*, also causes infections. This species has a more limited geographic distribution and is not associated with bird guano but with vegetation, for example red gum trees. In the United States, the organisms is found on the west coast with recent infections in the Pacific Northwest and infections with this species are reportable in Oregon and Washington. This species tends to infect competent hosts and CNS dissemination is most often seen as a cryptococcoma. The distinctive feature of *Cryptococcus* spp. yeast cells is the capsule. Other organisms that are found as yeast in host tissue have other distinguishing features such as the multiple budding form of *Paracoccidioides brasiliensis*, the small intracellular yeast cells of *Histoplasma capsulatum* and broad-base budding yeast cells of *Blastomyces dermatitidis*. *Aspergillus* spp. and agents of mucormycosis are examples of fungi that proliferate as hyphae in tissue.

341. The answer is d. (*Brooks, Ch 45. Levinson, Ch 48. Murray, Ch 71. Ryan, pp 721-722.*) Mycetoma is a slowly progressing disease of the subcutaneous tissues that is caused by a variety of fungi (eumycetoma or eumycotic mycetoma) or bacteria (actinomycetoma or actinomycotic mycetoma). The term *Madura foot* has been used to describe the foot lesion. While mycetoma of either fungal or bacterial etiology is progressive over years, eumycetoma progresses more slowly than actinomycetoma. A localized swollen lesion begins to develop at the site of traumatic inoculation, usually on the hand or foot. Lesions contain suppurative abscesses with sinuses that drain the abscess. Organisms coalesce into granules or grains. As infection advances there is swelling and distortion of the site of infection with sinus tracts waxing and waning. In this case, the infection has not reached the stage of draining sinus tracts. The agents of actinomycetoma also form filaments. A distinction between the two major etiologic groups can be made by observing the width of the filaments. Agents of actinomycetomas have filaments 0.5 to 1 μm in width while fungal hyaphe are greater than 1 μm. There are multiple bacteria or fungi that have been isolated from infection and specific etiology requires culture identification. Although several fungi have been isolated in the United States from persons who have mycetoma, *Pseudallescheria boydii* appears to be one of the most common. *P. boydii* is the teleomorph of *Scedosporium apiospermum* and *Graphium eumorpum*. In the other subcutaneous fungal infections, the organisms do not aggregate or coalesce into granules and have other features that may be useful in establishing etiology·of those infections.

342. The answer is d. (*Brooks, Ch 45. Levinson, Ch 49. Murray, Ch 72. Ryan, pp 743-746.*) Although pulmonary fungal infections in the healthy host are generally asymptomatic to subclinical, in some individuals they are symptomatic (see table on the next page). The degree and duration may be related to exposure or possibly strain. The fungi associated with these infections while found to varying degrees worldwide have endemic areas. In the United States, Kentucky is in the endemic area (heaviest along the Mississippi and Ohio Rivers) for histoplasmosis, an infection of *Histoplasma capsulatum*. Soil with high nitrogen content such as that containing bird or bat guano promotes growth of the organisms. Excavation or activity that disturbs soil can aerosolize organisms so outdoor activities such as construction work increase the risk of exposure. In its normal habitat, the organism grows in the mold form producing both tuberculate macroconidia and microconidia. The former are distinctive structures in culture identification and the later are small enough to be inhaled into the lungs. This is the most common of the pulmonary mycoses and more than 80% of individuals in the highly endemic area have evidence of exposure. Although men and women are equally exposed, men are more likely to get symptomatic disease than women (about 4:1). The primary pulmonary infection may disseminate. Examination and culture of sputum is often negative in pulmonary infection. In the host, the organism converts to a yeast growth form and can propagate intracellularly within macrophage. The endemic area for blastomycosis overlaps that of histoplasmosis but infection is much less common and is not associated with demolition and construction exposure. In the United States, the endemic area for coccidioidomycosis is in the desert southwest along the border with Mexico with

ENDEMIC MYCOSES	Coccidioidomycosis	Histoplasmosis	Blastomycosis	Paracoccidioidomycosis	Penicilliosis
Etiology	*Coccidioides immitis, C. posadasii*	*Histoplasma capsulatum var. capsulatum,*[a] *var. duboisii*	*Blastomyces dermatitidis*	*Paracoccidioides brasiliensis*	*Penicillium marneffei*
Habitat	Soil	Soil with high nitrogen content, for example enriched bat or avian droppings	Appears to be decaying organic matter	Not well-established, likely soil; endemic area has high humidity, rich vegetation, acidic soil, moderate temperature	Bamboo rat and habitat
Geographic distribution	Semiarid regions; *C. immitis* concentrated California; *C. posadasii* elsewhere southwestern USA, portions of Mexico, Central and South America	Global with endemic areas. In the USA var. *capsulatum* broad regions of Ohio and Mississippi River valleys; var. *duboisii*, African central west coast	In North America overlaps with histoplasmosis and includes southeastern and south central states, especially bordering Ohio and Mississippi Rivers, Midwest states, and Canadian provinces border Great Lakes and along St. Lawrence River Elsewhere most frequently Africa	Central and South America with greater prevalence the later, for example Brazil, Columbia	Southeast Asia, southern China, portion of an Indian state

Growth environment, ambient temperature	Hyaline septate hyphae and arthroconidia (barrel shaped 2-3 × 3-6 μm) that typically alternate disjunctor cells and released by lysis disjunctor cells	Hyaline septate hyphae, produce both tuberculate thick-wall macroconidia (8-16 μM) and round-oval smooth-walled microconidia (2-5 μM)	Hyaline septate hyphae producing pyriform to globose conidia (2-10 μm)	Hyaline septate hyphae; in the laboratory producing intercalary chlamydospores and in some conditions, round conidia (2-3 μm), and arthroconidia may also be observed	Hyaline septate hyphae producing typical *Penicillium* brush-like clusters of conidia (2.5-5 μM) chains at the tips of phialides; in culture colonies have bluish-gray-green center, white periphery and red diffusible pigment on the reverse
Infective form	Arthroconidia	Microconidia (small enough to reach alveoli)	Conidia	Presumed conidia and/or hyphal fragments	Conidia

(Continued)

ENDEMIC MYCOSES (CONTINUED)

	Coccidioidomycosis	Histoplasmosis	Blastomycosis	Paracoccidioidomycosis	Penicilliosis
Tissue form, 37°C	Thick-walled spherules (10-80 μM) filled with endospores (2-5 μm diameter) that rupture to release endospores to repeat cycle	Intracellular narrow-based oval budding yeast cells; var. *capsulatum* 2-6 μm and var. *duboisii* 12-15 μm	Thick-walled broad-based budding yeast (8-15 μm)	Large (15-30 μm) multiply budding yeast cells	Intracellular fission yeast cells elongated (1-8 μm) with transverse septum
Clinical manifestations (abbreviated)	Men and women equally exposed. Most cases (60%) asymptomatic, subclinical Primary pulmonary infection Chronic pulmonary infection Disseminated infection affects some groups more than others	Men and women equally exposed Most cases (90%) asymptomatic, subclinical Primary pulmonary infection Chronic pulmonary infection Disseminated disease	Many infections asymptomatic, subclinical Primary pulmonary infection Chronic pulmonary infection Disseminated infection with predilection for skin and bone but also other sites	Men and women equally exposed, symptomatic infection men (@11:1) Subclinical or symptomatic primary pulmonary infection self-limiting Chronic pulmonary infection May be dormant period and reactivate and disseminate any site with mucosal lesions prominent Young adults and immunocompromised, acute and subacute disease	Opportunistic infection that disseminates with skin lesions prominent

[a]Quite frequently when the var. *capsulatum* is discussed, the var. *capsulatum* is dropped, and the reference is only to *H. capsulatum* while discussion of var. *duboisii* makes clear that the topic is var. *duboisii*.

high endemicity in California and Arizona. The endemic area of paracoccidioidomycosis is in parts of South America. There is another species or variant of *Histoplasma*, *Histoplasma duboisii*. This species is found in some areas of Africa, and has a larger yeast cell in the host, and in infection, skin and skeleton are the organs most frequently affected.

343. The answer is d. (*Brooks, Ch 45. Levinson, Ch 48. Murray, Ch 71. Ryan, pp 719-720.*) Lymphocutaneous sporotrichosis, caused by *S. schenckii*, begins at the site of inoculation, usually on an extremity or the face. The organism is most often isolated from soil, plants, or plant products, for example straw. While the infection is global, it is more often reported from tropical and subtropical regions with areas of frequency, for example Mexico. Infection is usually associated with traumatic inoculation. Exposure is generally occupational or hobby. In the USA, the puncture is often associated with rose bush thorns. Recently the possibility of zoonotic transmission, particularly from infected cats, has received more attention. The initial lesion appears at the site of puncture. The lesion often ulcerates and may develop a raised erythematous border. Additional new lesions may appear along lymphatics that drain the primary lesion about 2 weeks after the primary lesion. Extracutaneous sporotrichosis is seen primarily in bones and joints. There is no evidence to suggest that any portal of entry besides skin is important. The primary lesion may become "fixed", may not spread, and may resemble a malignant process. *S. schenckii* is a thermally dimorphic fungus growing as a mold in its natural habitat and as a yeast in infected tissue. The organisms are often sparse in tissue complicating direct examination. Other species *Blastomyces, Coccidioides, Histoplasma,* and *Paracoccidioides* are also dimorphic but rarely cause primary cutaneous infection. *Fonsecaea pedrosoi* is the most common cause of another subcutaneous mycosis, chromomycosis. *Malassezia furfur* is a component of normal skin flora that may cause superficial disease, pityriasis versicolor while *Microsporum canis* is a zoophilic dermatophyte that can cause tinea corporis. *Stachybotrys chartarum* in recent years has been associated with growth on cellulose-rich materials in water damaged buildings.

344. The answer is a. (*Brooks, p 626. Levinson, pp 342-343. Murray, pp 718-724.*) The dermatophytes are a group of fungi that infect only superficial keratinized tissue (skin, hair, and nails; see the table in Question 338). Dermatophytes are probably restricted to nonviable skin because most are unable to grow at 37°C or in the presence of serum. Such lesions are among the most prevalent in the world. They are not life-threatening, but can be persistent and troublesome. The organisms form hyphae and arthroconidia in skin (see the image at the bottom of answer to Question 374). In hair, the hyphae and arthoconidia may be either inside (endothrix) or outside (ectothrix) the hair shaft. Infections by dermatophyte are termed tinea followed by the body site infected, for example tinea pedis for infection of the foot. More than one species may cause the same manifestation. In culture, macroscopic (color, texture, etc) observation of colonies and microscopic (conidia) morphology and nutritional requirements can be used in identification. The conidia that are formed are generally indicative of one of the three genera of dermatophytes. Identification of *Microsporum* spp. is aided by the appearance of macroconidia, *Trichophyton* spp. by microconidia, and *Epidermophyton floccosum* by distinctive macroconidia may sometimes described as "beaver tail" (see Question 358). Tinea pedis, or athlete's foot, is the most common dermatophytosis. The organism may be acquired from desquamated epithelial cells. Classically, this occurs in common bathing areas used by groups of individuals such as athletes and shared use of towels. Among prevention efforts in athletic facilities are maintaining cleanliness of shared facilities, daily washing of towels, education of athletes, and staff on infection control for skin diseases.

345. The answer is e. (*Brooks, Ch 45. Levinson, Ch 50. Murray, pp 754-756. Ryan, pp 723-729.*) *Candida albicans* is the most important species of *Candida* and is part of the normal flora of skin, mouth, GI tract, and vagina. When host defense is compromised it can cause opportunistic cutaneous and mucosal infections such as thrush (pseudomembranous candidiasis), vaginitis, skin, and nail infections as well as candidemia and deep-seated infection. As a commensal, it is generally in the yeast form while lesions in infection generally show the additional presence of hyphae and pseudohyphae. Material from a pseudomembrane will show host cells, bacteria and mass of yeast cells, pseudohyphae, and hyphae. Since the organisms can be present as a commensal, culture is not a confirmation of infection. The diagnosis is made by clinical presentation of the pseudomembrane and the microscopic observation. This patient has two risk factors for the development of pseudomembranous candidiasis; disturbance of the normal bacterial flora due to the use of penicillin and diabetes. *Candida* infection can be treated with topical nystatin or clotrimazole troches or oral fluconazole. Hyphae with acute angle branching is characteristic of *Aspergillus* spp., which may be recovered in sputum as may spherules containing endospores found in *Coccidioides* spp. But neither are associated with oral pseudomembranous lesions.

346. The answer is d. (*Brooks, Ch 45. Levinson, Ch 48. Murray, Ch 70. Ryan, Ch 44.*) Tinea nigra is a superficial infection of the stratum corneum that is usually a solitary lesion on the palms or sole that may range in color from tan to black. The lesion is chronic and asymptomatic. The infection is found most often in tropical climates and coastal regions in children and young adults with a greater incidence in women. The etiology is a dematiaceous fungus, *Hortaea werneckii* (previously *Cladosporium, Exophiala*, or *Phaeoannellomyces werneckii*). Dematiaceous (dark-colored) fungi produce melanin found in their cell walls. The melanin imparts a dark color to the organisms in host tissue as well as culture where colonies may appear dark brown, green-brown, or black. Microscopic examination of cultured organisms shows the pigmentation in the organism. The dark colorization of the lesion is from the fungus. The lesion may grossly resemble a malignant melanoma and more invasive procedures for this condition may be avoided by examination of skin scrapings of the lesion for fungal elements. The infection responds to topical treatment with keratolytic solutions or azole antifungal drugs. Although tinea manuum is an infection of the hand by fungi, the etiology is a dermatophyte. The other infections, tinea capitis, tinea corporis, and tinea pedis, are also infections by dermatophytes at other body sites (see the table in Question 336).

347. The answer is a. (*Brooks, Ch 45. Levinson, Ch 59. Murray, Ch 73. Ryan, Ch 44.*) Fungal infections are potentially serious in a bone marrow transplant unit (BMTU), *Candida* and *Aspergillus* are the most common causes of infection in BMT patients and both have a risk of mortality. However, the two differ in that *Candida* is a human commensal and cannot be excluded by construction practices and environmental air monitoring. On the other hand, aspergilli are ubiquitous in the environment. There are instances of multiple infections in new units that have not been monitored prior to opening or in units adjacent to construction projects. Strict precautions should be taken to exclude dust and debris from the BMTU area during construction, but in any event, the environment should be monitored for airborne microorganisms, especially *Aspergillus*, prior to opening the unit. Zygomycetes may also be present in the air but are a less frequent cause of opportunistic infection in the BMT patient. While *Penicillium* organisms are also frequent in air, the species associated with opportunistic infection, *P. marneffei*, is endemic in Southeast Asia where it causes disease in the AIDS patient. *Pneumocystis jiroveci* is an anthropophilic organism with a human reservoir and, like, *Candida* not excluded by construction practices. Although particularly recognized for opportunistic infection in AIDS patients, other immunocompromised patients may also have infection, including the occasional BMT patient.

348. The answer is b. (*Brooks, Ch 45. Levinson, Ch 49. Murray, Ch 72. Ryan, Ch 46.*) *Histoplasma capsulatum* is a thermally dimorphic fungus soil saprophyte that in the environment or room temperature grows as a mold that produces two types of conidia: tuberculate macroconidia and microconidia. Inhalation of the microconidia which are small enough to reach the lungs, initiates infection. Inhaled microconidia are engulfed by macrophages and develop into yeast forms. Most infections remain asymptomatic; small granulomatous foci heal by calcification. However, pneumonia can occur. In tissue, the yeasts are typically seen within macrophages since the organism is a facultative intracellular parasite. Arthrospores (arthroconidia) result from the fragmentation of hyphal cells. *Coccidioides* spp. produce arthroconidia in their natural habitat. In the infected host, this thermally dimorphic organism grows as spherules producing endospores. Another dimorphic fungus, *Blastomyces dermatitidis*, grows as yeast cells producing buds on a broad base in the human host. Yeast cells, hyphae, and pseudohyphae are associated with infections of *Candida albicans* (see the table in Question 342).

349. The answer is d. (*Brooks, Ch 45. Levinson, Ch 50. Murray, Ch 73. Ryan, Ch 45.*) This description is a typical picture of mucormycosis (also has been called zygomycosis) occurring in a diabetic patient. Etiologic agents of the genera *Rhizopus, Mucor, Lichtheimia* (former *Absidia*), *Rhizomucor*, and others belong to the order Mucorales. These organism have wide (10-15 μm), uneven thickness, and irregular branching hyphae that are aseptate or have rare septation. Hyphae may be sparse in infected tissue. The organisms do not contain melanin and are not dematiaceous. *Hortaea werneckii*, etiologic agent of tinea nigra, has dematiaceous hyphae in tissue. In skin some of the hyaline hyphae of dermatophytes may have arthroconidia. Among opportunistic molds, *Aspergillus* spp. have septate acute angle branching in tissue. Organisms that grow in yeast forms in the host include *Histoplasma* and *Blastomyces* while *C. albicans* generally has both yeast cells, hyphae, and pseudohyphae in lesions. Fungal hyphae are generally greater than 1 μm while narrow filaments are associate with bacteria such as *Nocardia* spp.

350. The answer is d. (*Brooks, Ch 45. Levinson, Ch 49. Murray, Ch 72. Ryan, Ch 46.*) Coccidioidomycosis is a primary pulmonary infection which is asymptomatic or subclinical in about 60% of infected individuals and is initiated from inhalation of arthroconidia (arthrospores) (see the table in Question 342). Coccidioidomycosis is endemic to the dessert southwest, parts of Mexico, and Central and South America. There are two species with *C. immitis* concentrated in California and *C. posadasii* elsewhere. The infection is the same regardless of species. The organism grows as a mold in soil. Some hyphae give rise to arthroconidia, which are produced in alternating cells. When the disjunctor cells separating the arthroconidia lyse, the barrel-shaped arthroconidia are released. These conidia can be aerosolized when the soil is disturbed. Subcutaneous fungal infections such as sporotrichosis are initiated by traumatic implantation. Some individuals with coccidioidomycosis have factors that increase the risk of dissemination and extrapulmonary infection. The most common site of dissemination is the skin. However, these skin lesions are not initiated by cutaneous contact or implantation but dissemination from the original primary pulmonary infection.

351. The answer is c. (*Brooks, Ch 45. Levinson, Ch 50. Murray, Ch 73. Ryan, Ch 45.*) *Aspergillus* can cause a variety of host infections or responses. In immunocompromised persons, invasive disease is the concern. Blood vessel invasion can result in thrombosis and infarction. Infection can progress rapidly and may disseminate. Invasive pulmonary infection is associated with mortality risk. The organism can infect wounds, for example burn wounds, cornea following trauma, or surgery. In pulmonary cavities (from preexisting conditions, eg, tuberculosis, histoplasmosis), "fungus ball" formation can occur, which can be seen on x-ray. Infection of the bronchi can result in allergic bronchopulmonary aspergillosis, characterized by asthmatic symptoms. Otomycosis is typically due to *A. niger* and is a superficial colonization with clinical features similar to other causes of external otitis.

352. The answer is a. (*Brooks, Ch 45. Levinson, Ch 49. Murray, Ch 72. Ryan, pp 749-753.*) Most individuals infected with *Coccidioides* spp. have asymptomatic or subclinical infections. Only about 40% have symptomatic primary pulmonary disease. In a small fraction of these individuals (about 5% of symptomatic individuals), the organism may disseminate and cause extrapulmonary disease. The risk of dissemination is greater among some population groups than others. Those at increased risk include infants and elderly, men, dark-skinned individuals, for example Filipinos, African Americans, and immunocompromised individuals including AIDS patients, and pregnant women. Women in the third trimester or immediate postpartum period are at very high risk of dissemination and death. Since the infection is self-limiting, in individuals without risk factors, antifungal therapy is not indicated although supportive therapy for symptoms may be offered. Those with risk factors or severe primary disease generally merit treatment to reduce risk of dissemination. Women in the third trimester require treatment. Amphotericin B and fluconazole are usually considered. Reports that several azoles possess teratogenic potential particularly early in pregnancy suggest that azoles should be used with care in pregnant women. A recent set of recommendations suggest amphotericin B during the first trimester and azoles later (Bercovitch et al. *Clin. Infect Dis* 2011;53(4):353–368.)

353. The answer is c. (*Brooks, Ch. 45. Levinson, Ch. 50, 52. Murray, Ch. 73, Ryan, Ch. 45.*) *Pneumocystis jiroveci* causes an interstitial pneumonia in immunocompromised patients and severely malnourished infants. The infection became more prominent with the AIDS epidemic as an AIDS-defining opportunistic infection in the United States. With current treatment strategies for HIV/AIDS and prophylaxis, there has been a decrease in those with access to treatment. However, it remains a leading cause of infection in those without access, who do not tolerate treatment, or who do not know of their HIV infection. Patients without HIV infection now account for the majority of cases in the developed world. These non-HIV immunocompromised patients include those with hematologic malignancies and organ transplants. Treatment-related risk factors for these patients include steroid and cytotoxic therapy. *P. jiroveci* (formerly *P. carinii*) was originally classified as a protozoan but has been reclassified in the fungal kingdom for many years. It is not a typical fungus as it lacks ergosterol in the plasma membrane, and thus antifungal drugs that target ergosterol or its biosynthesis are not effective. The organisms have not been maintained in culture and diagnosis depends on observing the organism in clinical specimens. The names of the forms that seem to be most commonly used still reflect the former protozoan designation. These are variously described as free trophic forms or trophozoites, which are haploid, and the diploid cyst that when mature may contain up to eight spores or intracystic bodies. *Pneumocystis* is found in humans and a variety of mammals and each fungal species appears to have host specificity so the *P. jiroveci* is isolated from humans and *P. carinii* from rats. Although the species infecting humans is now designated *P. jiroveci*, the name PCP (*P. carinii* pneumonia) has been retained by many for convenience. In AIDS patients, the onset of symptoms may be subtle with progression while in other immunocompromised patients the onset may be acute.

354 and 355. The answers are 354-c and 355-e. (*Brooks, Ch 45. Levinson, Ch 47. Murray, Ch 69. Ryan, Ch 43.*) See the answer for Question 336 and the below table). Several mechanisms of resistance to antifungal drugs have been identified. These include alterations in the drug target by mutation or overexpression, drug efflux pumps, changes in ergosterol or sterol content, and changes in uptake and metabolism. Alteration of the drug either through modification or degradation to inactive moieties has not been reported. Resistance to tolnaftate and allylamines that inhibit squalene epoxidase is not common but likely mechanisms include efflux pumps, mutation or overexpression of the enzyme and nonspecific stress adaptation. Resistance to flucytosine may occur via alteration of the permease that reduces entry into the fungal cell or at enzymatic steps, cytosine deaminase or uracil phosphoribosyl transferase, involved in metabolism of the drug to the active compounds. Resistance to azole class drugs may develop through expression of drug efflux pumps and alteration or overexpression of the drug target. In some resistant isolates, more than one mechanism may be operative. Resistance to polyenes may reflect a decrease in ergosterol content of the membrane or production of other non-polyene binding sterols.

356. The answer is e. (*Brooks, Ch 45. Levinson, Ch 47. Murray, Ch 69. Ryan, Ch 43.*) See the answer to Question 336 and the table in that question. Ergosterol in the fungal cell membrane is exploited by several drug classes. The squalene epoxidase is inhibited by both tolnaftate and allylamines.

A later step in the pathway, a cytochrome P450 enzyme 14-α-demethylase is inhibited by azole (imidazole, triazole) class drugs. Disruption of ergosterol biosynthesis results in aberrant cell membranes. Amphotericin B targets ergosterol by binding to the sterol.

357. The answer is e. (*Brooks, Ch 45. Levinson, Ch 50. Murray, Ch 72.*) *Penicillium marneffei* is a dimorphic fungus that causes opportunistic disseminated penicilliosis that develops following inhalation of conidia (see the table in Question 342). Infection is primarily seen in HIV-infected individuals, although it is also reported in other immunocompromised hosts. The organism is endemic in Southeast Asia (eg, Thailand, southern China, Viet Nam, a portion of India) and is associated with bamboo rats. A few imported cases have been reported elsewhere in patients with a travel history to the endemic region. A majority of patients have dissemination to the skin with rashes, papules, and pustules that are often located on the face. In the environment and culture at environmental temperature the organism grows as a mold with typical *Penicillium* morphology and produces a red diffusible pigment. In the host, the organism grows as a fission yeast unlike other infectious fungi with a yeast form that grow by budding. Microscopic detection of the fission yeast in clinical specimens such as smears from skin lesions is diagnostic.

358. The answer is a. (*Brooks, Ch 45. Levinson, Ch 50. Murray, Ch 70. Ryan, Ch 45.*) The presence of hyaline hyphae supports a diagnosis of a dermatophyte infection (see the table in Question 336). Dermatophyte infections may be exacerbated by the use of topical steroids. With such exposure the infection may not give the typical picture and may be called tinea incognito. This infection started in the groin region where such infections are known as tinea cruris or jock itch. Dermatophytes are identified in culture by the macroscopic morphology of the colony and the microscopic morphology of asexual production of conidia. Both macroconidia and microconidia may be produced but one is more abundant and used in identification while the other is rare. *Trichophyton* species produce numerous microconidia whose appearance and location are useful in their identification. *Microsporum* species (except *M. audouinii*) produce macroconidia that are borne singly and that have distinctive shapes and rough walls. *Epidermophyton floccosum* produces only macroconidia. These are usually produced in clusters and have a distinctive clavate shape sometimes described as "beaver-tail". The schematic shows clavate macroconidia with this shape, which is consistent with *E. floccosum*.

359. The answer is b. (*Brooks, Ch 45. Levinson, Ch 50. Murray, Ch 71. Ryan, Ch 44.*) Chromoblastomycosis also called chromomycosis is a subcutaneous fungal infection in which the etiologic agent gains entry to the host through traumatic implantation or inoculation. The recognized agents of this infection include *Phialophora verrucosa*, *Fonsecaea pedrosoi*, *Rhinocladiella aquaspersa*, *F. compacta*, and *Cladophialophora carrionii*. The agents of this infection, as indicated by the term "chromo," are all dematiaceous fungi that have pigmented cell walls due to the presence of melanin. The organism is also pigmented in tissue hence the presence of pigmented fungal structures. The characteristic feature is the presence of muriform cells known as sclerotic cells or Medlar bodies, which are thick-walled septated cells. The infection occurs mainly in the tropics and in males and more often on legs than on the upper body. The infection develops slowly and may have a history of many years development. In this case, the infection is in an early stage. When infection develops over a longer period, the lesion may become verrucous and warty and develop cauliflower-like lesions, which probably spread by autoinoculation or local lymphatic spread. Blastomycosis is initiated as primary pulmonary infection that may disseminate, with skin lesions being the most common extrapulmonary manifestation. *Blastomyces dermatitidis* is a thermally dimorphic fungus that in tissue is found in the yeast form with cells that have a broad base between mother and daughter cell. Lacaziosis (lobomycosis) is a subcutaneous mycosis caused by *Lacazia loboi* (formerly *Loboa loboi*) that is found primarily in South and Central American tropics. The infection is characterized by slowly developing nodules that vary in size, shape, and appearance, that may spread by autoinoculation, and that progress over decades. In tissue the organisms are found as large, thick-walled yeast cells that may appear as a chain of cells with narrow bridges. The organism has not been cultured. The infection is also found in dolphins and an aquatic habitat is postulated. Eumycetoma is another slow-developing subcutaneous fungal infection, frequently found on the legs or feet. The infection is more common in tropical areas and is present at higher frequency in some areas such as India, Africa, and Latin America. A number of fungal agents have been identified, many of them dematiaceous. There is localized swelling and abscess formation and draining sinuses. In tissue the organisms are found as granules that contain septate hyphae that may be distorted at the periphery. Granules may also be found in sinus tract exudate. A similar disease may have a bacterial etiology known as actinomycetoma with granules that also contain filaments that are narrower than fungal hyphae. Mycetoma is a term that covers both fungal and bacterial etiology. Sporotrichosis is yet another subcutaneous mycosis that, like the others, is initiated by traumatic implantation. The initial lesion appears at the site of trauma, and with disease development additional lesions may appear along the lymphatic draining the region (see the answer to 343). In tissue, the organism is a budding yeast that is sometimes described as cigar-shaped and there may be few present in a specimen.

360. The answer is e. (*Brooks, Ch 45. Levinson, Ch 48. Murray, Ch 70. Ryan, Ch 44.*) Onychomycosis is the most common nail disease in adults and the majority are attributed to dermatophytes and called tinea unguium (see the table in Question 338). Treatment for tinea unguium is prolonged. Without determining a fungal etiology, there may be expensive, ineffective treatment, and unnecessary drug exposure. The other infections are also dermatophyte infections at other body sites.

361. The answer is a. (*Brooks, Ch 45. Levinson, Ch 49. Murray, Ch 72. Ryan, Ch 46.*) Blastomycosis is a primary pulmonary infection that is frequently asymptomatic or subclinical as are the other infections, coccidioidomycosis, histoplasmosis, and paracoccidioidomycosis, with systemic dimorphic pathogens (see the table in Question 342). Infection may disseminate hematogenously with about two-thirds of extrapulmonary blastomycosis cases involving skin and bones. Pulmonary symptoms may not be present in disseminated disease. Infection is endemic in North America bordering the Mississippi and Ohio River basins, the Midwest and Canadian provinces around Great Lakes and St. Lawrence River, and in the Southeast. *Blastomyces dermatitidis* is a dimorphic fungus growing as mold in its normal habitat. The habitat has not been well characterized but may well involve patches of moist soil with abundance of organic material. The conidia of the environmental form are nondescript. They may be inhaled when the habitat is disturbed and initiate infection. The inhaled organism converts to a yeast phase, characterized by a broad base between mother and bud. The observation of these distinctive structures in a clinical specimen is a basis for diagnosis that should be confirmed by culture.

362. The answer is e. (*Brooks, Ch 45. Levinson, Ch 49. Murray, Ch 72. Ryan, Ch 46.*) In histoplasmosis, inhaled *H. capsulatum* conidia develop into yeast cells, which are engulfed by alveolar macrophages (see the table in Question 342). The yeast cells can replicate intracellularly. These may give rise to inflammatory reactions that become granulomatous. In culture at 25°C, *H. capsulatum* develops hyphae with microconidia and large, spherical macroconidia with peripheral projections of cell wall materials. The macroconidia are also called tuberculate macroconidia. The macroconidia are useful in culture identification, while the microconidia are small enough to be inhaled to initiate infection. Arthroconidia (arthrospores) result from the fragmentation of hyphal cells of *Coccidioides* spp. Spherules result when arthroconidia are inhaled and enlarge into larger bodies that contain endospores. Spherules can be produced in the laboratory using a complex medium. Sclerotic bodies are found in chromoblastomycosis infections. The agents of chromoblastomycosis reside in soil and vegetation and may cause infections when introduced into subcutaneous tissue. In tissue, the fungi appear as spherical brown cells termed muniform or sclerotic bodies that divide by transverse separation. Separation in different planes may give rise to a cluster of 4 to 8 cells.

363. The answer is b. (*Brooks, Ch 45. Levinson, Ch 50. Murray, Ch 73. Ryan, Ch 45.*) *Candida albicans* is a component of normal microbial flora of the skin and mucosal surfaces. *Candida* may reach the blood stream by translocation from the gut or more often via catheters. Candidemia has a high attributable mortality, and once in the blood the fungus can cause infection in any organ. Vascular catheters are an established risk factor for infection. Endogenous organisms or occasionally exogenous organisms (eg, from skin of health care worker) reach the lumen of the catheter and a biofilm develops. While planktonic organisms are organisms living alone, a biofilm is a community of organisms attached to a surface and surrounded by an extracellular matrix of its own production. Biofilms may have a complex species composition, for example tooth plaque, or be composed of a single species. As biofilms mature, planktonic organisms are released, and in the case of catheter biofilms, the released organisms continuously inoculate the blood. Organisms in biofilms acquire new phenotypic properties. One of the properties is reduced susceptibility to antifungal drugs (or antibacterial drugs in the case of bacteria). Drug concentrations that are effective against planktonic organisms are ineffective against biofilms. Consequently, a patient may receive a therapeutic drug dose that acts successfully against planktonic organisms in circulation or tissue but is not effective against the biofilm organisms. Biofilms can continue to release planktonic organisms to infect surrounding tissue or blood. As noted, the source of blood stream infection may be inoculation from a biofilm in the catheter. Therefore, the catheter is removed to eliminate a potential source of infection. While *Aspergillus* and *Cryptococcus*, as well as some other fungi can form biofilms on devices, the reports are still few and fungemia is uncommon. *Candida* is the most common cause of fungal biofilm-related infection and ranks high on the list of causes of nosocomial bloodstream infection.

364. The answer is a. (*Brooks, Ch 45. Levinson, Ch 49. Murray, Ch 72. Ryan, Ch 46.*) Coccidioidomycosis (also known as Valley fever) is caused by *C. immitis* or *C. posadasii* (see the table in Question 342). The infection is endemic in the semiarid regions of the southwestern United States, as well as Central and South America. Most *C. immitis* isolates are from California while *C. posadasii* has been found elsewhere. The species have few phenotypic differences and clinical manifestations appear the same. Hyphae form chains of arthroconidia (arthrospores), which often develop in alternate cells of a hypha. Individual arthroconidia are released from chains, become airborne, and are resistant to harsh environmental conditions. Following inhalation, arthroconidia become spherical, enlarge forming spherules that contain endospores. Such spherules have a thick, refractive cell wall and are diagnostic of *Coccidioides* spp. Blastospores represent conidial formation through a budding process, as seen in yeast. Sporangiospores are asexual structures characteristic of zygomycetes produced within an enclosed sporangium, often supported by one sporangiophore (*Rhizopus*, *Mucor*).

365. The answer is d. (*Brooks, Ch 45. Levinson, Ch 48. Murray, Ch 70. Ryan, Ch 44.*) Dermatophytoses are cutaneous mycoses caused by three genera of fungi: *Microsporum*, *Trichophyton*, and *Epidermophyton* (see the table in Question 338). Dermatophytes may have as their normal habitat the soil, animals (other than man), or man and are described, respectively, as geophilic, zoophilic, or anthropophilic organisms. Dermatophytes are found worldwide. Most isolates from infection today are anthropophilic with *Trichophyton rubrum* the most common isolate. There are differences in geographic distribution of species. Infection occurs in keratinized tissue. Infection can be transmitted by transfer of arthroconidia or hyphae or keratinous material containing the fungi. Some species remain viable in desquamated skin scales or hair for long periods and contact may be direct or indirect via fomites. There is a general correlation between normal habitat and infection with infections due to anthropophilic species, tending to be chronic, less responsive to treatment and recurrent while geophilic and zoophilic species are associated with more acute host response and respond to treatment. However, infection can reoccur, if the exposure continues. *Microsporum canis* is the most frequent zoophilic species isolated in the USA. Despite the name, there are more infected cats than dogs. In this case, the cat is likely infected, which may or may not be obvious to the household. As long as an individual continues in contact with the animal, there may be reinfection. To interrupt this cycle the pet will also need treatment. Many of the same drugs used to treat humans are used in the treatment of pets. Infection of the smooth skin is tinea corporis. The infection spreads outward, creating the round appearance indicated by ringworm. The lesion may have a cleared center and raised erythematous or vesicular border. Lesions may overlap giving a more irregular border and infections with anthropophilic isolates generally have a less inflammatory response.

366. The answer is b. (*Brooks, Ch 45. Levinson, Ch 49. Murray, Ch 72. Ryan, Ch 46.*) *Blastomyces dermatitidis*, the etiologic agent of blastomycosis, is a thermally dimorphic fungus (see the table in Question 342). In the environment, it grows as a mold producing conidia. The conidia are inhaled and convert to the yeast phase in the lung. The yeast phase is characterized by a broad base between the parent yeast cell and the daughter bud. At 25°C in the laboratory, the fungus grows as mold producing conidia. The conidia are not distinctive and look similar to conidia of other species. On the other hand, when grown on the appropriate medium at 37°C in the laboratory, the characteristic yeast form with broad-based budding is observed. Like *B. dermatitidis, Paracoccidioides brasiliensis* produces conidia in the mold form that are not distinctive in species identification, while the multiply-budding yeast form found in tissue and also grown in the laboratory is a distinctive structure in culture identification. Hyphae of the thermally dimorphic *Coccidioides* spp. can produce arthroconidia in nature and at room temperature in the laboratory. *Histoplasma capsulatum*, also one of the thermally dimorphic fungi that is an agent of systemic disease, produces both microconidia and macroconidia in nature and at room temperature in the laboratory. The macroconida are tuberculate and distinctive. In tissue the organism is a small budding yeast cell often found within macrophage. *Cryptococcus* spp. grow as encapsulated budding yeast in routine laboratory culture and also in tissue.

367. The answer is d. (*Brooks, Ch 45. Levinson, Ch 50. Murray, Ch 73. Ryan, Ch 5.*) *Candida albicans* is a component of normal human flora of mucosal (oral, gastrointestinal, and vaginal) and cutaneous surfaces. Most infections are of endogenous origin at or from these surfaces. There are occasional reports of infections traced to flora of health care workers. Because organisms can be isolated from normal locations in the absence of disease, isolation from these surfaces (or in contact with a surface, eg, sputum) must be correlated with clinical symptoms. On the other hand, isolation from a sterile site such as blood is significant. *C. albicans* is thought to reach the blood stream either by translocation from the gut or from a catheter in which a biofilm has developed after inoculation from skin organisms (see the answer to Question 363).

368. The answer is e. (*Brooks, Ch 45. Levinson, Ch 48. Murray, Ch 70. Ryan, Ch 44.*) Pityriasis versicolor is caused by species of *Malassezia* (this genus name is accepted over *Pityrosporum* that was sometimes used) that are normal skin flora. In 1996, seven taxa were recognized, of which *M. furfur* is only one. All seven species have been isolated from infection with geographical variation. Diagnosis is made by visualization of the fungal elements in epidermal skin scales treated with KOH with or without staining. Round yeast cells and hyphae, usually short, are present. The mixture of fungal elements has sometimes been described as "spaghetti and meatballs". Culture is usually not necessary for these normal flora species as they can be isolated in the absence of disease. Arthroconidia are distinctive structures used in culture identification of *Coccidioides* spp. In dermatophyte infections, infected skin and hair will show the presence of hyaline (clear) hyphae and arthroconidia with the later particular abundant in infected hair shaft specimens. Dematiaceous hyphae are found in skin scales removed from the superficial skin infection tinea nigra. Yeast cells with broad-based budding is observed in tissue infected with *Blastomyces dermatitidis.*

369. The answer is e. (*Brooks, Ch 45. Levinson, Ch 49. Murray, Ch 72. Ryan, Ch 46.*) The silver-stained structure is a parent yeast cell with multiple buds (see the table in Question 342). This is a distinctive structure found in tissue infected with *Paracoccidioides brasiliensis*, a dimorphic fungus. This is also the form observed in culture at 37°C. The mold phase is found in the environment and in culture at room temperature. The organism is found in areas of Central and South America. The skin test for exposure is about equal for men and women in the endemic areas. However, among adults symptomatic disease is more than 10:1 in men. After initial pulmonary infection, there may be a latent period that may be many years before additional pulmonary symptoms and potential dissemination. While dissemination may occur in any organ there is predilection for mucosal tissue and lesions are often seen in the mouth. The organism is assumed to grow in soil and exposure is by inhalation of conidia or hyphal fragments. While exposure could be by fomite transmission, the patient was most likely exposed during the period he was stationed in South America. Primarily in men this dimorphic fungus can convert to the yeast forms. Conversion can be inhibited by physiological levels of ergosterol in women. This failure to convert is the likely explanation for the sexual bias in symptomatic disease.

370. The answer is a. (*Brooks, pp 642-644. Levinson, pp 349-352. Murray, pp 751-759. Ryan, Ch 43.*) *Candida albicans* has several mechanisms of resistance or reduced susceptibility to azole class drugs (see the table in Question 336). These mechanisms include changes in or overexpression of the P450 14-α-demethylase and drug efflux pumps. Some resistant strains may have all three mechanisms. Resistance to flucytosine may reflect altered uptake or change in enzymes that are involved in metabolizing the drug to active structures. Resistance to echinocandins has been reported arising from mutation in a subunit in the β-1,3-glucan synthase complex. Resistance to amphotericin B, which binds to ergosteriol can arise from reduction in the amount of membrane ergosterol or change in membrane sterol composition.

371. The answer is b. (*Brooks, Ch 45. Levinson, Ch 50. Murray, Ch 73. Ryan, Ch 45.*) Vaginitis is one of the most frequent reasons for patient visits to a gynecologist. The most common cause of infectious vaginitis is bacteria (40%-50% cases) with yeast, vulvovaginal candidiasis, accounting for about 40%. *Candida albicans* is the most common cause of yeast vaginitis. It is estimated that about 75% of women in the United States will have one episode of yeast vaginal infection during childbearing years, which means millions of cases annually. Along with physical examination, preparation and examination of a wet mount of vaginal discharge is utilized. For *C. albicans* infection, both yeast cells and hyphae and potentially pseudohyphae (chains of elongated yeast cells that did not separate after cell division) should be observed. *C. albicans* is found as a component of normal flora of the vaginal mucosa in many women; thus the presence of the organism in culture of vaginal material is not sufficient for a diagnosis of infection. *Trichomonas vaginalis* accounts for 10% to 15% of infectious vaginitis case. Trichomoniasis is the most prevalent non-viral sexually transmitted disease (STD) in the United States in a 2013 report (Satterwhite et al. *Sex Transm Dis* 40:187). This parasite is usually a marker of high-risk sexual behavior and may be present with other sexually transmitted organisms. Vaginal smears are examined for trophozoites.

372. The answer is b. (*Brooks, Ch 45. Levinson, Ch 50. Murray, Ch 73. Ryan, Chs 45-46.*) Immunosuppressive agents have reduced the incidence of rejection of transplanted solid organs but have increased risk of opportunistic infection. Fungal infections, while not the majority of infections in these patients, carry a high risk of mortality. *Candida* and *Aspergillus* are responsible for most of these opportunistic infections that can occur within a month or after several months. *A. fumigatus* (most common species) infections are primary pulmonary infections that may be a rapidly necrotizing pneumonia with a potential to disseminate. The organism is a mold in the environment and in the host. The hyphae are septate with acute angle, dichotomous, branching. *Candida* infections generally start as candidemia, which may reach the blood stream by catheters or translocation from the gut. *C. albicans* is the most frequent *Candida* isolate. This component of normal flora is generally in the yeast form as a commensal and when infection occurs the additional presence of hyphae and pseudohyphae is observed. *C. glabrata*, which is seen with increasing frequency, does not form hyphae. *Cryptococcus neoformans* is an encapsulated yeast. Other fungi have been reported with less frequency.

373. The answer is a. (*Brooks, Ch 45. Levinson, Ch 47. Murray, Ch 69. Ryan, Ch 43.*) Polyenes, such as amphotericin B, bind to ergosterol in fungal membranes and generate ion channels that affect osmolarity, membrane integrity, and allow leakage of intracellular contents (see the table in Question 336). The polyene is not completely selective and binding to cholesterol in the mammalian membrane accounts for most of the toxicity.

374. The answer is c. (*Brooks, Ch 45. Levinson, Ch 47. Murray, Ch 65. Ryan, Ch 41.*) Asexual reproduction involves only mitosis and sexual reproduction includes meiosis. Meiosis is preceded by mating of two compatible mating types with protoplast and nuclear fusion. The form of a fungus with sexual reproduction is the teleomorph form, while the form that reproduces asexually is the anamorph. Some fungi can reproduce both sexual and asexual spores and in other fungi the teleomorph form has either disappeared or not been discovered. Normally, the teleomorph name has precedence. In numerous cases with agents of human disease, the anamorph was isolated from infection and named before the teleomorph was identified in the laboratory and also named. It can be confusing, particularly to nonmycologists, when an organism has two names. Even for a fungus that can reproduce sexually, it is practice in the clinical setting to refer to organisms by their asexual names as isolated from clinical material. Even with this practice, molecular taxonomy and further study have led to some name changes. For example, *Hortaea werneckii*, etiology of tinea nigra, has previously been known as *Cladosporium werneckii*, *Exophiala werneckii*, and *Phaeoannellomyces werneckii*.

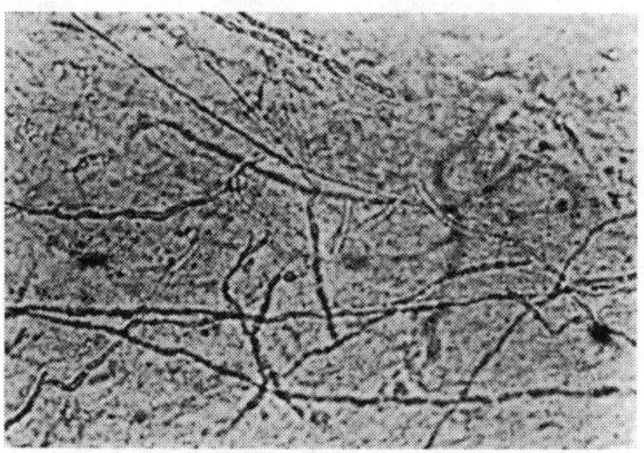

(Courtesy of *MG Rinaldi, San Antonio, Texas.*)

Parasitology

Questions

375. Babesiosis is a tick-borne disease, caused by intraerythrocytic parasites of the genus *Babesia*, resulting in affecting persons with malaise, nausea, fever, sweats, myalgia, and arthralgia and could be confused with *Plasmodium falciparum* ring form in red cells. Infection with Babesia has been most commonly observed in which of the following?

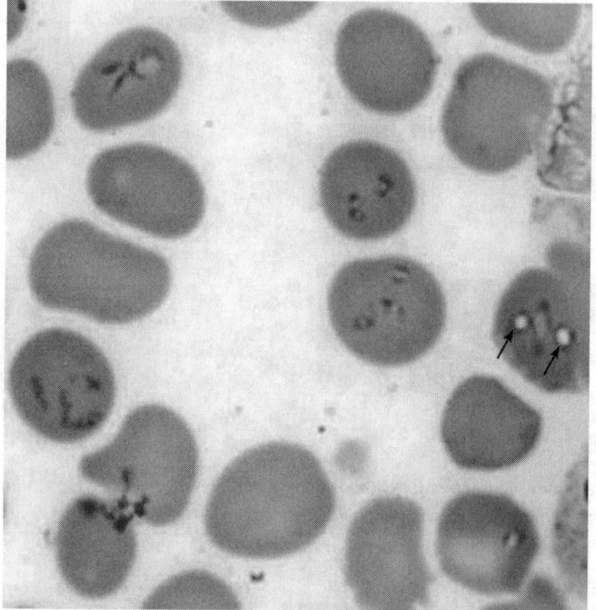

(Reproduced from the Centers for Disease Control and Prevention. http://www.dpd.cdc.gov/dpdx/html/babesiosis.htm.)

a. AIDS patients
b. Foresters
c. Splenectomized patients
d. Transfusion recipients
e. Transplant recipients

376. An AIDS patient (CD4 count < 200/μL) presents to his primary care physician with a 2-week history of watery, nonbloody diarrhea. Acid-fast staining demonstrates oocysts in fresh stool seen in the figure below. Which of the following is the most likely diagnosis?

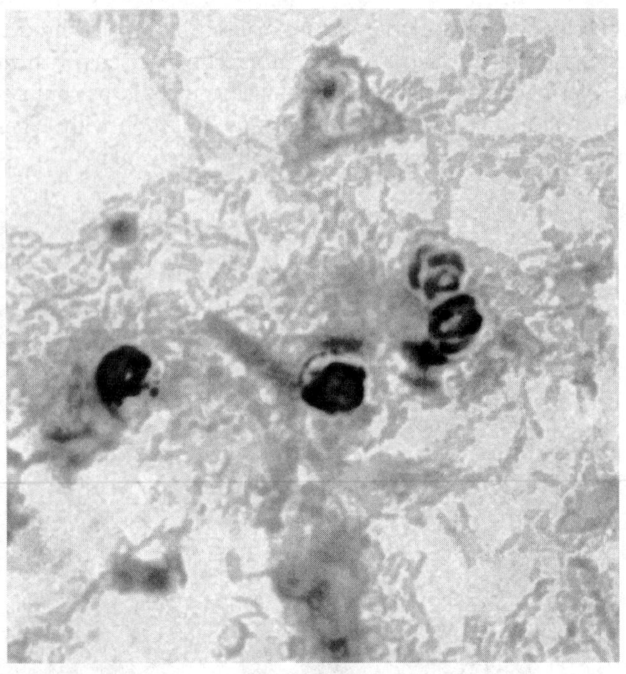

(Reproduced from the Centers for Disease Control and Prevention. Public Health Image Library, ID# 7829. http://phil.cdc.gov/phil/details.asp.)

a. Acid-fast bacilli
b. *Enterocytozoon*
c. *Cryptosporidium*
d. *Entamoeba histolytica*
e. Yeast

377. Flagellate parasite is the cause of vaginalis in women in temperate areas. It is a sexually transmittable disease. The prominent symptom is copious fowl-smelling yellow discharge that can be accompanied by cervical lesions and abdominal pain. What parasite does this represent?

a. *Entamoeba histolytica*
b. *Trichomonas vaginalis*
c. *Strongyloides stercoralis*
d. *Schistosoma mansoni*
e. *Balantidium coli*

378. A 30-year-old female stores her contact lenses in tap water. She notices deterioration of vision and visits an ophthalmologist, who diagnoses her with severe retinitis. Culture of the water as well as vitreous fluid would most likely reveal which of the following?

a. *Acanthamoeba*
b. *Babesia*
c. *Entamoeba coli*
d. *Naegleria*
e. *Pneumocystis*

379. A young nurse in a South American city located in the tropics develops classical symptoms of malaria. An accurate diagnosis of the *Plasmodium* species is necessary to provide the best treatment to insure recovery and prevent relapse. Sporozoites from a mosquito bite rapidly enter live cells where asexual merozoites enter the blood stream and RBCs are invaded. This erythrocytic stage provides a basis for laboratory diagnosis. Which of the diagnostic characteristics of *P. falciparum* is best described by the following?

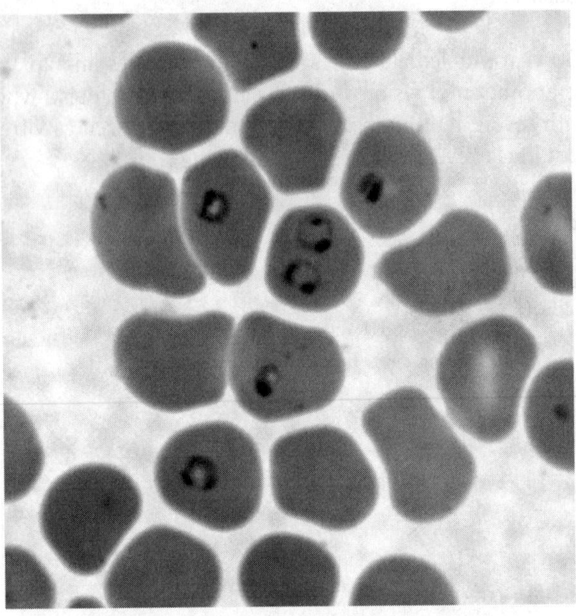

(Reproduced from the Centers for Disease Control and Prevention. http://www.dpd.cdc.gov/dpdx/html/Malaria.htm.)

a. An important diagnostic feature is the irregular appearance of the edges of the infected red blood cell
b. A period of 72 hours is required for the development of the mature schizont, which resembles a rosette with only 8 to 10 oval merozoites
c. Except in infections with very high parasitemia, only ring forms of early trophozoites and the gametocytes are seen in the peripheral blood
d. Schüffner dot stippling is routinely seen in red blood cells that harbor parasites
e. The signet-ring-shaped trophozoite is irregular in shape with amoeboid extensions of the cytoplasm

380. After returning from a wilderness camping outing, several children report watery, greasy, and foul-smelling stools. The life cycle of the parasite responsible for this outbreak consists of two stages: the cyst and the trophozoite. Which of the following is the most likely identification of this organism?

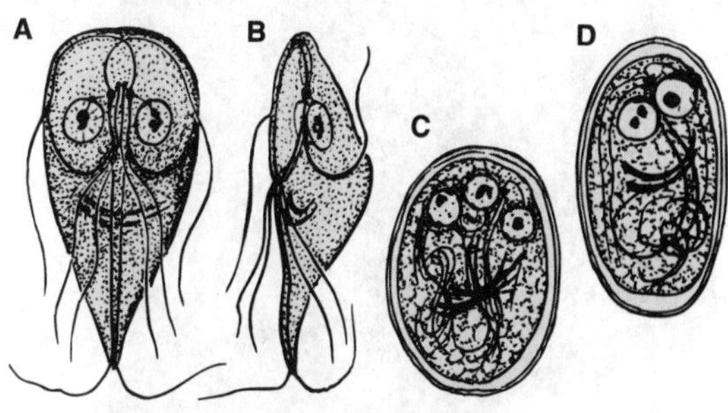

(**A**) "Face" and (**B**) "profile" of vegetative forms; (**C, D**) cysts (binucleate [D] and quadrinucleate stages). 2000×. *(Reproduced, with permission, from Brooks GF et al.* Jawetz's Medical Microbiology. *24th ed. New York, NY: McGraw-Hill; 2007:660.)*

a. *Clonorchis*
b. *Entamoeba*
c. *Giardia*
d. *Pneumocystis*
e. *Trichomonas*

381. A working mother takes her 4-year-old child to a day-care center. She has noticed that the child's frequent stools are nonbloody with mucus and are foul smelling. The child has no fever, but does complain of "tummy hurting." The increase of fat in the stool directs the pediatrician's concern toward a diagnosis of malabsorption syndrome associated with which of the following?

a. Amebiasis
b. Ascariasis
c. Balantidiasis
d. Enterobiasis
e. Giardiasis

382. The proglottid was purged from the intestinal tract of an individual who recently immigrated to United States from Nicaragua. The proglottid measured 10 mm in length. What species does it represent?

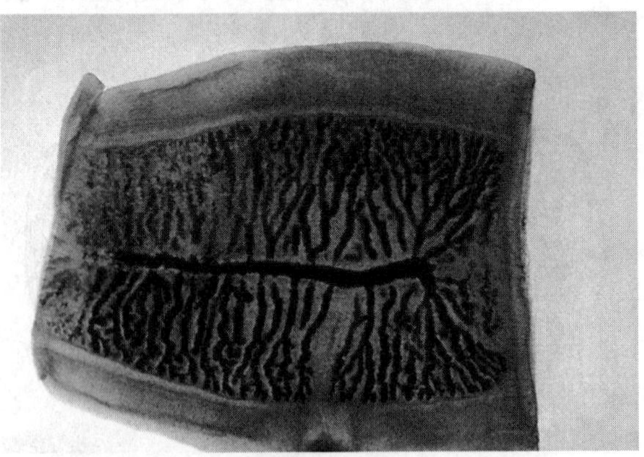

(Reproduced from the Centers for Disease Control and Prevention. Public Health Image Library, ID# 5259. http://phil.cdc.gov/phil/details.asp.)

a. *Diphyllobothrium latum*
b. *Dipylidium caninum*
c. *Taenia saginata*
d. *Taenia solium*
e. *Echinococcus granulosus*

383. Many of the POWs who were held captive in the Far East during the WWII contracted various parasitic infections, especially those prisoners who were forced to work on the infamous Thai-Burma railway. The tropical jungle environment of the Burma (Myanmar) railway project provided perfect conditions for development of the infective stage of a parasite larva, which infected the POWs through the soles of their poorly shod feet as they worked. In patients who have this chronic infection and are on chronic corticosteroid therapy, a syndrome can occur which results in high mortality rates. Which of the following parasites is most likely to be the culprit?

a. *Ancylostoma duodenale*
b. *Ascaris lumbricoides*
c. *Diphyllobothrium latum*
d. *Strongyloides stercoralis*
e. *Taenia solium*

384. Several diagnostic tests for antibodies to *Toxoplasma* are directly compared for sensitivity and specificity against the sera of 100 healthy adults. While differences are apparent in the accuracy of the tests, it is able to conclude that 80% of those tested have IgG antibodies against *Toxoplasma*. Which of the following is most compatible in helping to explain this finding?

a. A variety of parasitic infections induce the formation of *Toxoplasma* antibody
b. The IgM test is more reliable than the IgG test for determination of past infections; retesting for IgM would show that most people do not have *Toxoplasma* antibody
c. The potential for *Toxoplasma* infection is widespread, and the disease is mild and self-limiting
d. The test for *Toxoplasma* antibodies is highly nonspecific
e. Toxoplasmosis is caused by eating meat; therefore, all meat eaters have had toxoplasmosis

385. A 32-year-old homosexual man presents to his physician with nonbloody, foul-smelling, greasy stools 3 weeks after traveling to Mexico. While certain enteric protozoan and helminthic infections have been long related to contaminated food or water, sexual transmission of these diseases has produced a "hyperendemic" infection rate among homosexual males. Which of the following organisms is the most likely etiologic cause of this patient's diarrhea?

a. Amebiasis
b. Ascariasis
c. Enterobiasis
d. Giardiasis
e. Trichuriasis

386. Analysis of a patient's stool reveals small structures resembling rice grains; microscopic examination shows these to be proglottids. Which of the following is the most likely organism in this patient's stool?

a. *Ascaris lumbricoides*
b. *Enterobius vermicularis*
c. *Necator americanus*
d. *Taenia saginata*
e. *Trichuris trichiura*

387. An AIDS patient complains of headaches and disorientation. A clinical diagnosis of *Toxoplasma* encephalitis is made, and *Toxoplasma* cysts are observed in a brain section. Which of the following antibody results would be most likely in this patient?

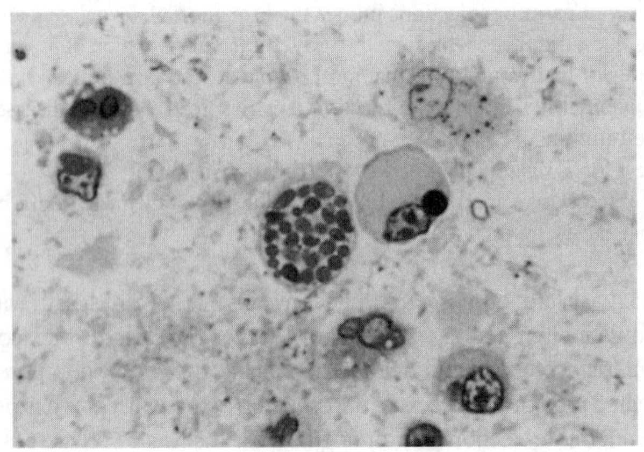

a. IgM nonreactive, IgG nonreactive
b. IgM nonreactive, IgG reactive (low titer)
c. IgM reactive (low titer), IgG reactive (high titer)
d. IgM reactive (high titer), IgG reactive (high titer)
e. IgM reactive (high titer), IgG nonreactive

388. A young boy from an impoverished area in Argentina presents to a public health clinic with Romana sign and a chagoma lesion. Several reduviid insects from the home are shown to the health care workers. In the chronic stage of this disease, where are the main lesions usually observed?

a. Digestive tract and respiratory tract
b. Heart and digestive tract
c. Heart and liver
d. Liver and spleen
e. Spleen and pancreas

389. A woman who recently returned from Africa complains of having paroxysmal attacks of chills, fever, and sweating. These attacks last a day or two at a time and recur every 36 to 48 hours. Examination of a stained blood specimen reveals ringlike and crescent-like forms within red blood cells. Which of the following is the most likely infecting organism?

a. *Plasmodium falciparum*
b. *Plasmodium vivax*
c. *Schistosoma mansoni*
d. *Trypanosoma gambiense*
e. *Wuchereria bancrofti*

Questions 390 and 391

390. A young man, who recently returned to the United States from Vietnam, has severe liver disease. Symptoms include jaundice, anemia, and weakness. Which of the following is the most likely etiologic agent shown in the figure below?

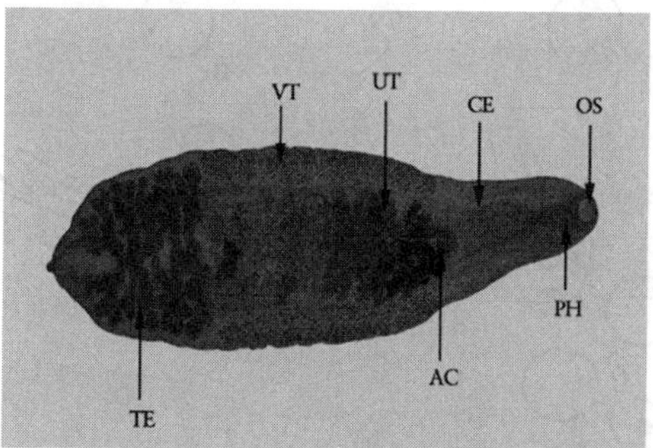

Oral sucker (OS), pharynx (PH), ceca (CE), acetabulum, or ventral sucker (AC), uterus (UT), vitellaria (VT) and testes (TE).

(Reproduced from the Centers for Disease Control and Prevention. http://www.dpd.cdc.gov/dpdx/html/clonorchiasis.htm.)

a. *Clonorchis sinensis*
b. *Diphyllobothrium latum*
c. *Plasmodium falciparum*
d. *Taenia saginata*
e. *Taenia solium*

391. An intermediate form of the organism shown in the photomicrograph (Question 390) lives in which of the following?

a. Cows
b. Mosquitoes
c. Pigs
d. Snails
e. Ticks

392. A woman who recently traveled through Central Africa now complains of severe chills and fever, abdominal tenderness, and darkening urine. Her febrile periods last for 28 hours and recur regularly. Which of the following blood smears would most likely be associated with the symptoms described?

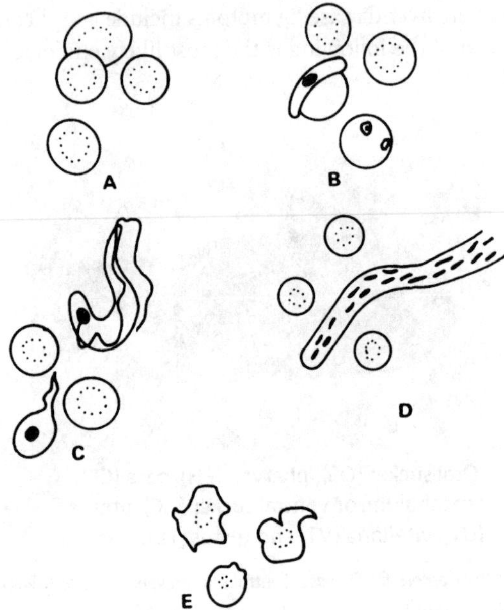

a. A
b. B
c. C
d. D
e. E

393. A young woman reports to her physician with possible urinary tract infection. The doctor finds the vagina and cervix tender, inflamed, and covered with a frothy yellow discharge. Which of the following protozoa described in this case is known to exist only in the trophozoite stage?

a. *Balantidium coli*
b. *Entamoeba histolytica*
c. *Giardia lamblia*
d. *Toxoplasma gondii*
e. *Trichomonas vaginalis*

394. An international photographer returns to the United States from a global picture assignment. He is seen by his physician, giving his major complaint as diarrhea. Which of the following can be ruled out?

a. *Echinococcus granulosus*
b. *Dientamoeba fragilis*
c. *Diphyllobothrium latum*
d. *Giardia lamblia*
e. *Leishmania donovani*

395. A medical technologist visits Scandinavia and consumes raw fish daily for 2 weeks. Six months after her return home, she has a routine physical and is found to be anemic. Her vitamin B_{12} levels were below normal. Which of the following is the most likely cause of her vitamin B_{12} deficiency anemia?

a. Cysticercosis
b. Excessive consumption of ice-cold vodka
c. Infection with *Diphyllobothrium latum*
d. Infection with Parvovirus B19
e. Infection with *Yersinia*

396. A renal transplant patient is admitted for graft rejection and pneumonia. A routine evaluation of his stool shows rhabditiform larvae. Subsequent follow-up reveals similar worms in his sputum. He has no eosinophils in his peripheral circulation. Which of the following is the most likely organism?

a. *Ascaris lumbricoides*
b. *Hymenolepis nana*
c. *Loa loa*
d. *Necator americanus*
e. *Strongyloides stercoralis*

397. A 56-year-old male immigrant from Bolivia complains of abdominal pain and cramping. He comments that 2 months previous to his current problems, he had numerous bloody stools every day. Physical findings include right upper quadrant pain over the liver with hepatomegaly, and a liver biopsy is performed. Which of the following parasites would most likely be identified in the liver biopsy?

a. *Acanthamoeba castellanii*
b. *Ascaris lumbricoides*
c. *Balantidium coli*
d. *Entamoeba histolytica*
e. *Taenia solium*

398. Human malarial infections start with the bite of a mosquito, and patients may experience the periodic paroxysms of this infection due to events that occur in the bloodstream. Up to one million deaths worldwide have been estimated annually. Which of the following control methods for this disease is currently most effective?

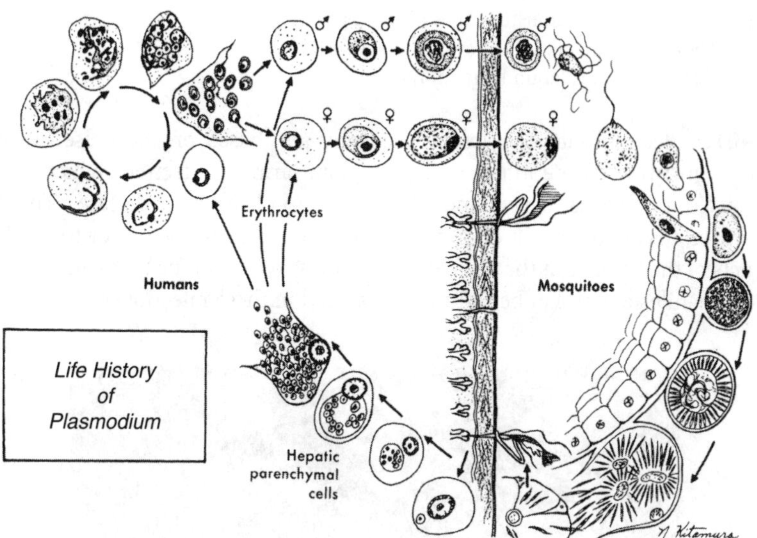

a. Antibiotics
b. A vaccine
c. Chemoprophylaxis
d. Tick repellents
e. White clothing

399. An African local clinic reports seeing increased cases of central nervous system (CNS) involvement in patients. Genetically induced changes in the glycoprotein coat of which one of the following organisms enhances its escape from the host's immune antibody response by having genes that encode multiple, variant surface glycoproteins?

a. *Trichinella spiralis*
b. *Trichomonas vaginalis*
c. *Toxoplasma gondii*
d. *Trypanosoma gambiense*
e. *Leishmania donovani*

400. Human parasitic amoebas are usually ingested for transmission. In less acute disease, patients may experience abdominal tenderness, abdominal cramps, nausea, vomiting, and diarrhea. Which of the following best describes these intestinal amebas?

a. Infection with *E. histolytica* is limited to the intestinal tract
b. They are usually nonpathogenic
c. They are usually transmitted as trophozoites
d. They can cause peritonitis and liver abscesses
e. They occur most abundantly in the duodenum

401. Infection with *Schistosoma haematobium*, based on the presence of eggs in urine, is identified in an Egyptian farmer's infection, which has caused dermatitis, fever, and chronic filero-obstructive disease. These symptoms are the result of granulomatous reactions to the ova or to products of the parasite at the place of oviposition. Which of the following clinical manifestations can be routinely observed in these infections?

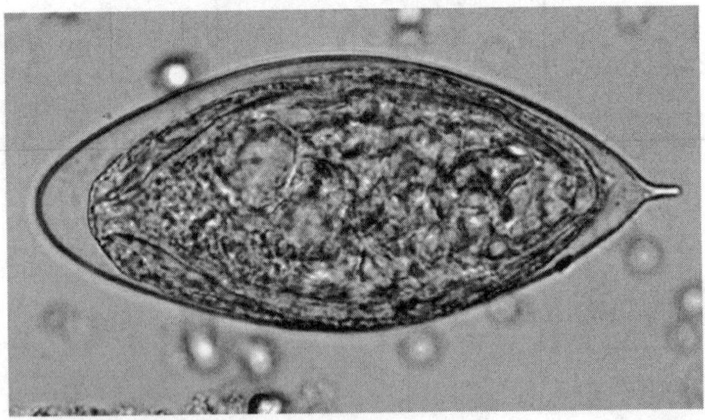

(Reproduced from the Centers for Disease Control and Prevention. http://www.dpd.cdc.gov/dpdx/html/Schistosomiasis.htm.)

a. Arthropathies
b. Bladder wall hyperplasia
c. Cardiac abnormalities
d. Pulmonary embolism
e. Hemorrhagic cystitis

402. A boy scout troop goes camping in a New England forest area in the late spring. Two weeks later, several of the boys present with erythema migrans lesions but no other clinical manifestations. *Borrelia burgdorferi*, the causative agent of Lyme disease, has been isolated from a variety of ticks such as *I. scapularis, Amblyomma, Dermacentor*, and *I. pacificus*. Which of the following statements most accurately describes Lyme disease?

a. *Dermacentor* and *Amblyomma* are significant vectors of *B. burgdorferi* to humans.
b. Dogs and cats are naturally immune to Lyme disease
c. *Ixodes scapularis* and *I. dammini* are different types of ticks
d. Only a small percentage of people who get bitten by a tick develop Lyme disease
e. White-tailed deer, an important reservoir for *I. scapularis*, are dying because of Lyme disease

403. A male patient in a tropical environment has eosinophilia during acute inflammatory episodes of his illness, but this is not considered to be the definitive diagnostic feature to determine what is causing his disease. Transmission of human parasites may occur via ingestion of contaminated food, water, snails, a variety of insects, and possibly even through pets or rat ectoparasites. Which of the following requires a mosquito for transmission?

a. Babesiosis
b. Bancroftian filariasis
c. Dog tapeworm
d. Guinea worm
e. Leishmaniasis

404. A Brazilian farmer presents to his medical clinic with hepatosplenomegaly with ascetic fluid in the peritoneal cavity. His liver is studded with white granulomas. He is treated with praziquantel. Which of the following organisms is endemic in Africa and South/Central America and is transmitted by skin penetration (by eggs with a large lateral spine), resulting in a dermatitis and katayama fever (serum sickness-like syndrome with fever, lymphadenopathy, and hepatosplenomegaly)?

a. *Clonorchis sinensis*
b. *Paragonimus westermani*
c. *Schistosoma haematobium*
d. *Schistosoma japonicum*
e. *Schistosoma mansoni*

405. The adults in a village in southern China suffer from fever, chills, mild jaundice, eosinophilia, and liver enlargement. Which of the following organisms may be ingested with raw fish, often resulting in an asymptomatic infection but, with a heavy infection, may cause biliary and bile duct obstruction and has an operculated egg?

a. *Clonorchis sinensis*
b. *Paragonimus westermani*
c. *Schistosoma haematobium*
d. *Schistosoma japonicum*
e. *Schistosoma mansoni*

406. Which of the following organisms is endemic in Asia, and has a small lateral egg spine, and in chronic disease may result in hepatosplenic disease, portal hypertension, and liver granulomas?

a. *Clonorchis sinensis*
b. *Paragonimus westermani*
c. *Schistosoma haematobium*
d. *Schistosoma japonicum*
e. *Schistosoma mansoni*

407. An African rice farmer, who depends on irrigation water from a regional lake, develops hematuria and dysuria severe enough to have concern for renal failure. Which of the following organisms has large terminal egg spines, may cause a chronic granulomatous bladder disease with urethral obstruction, chronic renal failure, and may be detected via eggs in the urine?

a. *Clonorchis sinensis*
b. *Paragonimus westermani*
c. *Schistosoma haematobium*
d. *Schistosoma japonicum*
e. *Schistosoma mansoni*

408. Campers in a European forest area drink unfiltered stream water and later experience abdominal cramps with foul-smelling and greasy stools. *Giardia lamblia* infection can occur by ingesting as few as 10 eggs, resulting in asymptomatic cyst passage, self-limited diarrhea, or chronic diarrhea with associated malabsorption and weight loss, This infection is best diagnosed by which of the following?

a. Baermann technique
b. Dilution followed by egg count
c. Enzyme immunoassay (EIA)
d. Using a scotch tape method
e. Sigmoidoscopy and aspiration of mucosal lesions

409. Patients with *E. histolytica* have an asymptomatic carrier rate greater than 90%. Chronic disease (intermittent bloody diarrhea and abdominal pain from months to years) is often difficult to distinguish from inflammatory bowel disease. *E. histolytica* infection is best diagnosed by which of the following?

a. Baermann technique
b. Dilution followed by egg count
c. EIA
d. Examination of a cellophane tape swab
e. Sigmoidoscopy and aspiration of mucosal lesions

410. Many patients with *Strongyloides* low worm burden are asymptomatic. Initial infection occurs by skin penetration and a pulmonary migration occurs. Patients demonstrate dry cough, wheezing, low-grade fever, dyspnea, and hemoptysis. Treatment is available for parasite eradication. Which is the best method listed below for detecting *Strongyloides* larvae?

a. Baermann technique
b. Dilution followed by egg count
c. EIA
d. Examination of a cellophane tape swab
e. Sigmoidoscopy and aspiration of mucosal lesions

411. *Ascaris lumbricoides* are large worms that have a complex life cycle in human hosts involving the digestive system, bloodstream, heart and liver, pulmonary circulation, and back to the small intestine. Serious medical complications may occur in any of these sites making diagnosis critical. *Ascaris* is best observed in human specimens by which one of the following?

a. Baermann technique
b. Dilution followed by egg count
c. EIA
d. Examination of a cellophane tape swab
e. Sigmoidoscopy and aspiration of mucosal lesions

412. A butcher develops a questionable habit of eating various kinds of raw, ground meat over several years. He eventually starts suffering from fatigue and lymphadenopathy. In his extensive physical examination, intensely white focal retinal lesions with vitritis are observed. Chorioretinitis is diagnosed, even though an older laboratory test, the Sabin–Feldman dye test, is found positive. This patient is found to be infected with which of the following?

a. Giardiasis
b. Schistosomiasis
c. Toxoplasmosis
d. Trichinosis
e. Visceral larva migrans

413. One week after eating bear meat, a fur trapper develops diarrhea, nausea, and vomiting. The next week, he experiences systemic symptoms of fever, myalgias, and malaise. His doctor notes periorbital edema and swollen eyelids, and laboratory tests report an eosinophilia. He is diagnosed with which of the following?

a. Giardiasis
b. Schistosomiasis
c. Toxoplasmosis
d. Trichinosis
e. Visceral larva migrans

414. A newspaper correspondent is sent to St Petersburg, Russia, to cover political events occurring there. She drinks only bottled water except on a side trip to the countryside to visit an old monastery. Two weeks later and at home, she develops a chronic diarrhea where the stools are watery, greasy, and foul smelling. Which of the following is the most likely diagnosis?

a. Giardiasis
b. Schistosomiasis
c. Toxoplasmosis
d. Trichinosis
e. Visceral larva migrans

415. A retired air force colonel has had abdominal pain for 2 years; he makes yearly freshwater fishing trips to Puerto Rico and often wades with bare feet into streams. Which of the following should be included in the differential diagnosis?

a. Giardiasis
b. Schistosomiasis
c. Toxoplasmosis
d. Trichinosis
e. Visceral larva migrans

416. A teenager who works in a dog kennel after school for 2 years has had a skin rash, eosinophilia, and an enlarged liver and spleen. Which of the following is the most likely cause of this infection?

a. Giardiasis
b. Schistosomiasis
c. Toxoplasmosis
d. Trichinosis
e. Visceral larva migrans

417. A young woman goes to her doctor with a variety of medical complaints. Her mucosal surfaces are tender, inflamed, eroded, and covered with a yellow discharge. For one problem, the laboratory reports the isolation of a pear-shaped protozoan with a jerky motility. This organism is observed in which of the following?

a. Biopsied muscle
b. Blood
c. Duodenal contents
d. Sputum
e. Vaginal secretions

418. A hunter, successful in his first black bear hunt, takes the meat home to eat. After consuming meals including bear meat over several weeks, two family members develop a flu-like syndrome and mild diarrhea. Several weeks later, two others have fever, GI distress, eosinophilia, muscle pain, and periorbital edema. Which of the specimens listed below would most easily detect the organism responsible for the clinical presentations described?

a. Biopsied muscle
b. Blood
c. Duodenal contents
d. Sputum
e. Vaginal secretions

419. A family of four goes on a vacation for 3 weeks to Central and South America. They consume the usual diets in all the areas they visit, including raw and pickled crustacean. Weeks later, two members produce brown sputum when coughing, hemoptysis, and eosinophilia, while the others are asymptomatic. A tissue-dwelling trematode causing this may be found in feces and which of the following?

a. Biopsied muscle
b. Blood
c. Duodenal contents
d. Sputum
e. Vaginal secretions

420. A forest ranger who routinely drinks untreated stream water and develops minor, intermittent diarrhea, which becomes chronic. Laboratory examination of several stools fails to determine any specific organism. Her physician decides to use the Entero-Test to try to discover the agent causing the symptoms. Cysts of a protozoan adhere to a piece of nylon yarn coiled in a gelatin capsule, which is swallowed. These cysts are usually found in which of the following?

a. Biopsied muscle
b. Blood
c. Duodenal contents
d. Sputum
e. Vaginal secretions

421. A person from Nantucket Island, Massachusetts, develops fever, fatigue, sweats, and arthralgia after hiking with friends in a forest. His physician finds evidence of tick bites that had not been noticed. A parasite resembling malaria that infects both animals and humans and is carried by the same tick that transmits *B. burgdorferi* (the Gram-negative spirochete that causes Lyme disease) would most likely be observed in which of the following?

a. Biopsied muscle
b. Blood
c. Duodenal contents
d. Sputum
e. Vaginal secretions

422. A patient with AIDS returns from Haiti with acute diarrhea. The stool reveals an oval organism (8-9 μm in diameter) that is acid-fast and fluoresces blue under ultraviolet light. The most likely identification of this organism is which of the following?

a. *Cryptosporidium hominis*
b. *Cyclospora cayetanensis*
c. *Enterocytozoon bieneusi*
d. *Giardia lamblia*
e. *Prototheca wickerhamii*

423. A 64-year-old sheepherder from the farming region of central California is rushed to the emergency room in anaphylactic shock. The history, as told by the ambulance medic, is that the man was hit in the abdomen during a barroom brawl. Ultrasound reveals a large cyst mass in the liver. A cautious needle aspiration of the liver mass reveals "hydatid sand." Which of the following is the most likely agent involved?

a. *Ascaris lumbricoides*
b. *Clonorchis sinensis*
c. *Echinococcus granulosus*
d. *Fasciolopsis hepatica*
e. *Schistosoma mansoni*

424. In a boy from Iraq, a lesion shown below was found to be irritated, with intense itching and begins to enlarge and ulcerate but did heal spontaneously. However, a permanent scar was left at the site. What would be your diagnosis?

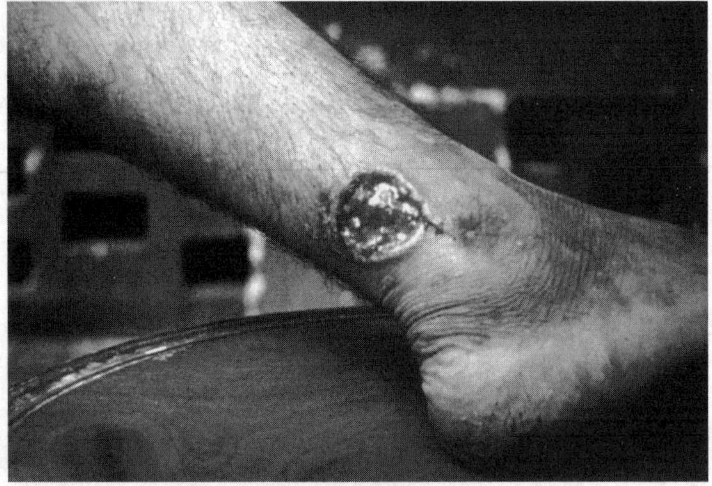

(Reproduced from the Centers for Disease Control and Prevention. Public Health Image Library, ID# 15069. http://phil.cdc.gov/phil/details.asp.)

a. *Schistosoma mansoni* infection
b. Cutaneous leishmaniasis (*L. tropica*)
c. Mucocutaneous leishmaniasis (*L. braziliensis*)
d. American trypanosomiasis (*T. cruzi*)
e. Inflammation due to a tick bite

425. A tiny worm was passed in the stool of a 6-year-old child. The child reported perianal pruritus, especially at night. The worm measured 10 mm in length and had a pointed tail. The eggs recovered by "Scotch tape" method. What species does it represent?

a. *Ascaris lumbricoides*
b. *Enterobius vermicularis*
c. *Necator americanus*
d. *Schistosoma mansoni*
e. *Trichuris trichiura*

426. A 12-year-old boy, a recent immigrant from Ethiopia, presented with abdominal pain associated with abdominal distention, nausea, and vomiting. The physician noted an enlarged liver with a palpable mass in the right upper quadrant of abdomen. Radiology was ordered; ultrasonography and computed tomography (CT) revealed a hepatic cyst. Microscopic examination of a biopsy specimen confirmed the diagnosis of a parasitic infection. What is the causative agent of this disease?

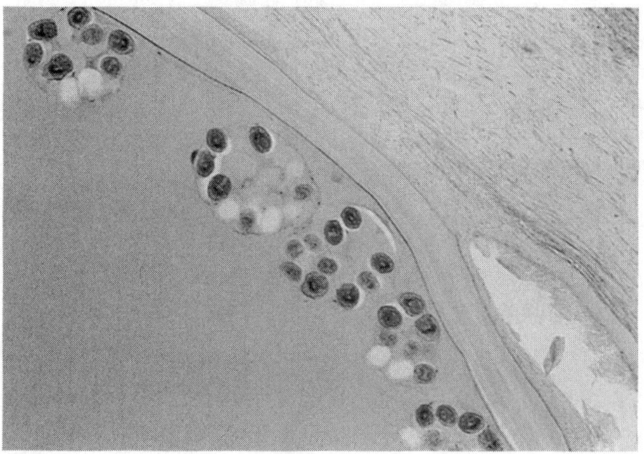

(Reproduced from the Centers for Disease Control and Prevention. Public Health Image Library, ID# 1452. http://phil.cdc.gov/phil/details.asp.)

a. *Hymenolepis nana*
b. *Schistosoma haematobium*
c. *Echinococcus granulosus*
d. Cysticercosis
e. *Schistosoma japonicum*

427. A 23-year-old woman who was a pig farmer in Peru but had lived in the United States for over 15 years presented with a 2-month history of left-side weakness and onset of seizures. An MRI of the patient's head revealed cysts in parietal lobe. What is your diagnosis?

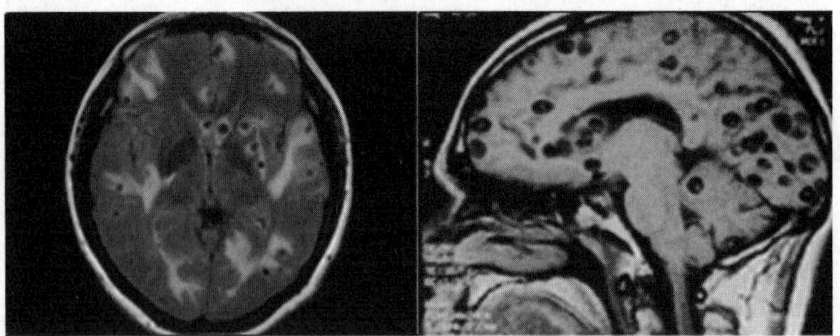

(Reproduced from the Centers for Disease Control and Prevention. http://www.cdc.gov/parasites/cysticercosis/.)

a. *Toxoplasma gondii*
b. *Entamoeba histolytica*
c. Neurocysticercosis
d. *Strongyloides stercoralis*
e. *Acanthamoeba castellanii*

Parasitology

Answers

375. The answer is c. (*Brooks, p 680. Levinson, pp 355, 371. Murray [2009], pp 840-841. Garcia [2007], pp 180-185.*) *Babesia* is transmitted by ticks of the genus *Ixodes*. *Babesia* can be mistaken for *Plasmodium* spp. (causative organism of malaria) in a blood smear. *Babesia* has several distinct characteristics including that the parasites are pleomorphic, often vacuolated, and unlike malarial parasites they are not pigment-producing organisms. Often a dividing tetrad form another distinguishing feature of *Babesia* can also be seen in the blood smears. Patients become anemic and develop hepatosplenomegaly, but patients who are asplenic are at a much greater risk. Transfusion recipients, foresters, immunosuppressed, and elderly patients may be at risk of acquiring disease but not to the same extent as those patients who have been splenectomized.

376. The answer is c. (*Brooks, p 681. Levinson, pp 358-359. Murray [2009], pp 829-830. Ryan, p 702. Garcia [2007], pp 57-73.*) The figure presented in the question shows *Cryptosporidium* oocysts stained with a modified acid-fast stain and they are not acid-fast bacilli. *Cryptosporidium* oocysts are rounded and measure 4.2 to 5.4 μm in diameter. Worldwide, the prevalence of Cryptosporidiosis is 1% to 4.5% in developed countries and 3% to 20% in developing countries. Estimated infection rates in AIDS patients range from 3% to 20% in the United States and 50% to 60% in Africa and Haiti. Acid-fast staining methods, with or without stool concentration, are most frequently used in clinical laboratories. Infection with *Cryptosporidium* sp. results in a wide range of manifestations, from asymptomatic infections to severe, life-threatening illness. Symptoms can be chronic and more severe in immunocompromised patients, especially those with CD4 counts <200/μL.

377. The answer is b. (*Garcia [2007], pp 123-130.*) *Trichomonas vaginalis* is an important sexually transmitted flagellate. An estimated 250 million new cases of Trichomoniasis occur around the world with nine million new cases in the United States every year. The parasite inhabits predominately the female lower genital tract and can also be found in the male urethra and prostate. The parasite divides by binary fission and does not have a cyst form and is transmitted human to human primarily by sexual intercourse. *T. vaginalis* infection in women is frequently symptomatic. Vaginalis with a profuse fowl-smelling yellow discharge is the prominent symptom and can be accompanied by cervical lesions and abdominal pain. Growth of the organism is favored by high pH >5.9 (normal pH in vagina = 3.5-4.5). In males, the infection is often asymptomatic but urethritis, epididymitis, and prostatitis can occur. This is a case of *Trichomonas vaginalis* showing a profuse discharge stemming from the cervical os.

378. The answer is a. (*Brooks, pp 672, 674. Levinson, pp 355, 371. Murray [2009], pp 803, 844-845. Ryan, p 733.*) *Acanthamoeba* is a free-living ameba, as is *Naegleria. Naegleria* usually causes severe, often fatal, meningoencephalitis, while *Acanthamoeba* is isolated from contact lens fluid and patients with retinitis who do not store their lenses under sterile conditions. Entry of *Acanthamoeba* into the CNS can occur from skin ulcers or traumatic penetration. Diagnosis is by examination of the CNS, which contains trophozoites and RBCs but no bacteria. *Naegleria,* also a free-living amoeba, produces an explosive, rapid brain infection. *Babesia* are widespread animal parasites, transmitted by ticks. *Entamoeba coli* is ingested and invade the intestinal epithelium. *Pneumocystis jiroveci* (not *P carinii*) causes pneumonia in immunocompromised patients. This agent may be an obligate member of the normal flora.

379. The answer is c. (*Brooks, pp 674-679. Levinson, pp 361-365. Murray [2009], pp 838-839. Ryan, p 712.*) *Plasmodium falciparum* infection is distinguished by the appearance of ring forms of early trophozoites and gametocytes, both of which can be found in the peripheral blood. The size of the RBC is usually normal. Double dots in the rings are common. Irregular edges of the infected RBC do not appear to be a reliable or important diagnostic feature. There are usually more than 12 merozoites in *P. falciparum*-infected RBCs, and these are rare in peripheral blood. Schüffner dots are found in *P. vivax* and *P. ovale* infections. *Plasmodium falciparum* peripheral smears show small, delicate-appearing

ring trophozoites. *P. vivax* and *P. ovale* produce thicker and larger ring trophozoites.

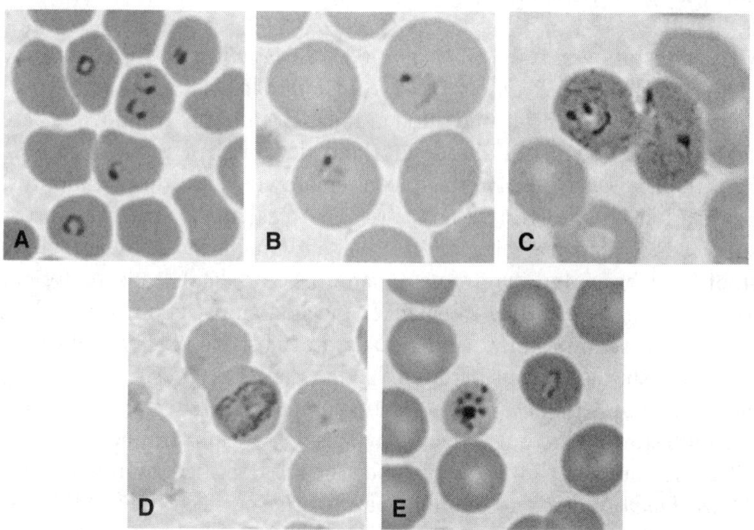

(**A**) Ring-form trophozoites of *P. falciparum* in a thin blood smear (**B**) Ring-form trophozoites of *P. vivax* in a thin blood smear. (**C**) Trophozoites of *P. ovale* in a thin blood smear. (**D**) Band-form trophozoites of *P. malariae* in a thin blood smear. (**E**) Schizont and ring-form trophozoite of *P. knowlesi* in a thin blood smear. *(Reproduced from the Centers for Disease Control and Prevention. http://www.dpd.cdc.gov/dpdx/html/Malaria.htm.)*

380. The answer is c. (*Brooks, p 660. Levinson, pp 355-358. Murray [2009], pp 824-826. Ryan, pp 745-748.*) *Giardia* exists in both trophozoite and cyst form. The "trophs" are fragile and not commonly seen in stools. The cysts are infectious. *Giardia* is the most common parasitic disease in the United States. It is commonly contracted from drinking cyst-contaminated water. Chlorine does not kill *Giardia* cysts, but contaminated water can be made cyst-free by filtration. *Clonorchis* is a trematode and has a soft-bodied syncytial shape (flatworms) and are called flukes. *Clonorchis sinensis* is a liver fluke with a snail host in its life cycle. *Entamoeba* are common parasites of the human large intestine and have no flagella on the active amoeba. *Pneumocystis* was thought to be a protozoan but molecular biology studies have proved it to be a fungus. *Trichomonas* are flagellar protozoa with 3 to 5 anterior flagella and an undulating membrane.

381. The answer is e. (*Brooks, p 660. Levinson, pp 357-358. Murray [2009], pp 824-826. Ryan, pp 745-748.*) *Giardia lamblia* is the only common protozoan found in the duodenum and jejunum. Trophozoites are commonly found in the duodenum and do not penetrate the tissues. Four nuclei cysts (infective stage) can remain viable for up to 4 months. Excystation is via digestive enzymes. The mechanical irritation to tissues leads to diarrhea, with increased fat and mucus in the foul-smelling stool. Malabsorption syndrome (vitamin A and fats) leads to weight loss, anorexia, electrolyte imbalance, and abdominal cramps. Children and immunocompromised individuals are most significantly affected. Giardiasis should be considered in the differential diagnosis of any "traveler's diarrhea." *Entamoeba* species are common parasites of the human large intestines. Mucosal surfaces have discrete ulcers. Trophozoites and RBCs are found in liquid stools and can be identified by microscopy. *Ascaris lumbricoides* is a common roundworm found in the small intestine with larvae in the lungs. *Balantidium coli* is the largest intestinal protozoan found in humans. It is a ciliated, oval organism 60 × 45 μm or larger. Cysts are passed in human stools and infections occur in areas of poor sanitation and crowding. *Enterobius vermicularis* is the common pinworm, with an anal–oral transmission (self-contamination occurs regularly in children).

382. The answer is c. (*Garcia [2007], pp 357-380.*) A number of branches in the uterus are diagnostic for *T. saginata* (beef tapeworm) and *T. solium* (pork tapeworm). *T. saginata* has 15 to 20 branches on each side (A) and *T. solium* has 7 to 13 (B). Humans acquire the *T. saginata* infection by ingesting undercooked beef containing infective larval cysts (cysticerci). *T. solium* infection is contracted by humans when they eat undercooked pork containing cysticerci. Both beef tapeworm and pork tapeworm can, in the adult form, cause disturbances of intestinal function. In addition, *T. saginata*, because of its large size, may produce acute intestinal blockage. Unlike *T. saginata*, *T. solium* produces cysticercosis, which could result in serious disease in humans. In *T. saginata*, the cysticercus—encysted larvae stage—develops only in cattle.

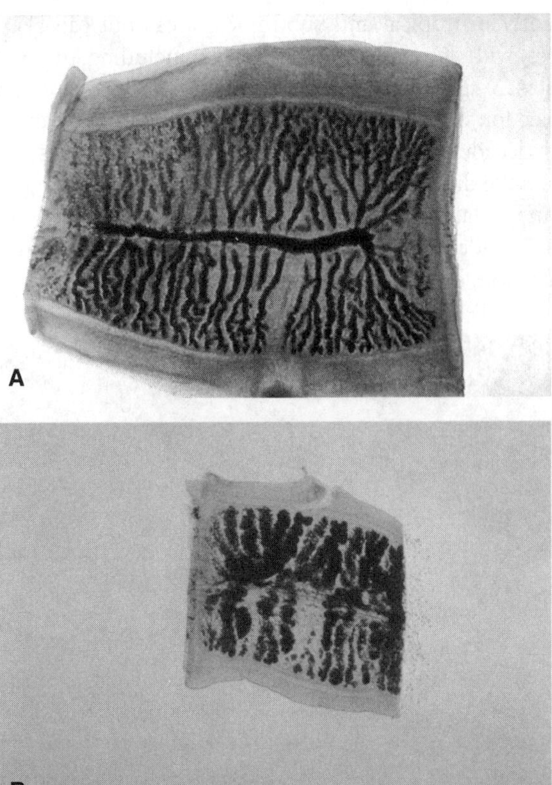

(Reproduced from the Centers for Disease Control and Prevention. Public Health Image Library, (A) ID# 5259 and (B) ID #4835. http://phil.cdc.gov/phil/details.asp.)

383. The answer is d. (*Garcia [2007], pp 271-282.*) The tropical jungle environment of the Burma railway project provided perfect conditions for development of the filariform *Strongyloides* larvae, which infected the POWs through the soles of their poorly shod feet as they worked. This roundworm has a complex life cycle and the parasite can complete its life cycle via a free-living cycle or one of the two kinds of parasitic cycles. The principal definitive hosts of *S. stercoralis* are humans but infection in dogs can also be established. As long as the patient is infected, which can be for several decades, the infection remains transmissible. Transmission occurs predominantly in tropical and subtropical areas but can also be found in countries with temperate environments including the Southeastern United States. *S. stercoralis* in humans usually produces an asymptomatic chronic infection of the gastrointestinal tract that can remain undetected for several decades. In some patients, a hyperinfection syndrome can develop with the dissemination of larvae to extraintestinal organs and that can result in mortality rates exceeding 80%. Risk factors and predisposing conditions include: immunosuppressive therapies with corticosteroids, HTLV-1 infection, organ transplantation, and malnutrition.

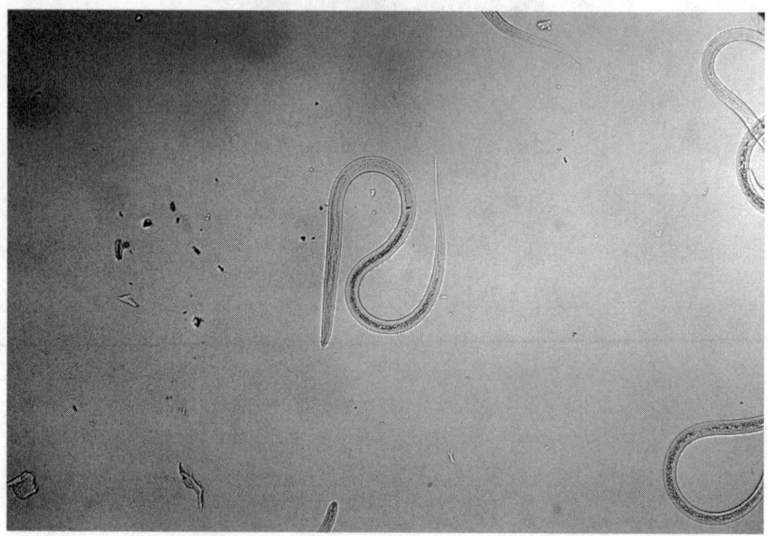

(Reproduced from the Centers for Disease Control and Prevention. Public Health Image Library, ID# 1547. http://phil.cdc.gov/phil/details.asp.)

384. The answer is c. (*Brooks, pp 682-683. Levinson, pp 365-366, 518. Murray [2009], pp 841-844. Ryan, pp 722-727.*) Serologic tests, such as the Sabin–Feldman dye test and indirect immunofluorescence, have shown that a high percentage of the world's population has been infected with *T. gondii*. In adults, clinical toxoplasmosis usually presents as a benign syndrome resembling infectious mononucleosis. However, fetal infections are often severe and associated with hydrocephalus, chorioretinitis, convulsions, and death. Acute toxoplasmosis is best diagnosed by an IgM capture assay. In most patients, specific IgM antibody disappears within 3 to 6 months. Obviously, *Toxoplasma* infection is widespread in animal and bird hosts but does not appear to cause disease in them. Congenital infection occurs only when the nonimmune mothers are infected during pregnancy. Most human infections are asymptomatic. Fatal infections may develop in AIDS patients. *Toxoplasma* antigens do not appear to cross-react with many of the other parasites' antigens. IgM and IgG antibodies can be detected with equal reliability. IgM levels drop eventually while IgG antibodies may be measured for years. The diagnostic test for *Toxoplasma*, in order to be approved for use, must be highly specific and sensitive. There is no evidence that *Toxoplasma* is spread by water.

385. The answer is d. (*Brooks, p 660. Levinson, pp 357-358. Murray [2009], pp 824-826. Ryan, pp 745-748. Toy, p 314.*) The infection rate with *G. lamblia* in male homosexuals has been reported to be from 21% to 40%. These high-prevalence rates are probably related to three factors: the endemic rate, the sexual behavior that facilitates transmission (the usual barriers to spread have been interrupted), and the frequency of exposure to an infected person. Amebiasis is infection with amoebas and asymptomatic cyst carriers exist, forming part of a pool that potentially could contribute to this problem. However, the foul-smelling greasy stools point to *Giardia*. *Ascaris* is a nematode worm that also inhabits the intestine of vertebrates. This life cycle includes swallowing eggs (from contaminated water), hatching of eggs in the intestine, migration of nematode to the lungs, and finally reaching the duodenum. Diarrhea episodes do not appear to be routinely reported in this infection. *Enterobius vermicularis* infections are noted for perirectal irritation and pruritis, not diarrhea episodes. Trichuriasis (whipworm) transmission is via fecally contaminated soil, not person to person.

386. The answer is d. (*Brooks, pp 686, 690. Levinson, pp 373-376. Murray [2009], pp 881-884. Ryan, pp 793-795. Toy, pp 314, 332.*) *Enterobius* (pinworm), *Ascaris* (roundworm), *Necator* (hookworm), and *Trichuris* (whipworm) are roundworms, or nematodes. *Taenia saginata* (tapeworm), a segmented flatworm, affects the small intestine of humans. Tapeworm segments, called *proglottids*, appear in the stool of infected persons. The *Taenia* group of tapeworms are considered to be the large (3-10 m in length) ones that infect humans. "Measly pork" contains bladderlike larvae (cysticerci) which are the size of rice grains. These develop into giant tapeworms in the intestine and egg-filled terminal proglottids break off and are eliminated in the feces. *Ascaris lumbricoides*, the giant roundworm of humans, infects more than one billion people. *Enterobius vermicularis* is the pinworm, where anal irritation causes anal–oral transmission by contaminated fingers. *Necator* species are hookworms which enter skin directly from infected soil; the other important species of hookworms is *Ancylostoma duodenale*. Hookworms infect over a billion people worldwide. Iron deficiency anemia (caused by blood loss at the site of intestinal attachment of the adult worms) is the most common symptom of hookworm infection. *Trichuris* (whipworm) also is transmitted by ingestion of eggs from feces-contaminated soil.

387. The answer is b. (*Brooks, pp 682-683. Levinson, pp 365-366, 518. Murray [2009], pp 841-844. Ryan, pp 722-727.*) One of the leading causes of death among AIDS patients is CNS toxoplasmosis. It is thought that *Toxoplasma* infection is a result of reactivation of old or preexisting toxoplasmosis. Occasionally, the infection may be acquired by needle sharing. Because the disease is a reactivation of old or preexisting toxoplasmosis, routine quantitative tests for IgM antibody are usually negative, and IgG titers are low (≤1:256, IFA). More sophisticated methods, such as IgM capture or IgG avidity, may reveal an acute response.

388. The answer is b. (*Brooks, pp 663-666. Levinson, pp 366-368. Murray [2009], pp 850-852. Ryan, pp 695, 757-760.*) American trypanosomiasis (Chagas disease) is produced by *T. cruzi*, which is transmitted to humans by the bite of an infected reduviid bug. They are introduced when infected bug feces are rubbed into the conjuctiva, the bug bite, or a break in the skin. Infants are often infected and demonstrate a unilateral swelling of the eyelids (Romana sign). Romana sign is a marker of acute Chagas disease. The swelling is due to bug feces being accidentally rubbed into the eye, or because the bite wound was on the same side of the child's face as the swelling. After multiplication, the tissues most likely to be affected in the chronic stage of the disease are the cardiac muscle fibers and the digestive tract. A diffuse interstitial fibrosis of the myocardium results and may lead to heart failure and death. The inflammatory lesions in the digestive tract that are seen in the esophagus and colon produce considerable dilatation. Chagas disease has not been an important disease in the United States; most cases have been imported, although there are a few reports of endogenous disease in the southern United States. The other organs may be affected, but not at the rate the heart and digestive tract are invaded.

389. The answer is a. (*Brooks, pp 674-679. Levinson, pp 361-365. Murray [2009], pp 835-839. Ryan, p 712.*) The febrile paroxysms of *Plasmodium malariae* malaria occur at 72-hour intervals; those of *P. falciparum* and *P. vivax* malaria occur every 48 hours. The paroxysms usually last 8 to 12 hours with *P. vivax* malaria but can last 16 to 36 hours with *P. falciparum* disease. In *P. vivax, P. ovale,* and *P. malariae* infections, all stages of development of the organisms can be seen in the peripheral blood; in malignant tertian (*P. falciparum*) infections, only early ring stages and gametocytes are usually found. *Schistosoma, Trypanosoma,* and *Wucheria* infections do not present with periodic symptoms in their disease progressions.

390. The answer is a. (*Brooks, pp 692-693. Levinson, p 382. Murray [2009], pp 874-875. Ryan, pp 807-808.*) The Chinese liver fluke, *C. sinensis*, is a parasite of humans that is found in Japan, China, Korea, Taiwan, and Indochina. An estimated 25 million people in the Far East are infected. Up to one fourth of Chinese immigrants to the United States harbor this fluke. Ingestion of contaminated raw, undercooked, frozen, salted or dried fresh water fish is the source of infection—cooking contaminated fish is the most effective way of eliminating the parasite on individual basis. Most pathologic manifestations result from inflammation and intermittent obstruction of the biliary ducts.

In the acute phase, abdominal pain, nausea, diarrhea, and eosinophilia can occur. In long-standing infections, gall bladder/biliary duct involvement is common (eg, cholangitis, cholelithiasis), pancreatitis, and cholangiocarcinoma can develop, which may be fatal. Praziquantel is the drug of choice. *Diphyllobothrium latum*, the fish tapeworm, travels from copepod to frog to water snail or rodent to a carnivore. *D. latum* absorbs vitamin B_{12}, causing a host vitamin deficiency. *Plasmodium* species are transmitted via a mosquito vector. *Taenia* species are transmitted by ingestion of undercooked, larvae-containing beef or pork.

391. The answer is d. (*Brooks, pp 692-693. Levinson, p 382. Murray [2009], pp 874-875. Ryan, pp 807-808.*) The life cycle of *C. sinensis* is similar to that of other digenetic trematodes. A snail is characteristically the first intermediate host of trematodes. Cows and pigs are intermediate hosts for

Taenia species. Mosquitoes serve as intermediate hosts for *Plasmodium* species. Ticks are not intermediate hosts for *Clonorchis* species.

392. The answer is b. (*Brooks, pp 674-679. Levinson, pp 361-365. Murray [2009], pp 838-839. Ryan, pp 711-722.*) The case history presented in the question is characteristic of infection with *P. falciparum*, the causative agent of malignant tertian malaria. The long duration of the febrile stage rules out other forms of malaria. The presence of ringlike young trophozoites and crescent-like mature gametocytes—as represented in the illustration below—as well as the absence of schizonts is diagnostic of *P. falciparum* malaria. Answer option A represents only RBCs and C represents trypanosomes and RBCs. Choice D represents a microfilarium and RBCs while E exhibits crenellated RBCs (round RBCs into shrunken, starry forms).

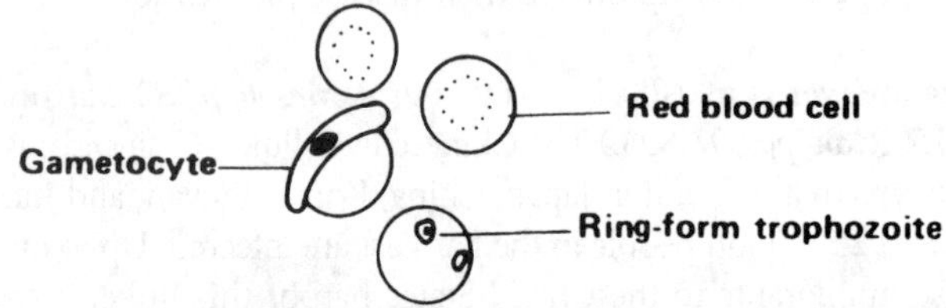

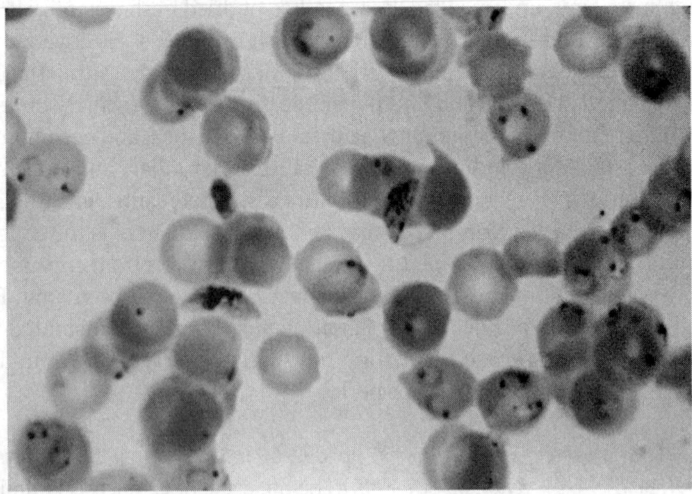

(Reproduced from the Centers for Disease Control and Prevention. Public Health Image Library, ID# 5856. http://phil.cdc.gov/phil/details.asp.)

393. The answer is e. (*Brooks, pp 661-662. Levinson, pp 356-360. Murray [2009], pp 826-827. Ryan, pp 742-745.*) *Trichomonas vaginalis* is the only protozoan listed where the trophozoite is the diagnostic and infective stage that feeds on the mucosal surface of the vagina (bacteria and leukocytes). The trophozoite possesses a short, undulating membrane (one-half of the body) and four anterior flagella. No cyst stage exists. A persistent vaginalis with a frothy and foul-smelling discharge with burning, itching, and increased frequency of urination is common. *Balantidium coli* is a large ciliated protozoan parasite. *Entamoeba histolytica* is an intestinal amoeba. *Giardia lamblia* is a flagellated protozoan found in the duodenum and jejunum of humans. *Toxoplasma gondii* is a coccidian protozoan especially important in congenital infections when the pregnant woman becomes infected during pregnancy.

394. The answer is a. (*Brooks, pp 686t, 694. Levinson, pp 378-382. Murray [2009], pp 886-887. Ryan, pp 799-801.*) *Echinococcus granulosus* causes hydatid disease. The definitive hosts are dogs. Sheep, cattle, and humans are intermediate hosts. The adult tapeworm does not occur in humans. In the herbivores (infected by grazing where eggs have been deposited by carnivore feces) the eggs hatch and release hexacanths. These penetrate the gut and pass to other tissues (liver, viscera, muscle, and brain). Humans are only infected from dog feces and develop hydatid cysts, as described for herbivores. Diarrhea, therefore, does not occur with *E. granulosis* human infections, whereas the other four choices can routinely present with diarrhea.

395. The answer is c. (*Brooks, pp 695. Levinson, pp 376-377. Murray [2009], pp 884-886. Ryan, pp 797-798.*) Consumption of raw fish causes endemic diphyllobothriasis in Scandinavia and the Baltic countries. While most people do not become ill, a small percentage (2%) develops vitamin B_{12} deficiency anemia. The adult fish tapeworm has an affinity for vitamin B_{12} and may induce a serious megaloblastic anemia. Parvovirus B19 causes acute hemolytic anemia primarily in immunosuppressed patients. *Yersinia* infection is common in Scandinavia but is not fish-borne and does not cause anemia. The larval stage of *T. solium* is called *cysticercus*. Humans usually acquire cysticercosis by ingestion of food and water contaminated by infected human feces. Excessive consumption of ice-cold vodka may lead to headaches and memory loss, but otherwise has nothing to do with parasitemia.

396. The answer is e. (*Brooks, pp 688-691. Levinson, pp 387, 390. Murray [2009], pp 860-862. Ryan, pp 763, 774-777. Toy, p 314.*) Strongyloidiasis is endemic in Southeast Asia, Latin America, sub-Saharan Africa, and parts of the southeastern United States. Hyperinfection occurs when the rhabditiform larvae transform into filariform larvae in the gastrointestinal tract, which then penetrate the perirectal skin or the wall of the intestine and gain access to the bloodstream. Dissemination to the lungs, liver, CNS, and other organs leads to severe inflammation and organ dysfunction. The prognosis for patients with hyperinfection syndrome is poor, with mortality rates exceeding >80% in some reports. Definitive diagnosis depends on the demonstration of *S. stercoralis* larvae in stool, duodenal fluid, or tissue specimens. Gram staining of sputum and/or bronchoalveolar lavage fluid samples may be useful for patients with hyperinfection syndrome. *Necator* must be distinguished from *Strongyloides* by microscopy. Gross appearances are similar. *Ascaris* is a common roundworm which can be found in the small intestine and lungs, but not in all body fluids. *Hymenolepis* species are tapeworms, found only in the small intestine. Loiasis is an infection transmitted by the bite of deer flies found in equatorial Africa. They invade subcutaneous tissue and are migratory. Microfilariae are also found in the blood.

397. The answer is d. (*Brooks, pp 669-672. Levinson, pp 354-357, 517. Murray [2009], pp 822-824. Toy, p 314.*) *Entamoeba histolytica* is a pathogenic species that is capable of causing disease, such as colitis or liver abscess, in humans. *Entamoeba dispar* is indistinguishable from *E. histolytica* by usual laboratory tests but only exists in humans as an asymptomatic carrier state and does not cause colitis. Infection with *E. histolytica* is prevalent in Central and South America, southern and western Africa, the Far East, and India. Poor sanitation and lower socioeconomic conditions favor the spread of the disease. In the United States, those who travel to endemic areas, homosexual males, and institutionalized persons are at increased risk of infection. *Acanthamoeba* species are free-living amebas in soil and water and usually cause infections of skin, encephalitis, and keritits. *Ascaris* is a nematode and is transmitted by ingestion. They hatch in the small intestine, and larvae migrate to the pulmonary alveoli. From here, they induce a cough and are swallowed by the host, maturing in the small intestine. *Balantidium coli* is a ciliate, infecting the lining of the large intestine, cecum, and terminal ilium. *Taenia* species (beef and pork) are ingested in undercooked meat. Only *T. solium* (pork) may occasionally involve liver if cysticercosis occurs.

398. The answer is c. (*Brooks, pp 674-680. Levinson, pp 361-365. Murray [2009], pp 835-838. Ryan, pp 711-722.*) Prophylaxis for malaria should be considered whenever a person is traveling in a malaria-endemic area. Most drugs used in treatment are active against the parasite forms in the blood (the form that causes disease) and include: chloroquine, sulfadoxine-pyrimethamine, mefloquine, atovaquone-proguanil, quinine, artemisinin derivatives (not licensed for use in the United States, but often found overseas). The WHO recommends intravenous artesunate as the treatment of choice for severe malaria in adults and children in areas of low transmission. Other control measures such as draining swamps, protective clothing and netting, and insect repellents are also effective. There is no currently available vaccine for malaria. Tick repellents would not be useful since only mosquitoes are malarial vectors.

399. The answer is d. (*Brooks, pp 663-668. Levinson, pp 366-369. Murray [2009], pp 848-852. Ryan, p 902.*) African trypanosomiasis (sleeping sickness) is caused by *T. brucei gambiense* and *T. brucei rhodesiense* and transmitted by tsetse flies. From the fly's salivary glands, the trypomastigotes enter the host's blood and lymph and eventually the CNS. The trypomastigotes reproduce by binary fission and are infective for biting tsetse flies. During the course of trypanosome infection, the number of parasites in the blood and lymph tissues fluctuates according to the host's immune response. An increase in parasite number is related to the proliferation of parasite subpopulations that express an antigenically new or variant glycoprotein coat. Each parasite carries genes encoding multiple, variant surface glycoproteins (VSG) with only one VSG being expressed at any one time. These changes lead to evasion of the immune system and produce challenges for vaccine development. The other parasites listed do not exhibit this ability to change surface glycoproteins.

400. The answer is d. (*Brooks, pp 669-671. Levinson, pp 354-357, 517. Murray [2009], pp 822-824. Ryan, pp 733-738.*) Of the intestinal amebas, *E. hartmanni, E. coli, E. polecki*, and *E. nana* are considered nonpathogenic. *Entamoeba histolytica* is distinctively characterized by its pathogenic potential for humans, although infection with this protozoan is commonly asymptomatic (causing "healthy carriers"). Symptomatic amebiasis and dysentery occur when the trophozoites invade the intestinal wall and produce ulceration and diarrhea. Peritonitis can occur, with the liver the most common site of extraintestinal disease. The life cycle of the *ameba* is simple by comparison. There is encystment of the troph, followed by excystation in the ileocecal region. The trophs multiply and become established in the cecum, where encystation takes place and results in abundant amebas, cysts, and trophozoites. Infection is spread by the cysts, which can remain for weeks or months in appropriately moist surroundings.

401. The answer is e. (*Brooks, pp 665, 688. Levinson, pp 379-382. Murray [2009], pp 876-879. Ryan, pp 803, 808-813.*) Three major species of blood flukes (*Schistosoma mansoni, S. japonicum*, and *S. haematobium*) cause the disease schistosomiasis. The position of spines in their eggs is specific for each schistosome species. This disease is endemic in 74 developing countries and an estimated 200 million infected and 800 million people are at risk of acquiring schistosomiasis. Intestinal schistosomiasis is caused by *S. mansoni.* Oriental or Asiatic intestinal schistosomiasis is caused by the *S. japonicum* and urinary schistosomiasis, caused by *S. haematobium*. Major Pathology of schistosomiasis is due to immunological reactions to *Schistosoma* eggs trapped in tissues. Antigens released from the egg stimulate a granulomatous reaction comprised of T cells, macrophages, and eosinophils that results in clinical disease. Continuing infection may cause granulomatous reactions and fibrosis in the affected organs, which may result in manifestations that include: portal hypertension and hepatosplenomegaly (*S. mansoni, S. japonicum*). Cystitis and urethritis (*S. haematobium*) with hematuria, which can progress to bladder cancer. Control strategies for schistosomiasis include: mass treatment with praziquantel in the community, introduction of public hygiene programs (safe water supply, sanitary disposal of excreta, flushable toilets) and snail eradication programs. Currently there is no vaccine against this disease.

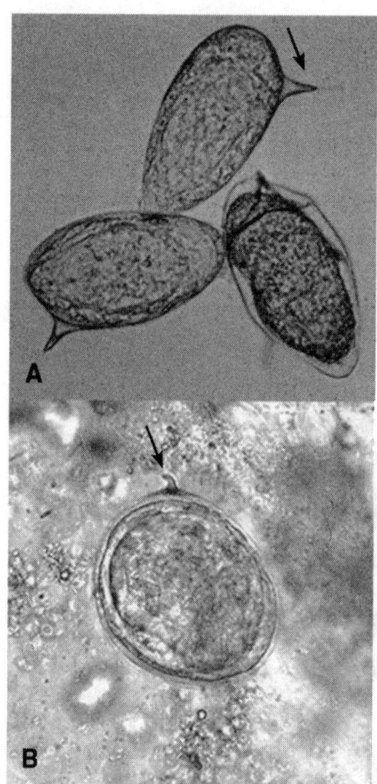

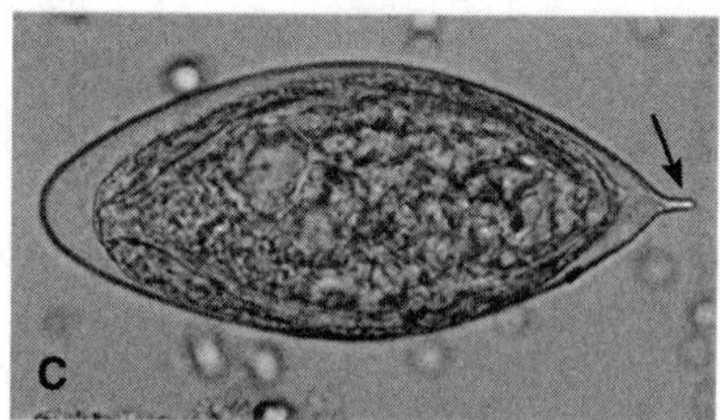

(A) Eggs of *S. mansoni* (found in feces)
(B) Egg of *S. japonicum* (found in feces)
(C) Egg of *S. haematobium* (found mostly in urine)
Note the position of spines – a diagnostic characteristic

(Reproduced from the Centers for Disease Control and Prevention. http://www.dpd.cdc.gov/dpdx/html/Schistosomiasis.htm.)

402. The answer is d. (*Brooks, pp 337-339. Levinson, pp 176-177. Murray [2009], pp 411-414. Ryan, pp 434-437.*) In the United States, *B. burgdorferi*, the causative agent of Lyme disease, has two principal vectors: *I. scapularis* in the eastern and midwestern United States and *I. pacificus* in the western United States. The ticks are tiny and can easily be missed. Fortunately, relatively few people who are bitten by ticks develop Lyme disease. Lyme disease, usually with joint involvement, is also seen in veterinary patients such as dogs, cats, and horses. White-tailed deer and small rodents are an important reservoir for these ticks. *B. burgdorferi* has been isolated from mosquitoes and *Dermacentor* and *Amblyomma* ticks, as well as from several *Ixodes* species. However, the isolation of the bacterium from these ticks is not sufficient evidence to indicate that they transmit the disease to humans.

403. The answer is b. (*Brooks, pp 687, 692. Levinson, pp 392-393. Murray [2009], pp 863-865. Ryan, pp 695-779, 784-785.*) *Wuchereria bancrofti* is the cause of bancroftian filariasis or filarial elephantiasis. Control of the mosquito vectors (culex, anopheles, and Aedes) is the most significant mechanism to control human infections. A disease of the tropics and subtropics, adults live in the lymphatics of a host and cause lymph blockage of the feet, arms, genitals, and breasts. Enlargement of the affected body part (elephantiasis) can then occur. Babesiosis is caused by tick-borne *Babesia microti*. Leishmaniasis is spread by a sandfly (Phlebotomus) vector. Guinea worms (*Dracunculus medinensis*) has an aquatic life cycle involving copepods (water fleas). Dog tapeworms would routinely be transmitted by fecal contamination.

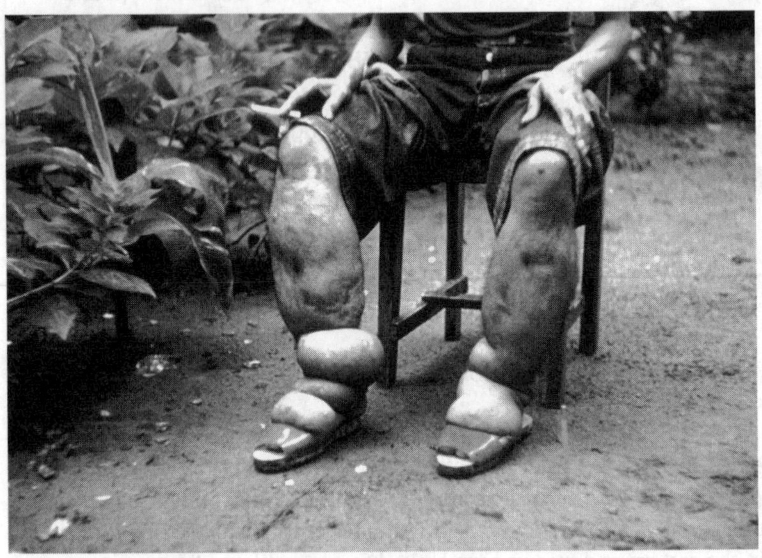

(Reproduced from the Centers for Disease Control and Prevention. Public Health Image Library, ID# 373. http://phil.cdc.gov/phil/details.asp.)

404 to 407. The answers are 404-e, 405-a, 406-d, and 407-c. (*Brooks, pp 685, 688, 693. Levinson, pp 379-382. Murray [2009], pp 871-880. Ryan, pp 803, 809-813.*) The life cycle of the medically important trematodes (or flukes) involves a sexual cycle in humans and an asexual cycle in snails. The schistosomes can penetrate the skin, whereas *Clonorchis* and

Paragonimus are ingested, usually in fish or seafood. These flukes can be easily differentiated morphologically by the appearance of the egg. Schistosome eggs have an identifiable spine, and both *Clonorchis* and *Paragonimus* eggs are operculated; that is, they have what appears to be a cover that opens. Serological tests are not useful. Many patients with schistosomiasis are asymptomatic, but disease may become chronic, resulting in malaise, diarrhea, and hepatosplenomegaly (an enlarged liver and spleen). *Clonorchis* infection usually causes upper abdominal pain but can also cause biliary tract fibrosis. Paragonimiasis is characterized by a cough, often with bloody sputum, and pneumonia. Praziquantel is the treatment of choice for these flukes.

408 to 411. The answers are 408-c, 409-e, 410-a, and 411-b. (*Brooks, pp 660-662, 669-674. Levinson, pp 357-358, 390. Murray [2009], pp 821-826, 853-855, 860-862. Ryan, pp 695-696, 733-738, 745-748, 769-771, 774-777. Toy, p 332.*) It is not uncommon that repeated stool specimens do not reveal the suspected parasite. Also, microscopic analysis of stool may not reveal parasite load when such data are necessary. For these reasons, other techniques are available to identify parasites as well as to quantitate them. A Scotch Tape method is used for diagnosis of *Enterobius vermicularis* (pinworms).

The diagnosis of giardiasis is usually made by detecting trophozoites and cysts of *G. lamblia* in consecutive fecal specimens. Alternatively, a gelatin capsule on a string (enterotest) can be swallowed, passed to the duodenum, and then retrieved after 4 hours. The string is then examined for *Giardia*. A recent innovation is the introduction of an EIA for *G. lamblia*. The EIA is more sensitive than microscopy, can be performed on a single stool specimen, and does not depend on the presence of entire trophozoites and cysts.

During sigmoidoscopy, a curette or suction device may be used to scrape or aspirate material from the mucosal surface. A direct mount of this material should immediately be examined for *E. histolytica* trophozoites, and then a permanent stain made for subsequent examination.

The Baermann technique may be helpful in recovering *Strongyloides* larvae (See Figure on the next page). The picture is of a rhabditoid larva of *S. stercoralis* in an unstained wet mount of stool. Notice the rhabditoid esophagus (*white arrow*) and prominent genital primordium. Essentially, fecal material is placed on damp gauze on the top of a glass funnel that is three-quarters filled with water. The larvae migrate through the damp gauze and into the water. The water may then be centrifuged to concentrate the *Strongyloides*.

Worm burdens may be estimated by a number of microscopic methods. While not often done, such procedures may provide data on the extent of infection or the efficacy of treatment of hookworms, *Ascaris*, or *Trichuris*. Thirty thousand *Trichuris* eggs per gram, 2000 to 5000 hookworm eggs per gram, and one *Ascaris* egg are clinically significant and suggest a heavy worm burden.

A cellophane tape swab is used to trap pinworms crawling out of the anus during the night. The tape is then examined microscopically for *Enterobius*.

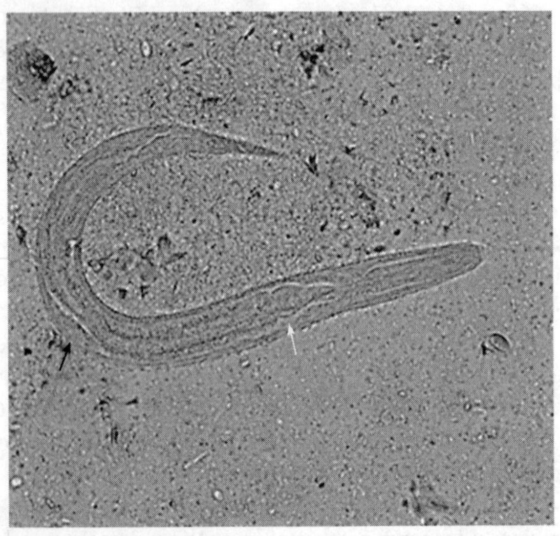

(Reproduced from the Centers for Disease Control and Prevention. http://www.dpd.cdc.gov/dpdx/html/Strongyloidiasis.htm.)

412. The answer is c. (*Brooks, pp 682-684. Levinson, pp 365-366. Murray [2009], pp 841-844. Ryan, pp 695-696, 723-727, 746-748, 779-784, 809-813.*) Toxoplasmosis is generally a mild, self-limiting disease; however, severe fetal disease is possible if pregnant women ingest *Toxoplasma* oocysts. Consumption of uncooked meat may result in either an acute toxoplasmosis or a chronic toxoplasmosis that is associated with serious eye disease. Most adults have antibody titers to *Toxoplasma*, and thus would have a positive Sabin–Feldman dye test. The Sabin–Feldman dye test measures antibodies that render the membrane of living *T. gondii* impermeable to methylene blue (no staining occurs). It is being replaced by IFA and ELISA tests. While we usually think of in utero infections of a developing fetus and the subsequent medical difficulties of the newborn infant, an equally important source of human exposure is raw or undercooked meat in which infective tissue cysts are frequently found. When a tissue cyst ruptures, numerous bradyzoites are released and grow, causing chorioretinitis, myocarditis, and polymyositis. Treatment is with pyrimethamine and sulfadiazine. Schistosomiasis is caused by blood flukes whose cercariae (larvae) penetrate skin in snail-infested water. Trichinosis is caused by the trichina worm whose larvae are found in uncooked pork. Cutaneous larva migrans consists of subcutaneous migrating larvae of hookworms. Visceral larva migrans is a condition in humans caused by the migratory larvae of certain nematodes, humans being a terminal host. Nematodes causing such zoonotic infections are *Toxocara canis, Toxocara cati*, and *Ascaris suum*. Larva currens is an itchy, cutaneous condition caused by infections with *Strongyloides stercoralis* that intermittently comes and goes every few hours.

413 to 416. The answers are 413-d, 414-a, 415-b, and 416-e. (*Brooks, pp 660, 685, 687t, 691. Levinson, pp 357-358, 379-382, 390-391. Murray [2009], pp 824-826, 855-856, 862-863, 876-879. Ryan, pp 695-696, 723-727, 746-748, 779-784, 809-813.*) Trichinosis most often is caused by ingestion of contaminated pork products. However, eating undercooked bear, walrus, raccoon, or possum meat also may cause this disease. Symptoms of trichinosis include muscle soreness and swollen eyes. The described symptoms of the fur trapper would not fit the clinical presentations of giardiasis, schistosomiasis, toxoplasmosis, or visceral larva migrans.

Although giardiasis has been classically associated with travel to endemic areas many cases of giardiasis caused by contaminated water have been reported in the United States as well. Diagnosis is made by detecting cysts in the stool. In some cases, diagnosis may be very difficult because of the relatively small number of cysts present. Alternatively, an EIA may be used to detect *Giardia* antigen in fecal samples. The symptoms that were experienced by the correspondent would not fit the clinical presentation of schistosomiasis, toxoplasmosis, trichinosa, or visceral larva migrans.

Schistosomiasis is a worldwide public health problem. Control of this disease entails the elimination of the intermediate host snail and removal of streamside vegetation. Abdominal pain is a symptom of schistosomiasis. The symptoms that were experienced by the colonel would not fit the clinical presentation of giardiasis, toxoplasmosis, trichinosa, or visceral larva migrans.

Visceral larva migrans is an occupational disease of people who are in close contact with dogs and cats. The disease is caused by the nematodes *Toxocara canis* (dogs) and *Toxocara cati* (cats) and has been recognized in young children who have close contact with pets or who eat dirt. Symptoms include skin rash, eosinophilia, and hepatosplenomegaly. The symptoms that were experienced by the teenager would not fit the clinical presentation of giardiasis, toxoplasmosis, trichinosa or schistosomiasis.

417 to 421. The answers are 417-e, 418-a, 419-d, 420-c, and 421-b. (*Brooks, pp 660-662, 680, 690, 693. Levinson, pp 357-360, 382-383, 390-391. Murray [2009], pp 824-827, 862-863, 875-876. Ryan, pp 695-696, 741-748, 779, 781-784, 803, 805-807.*) *Trichomonas vaginalis*, an odd-looking protozoan, moves with a jerky, almost darting motion. Trichomoniasis, a bothersome vaginal infection, can be diagnosed by observing this organism in a wet mount of vaginal secretions. It may be washed out in the urine as well. *Trichomonas vaginalis* can be grown in special media, and there are now several products available for direct detection of the organism.

Trichinella spiralis causes trichinosis, a parasitic disease that is usually mild and results in muscle pain and a mild febrile illness. However, fulminant fatal cases have been described. Humans, who are accidental hosts, become infected by ingesting cysts that are in the muscle of animals. Most infections still come from pork, although regulations on pig feeding have markedly reduced the incidence. Laboratory diagnosis is by serology or demonstration of the larvae in the muscle tissue.

Paragonimus westermani is a lung fluke. This trematode infects lung tissue and is seen not only in sputum but also in feces because infected patients swallow respiratory secretions. Paragonimiasis is contracted by ingesting the metacercariae that are encysted in crabs or crayfish.

Giardia infection may be difficult to diagnose by stool examination, as patients may shed the cysts intermittently. When symptoms persist and the stool examination is negative, then duodenal contents may be sampled directly with the enterotest. The patient swallows a gelatin capsule that contains a coiled string. The other end is attached to the patient's face. The gelatin capsule dissolves, and *Giardia* organisms, if present, adhere to the string within a 4-hour period. The string is retrieved and examined microscopically. Alternatively, an enzymatic immunoassay can detect *Giardia* antigen directly in a single specimen of feces.

Babesia is a sporozoan parasite transmitted by the bite of *I. scapularis*, the same tick that carries *B. burgdorferi*. Reproduction of this parasite occurs in erythrocytes and may resemble *Plasmodium* species when blood smears are examined. *Babesia* is endemic in the northeastern United States, particularly in the islands of Massachusetts. Laboratory diagnosis is made by examining blood smears for this parasite, or by detection of specific antibody. Babesiosis clinically resembles malaria.

422. The answer is b. (*Brooks, p 680. Levinson, pp 371-372. Murray [2009], pp 830-832.*) Coccidian-like bodies have been identified in stools of some patients with diarrhea. These organisms appear to be similar to blue-green algae and were referred to as *Cyanobacterium*-like until they were recently reclassified as *Cyclospora*. They are larger than the microsporidia and resemble neither *Giardia* nor *Prototheca* nor other algae-like organisms. Unlike *Cryptosporidium* (4-5 μm), these organisms fluoresce under ultraviolet light. The diarrhea can be prolonged and relapsing, and the treatment is usually trimethoprim–sulfamethoxazole. See the figure for an illustration of *G. lamblia*.

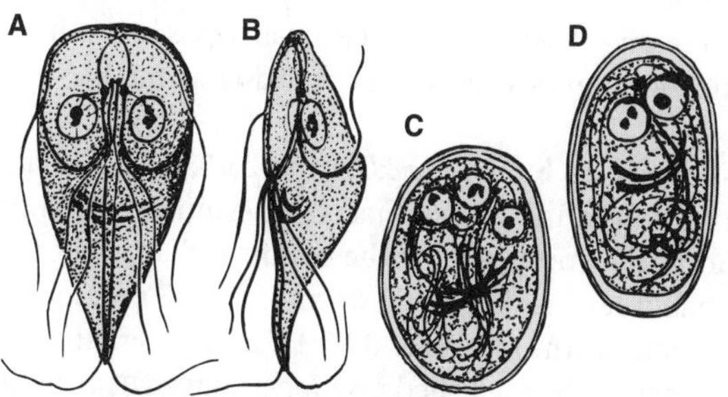

Giardia lamblia. (**A**) "Face" and (**B**) "profile" of vegetative forms; (**C, D**) cysts (binucleate [D] and quadrinucleate stages). 2000×. *(Reproduced, with permission, from Brooks GF et al.* Jawetz's Medical Microbiology. *24th ed. New York, NY: McGraw-Hill; 2007:660.)*

423. The answer is c. (*Brooks, p 694. Levinson, p 377. Murray [2009], pp 886-889. Ryan, pp 799-801.*) *Echinococcus* is a small, three-segmented tapeworm found only in the intestines of dogs and other carnivores. Eggs leave these hosts and infect grazing animals. In the herbivore gut, the eggs hatch and the released forms penetrate the gut. Various organs (especially the liver) develop huge, fluid-filled cysts in which future scoleces form (hydatid sand). Dogs become infected when they feed on viscera of diseased sheep or cows. Hydatid disease in humans occurs only through ingestion of dog feces. Humans are only an intermediate host of this organism and never the final host. None of the other answer options are cestodes, or tapeworms.

424. The answer is b. (*Garcia [2007], pp 190-217.*) Leishmaniasis is caused by three major species of parasites. Cutaneous leishmaniasis is caused by *L. tropica* (Baghdad Sore) is found in the Mediterranean region; mucocutaneous leishmaniasis is caused by *L. braziliensis* (American leishmaniasis) and is endemic in South/Central America; visceral leishmaniasis is caused by *L. donovani* (Kala-azar) and is wide spread in Asia. In cutaneous disease, centrifugally growing papular lesion with central crusting is seen which heals spontaneously but leaves a permanent scar. Mucocutaneous leishmaniasis which involves the skin and mucoid tissue, initially same as cutaneous lesion but it does not heal and leads to necrosis of mucoid tissue, metastasis to distant mucoid tissues and is very disfiguring. Visceral leishmaniasis involves liver, spleen, bone marrow, lymph nodes, skin, there is no bite reaction and results in lymphadenopathy, splenomegaly and hepatomegaly, chills and fever, and darkening of skin. Visceral leishmaniasis is becoming an important opportunistic infection in areas where it coexists with HIV.

425. The answer is b. (*Garcia 2007, pp 258-260.*) The most common helminth infection in the United States (an estimated 40 million persons infected). Adult pinworms inhabit the cecum and adjacent portions of the large and small intestine. The male worm is 2 to 5 mm long and 0.2 mm wide. The female worm measures 8 to 13 mm in length and 0.5 mm in width. The female is distinguished by a long, thin sharply pointed tail. The female when fully gravid, migrate down the intestinal tract to pass out the anus and deposit their eggs. Diagnosis of *Enterobius vermicularis* is made by using a Scotch Tape Test. Eggs are thin-walled eggs and measure 50 to 60 mm × 20 to 30 mm and are ovoid and flattened on one side.

426. The answer is c. (*Garcia 2007, pp 381-410.*) The photomicrograph is showing a number of *Echinococcus* protoscolices in a cut section of a hydatid cyst. Hydatid disease is caused by the larval stages of cestodes of the genus *Echinococcus. E. granulosus* (dog tapeworm) causes cystic disease, the form most frequently encountered. *E. multilocularis* (fox tapeworm) causes alveolar disease. *E. vogeli* and *E. oligarthrus* are the causative agents of polycystic hydatidosis. The diagnosis of hydatid disease relies mainly on findings by ultrasonography and/or other imaging techniques supported by positive serologic tests. In *E. granulosus* infections hepatic involvement can result in abdominal pain, a mass in the hepatic area, and biliary duct obstruction. Most importantly, the break/leakage from the cyst can lead to fever, urticaria, eosinophilia, and anaphylactic shock, as well as spreading of cysts to other areas. Furthermore, other organs (lungs, brain, bone, and heart) can also be involved with *E. granulosus* hydatid infection. Hydatidosis with *E. multilocularis* affects the liver as a slow growing tumor, with abdominal pain, biliary obstruction often with metastatic lesions into the lungs and brain. *E. vogeli* cysts are normally found in the liver, where it acts as a slow growing tumor; secondary cystic development is also normal.

427. The answer is c. (*Garcia [2007], pp 363-371.*) Cysticerci cysts of *T. solium* (pig tapeworm) are larval cysts that infect brain, muscle, or other tissue, and are a major cause of adult-onset seizures in most low-income countries. Cysticercosis is acquired by ingesting eggs excreted by a person who is carrying an intestinal pig tapeworm. In case of neurocysticercosis, CT and MRI provide evidence on number and location of cysticerci as well as on their viability and the acuteness of the host inflammatory response. Neurocysticercosis can cause a wide variety of manifestations including seizures, mental disturbances, focal neurological deficits, and signs of space-occupying intracerebral lesions.

Immunology

Questions

Questions 428 to 431

Hypersensitivity reactions are excessive or uncontrolled immune responses that can sometimes result in damage to the host instead of providing protection. The four main types are represented below. Use these reactions to answer the following questions.

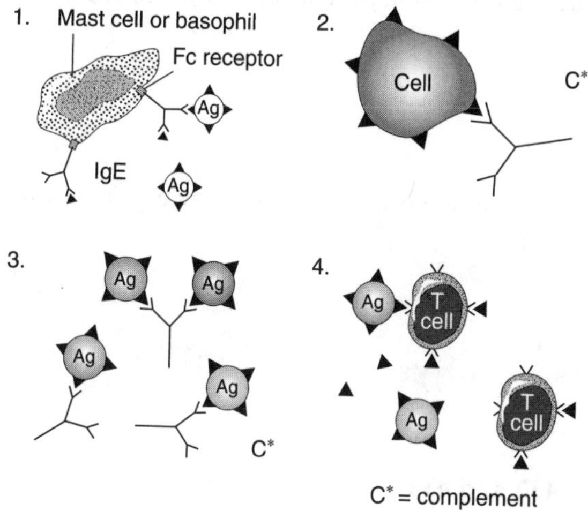

428. A 13-year-old male with cystic fibrosis develops repeated episodes of pneumonia resulting in multiple hospitalizations. Previous antibiotic treatment resulted in severe rash, fever, and systemic anaphylaxis almost immediately. A penicilloyl polylysine skin test yields positive results. Which of the following best illustrates the type of hypersensitivity reaction associated with this clinical scenario?

a. Type I
b. Type II
c. Type III
d. Type IV

429. After playing in the bushes during a camping trip, a 7-year-old girl complains of intense itching and blistering of the hands, arms, and legs. Which of the following are the most likely medical condition and the correct hypersensitivity diagram from those presented?

a. Contact dermatitis and type II
b. Contact dermatitis and type III
c. Contact dermatitis and type IV
d. Arthus reaction and type I
e. Arthus reaction and type II
f. Arthus reaction and type III

430. Skin testing is useful in the diagnosis of which of the following?

a. Type I and II
b. Type I and III
c. Type I and IV
d. Type II, III, and IV

431. Rh disease and Goodpasture syndrome are best represented by which of the following?

a. Type I and II
b. Type II and III
c. Type II and IV
d. Type II only
e. Type III only

Questions 432 and 433

432. A 7-month-old male infant presents to the emergency department with severe middle ear and upper respiratory tract infections, which respond promptly to antibiotics. Two months later he is again admitted, this time with *Streptococcus pneumoniae* pneumonia. After several more episodes of bacterial infections, genetic testing is done and the presence of a defective B-cell tyrosine kinase gene (*btk* gene or *X-LA* gene) is revealed. In addition, physical examination detects very small tonsils. Which of the following is the most likely diagnosis?

a. Ataxia-telangiectasia
b. Bruton agammaglobulinemia
c. Chronic granulomatous disease
d. Late (C5, C6, C7, C8, C9) complement deficiency
e. Thymic aplasia (DiGeorge syndrome)

433. Which of the following pathogens presents the most serious threat to this child?

a. *Chlamydia trachomatis*
b. Measles virus
c. *Mycobacterium tuberculosis*
d. Varicella-zoster virus (VZV)

Questions 434 and 435

Flow cytometry of blood from an HIV-positive patient yielded a CD4:CD8 ratio less than 1.

434. This ratio best represents a major decline in which of the following cell types and its associated cell surface proteins?

a. B lymphocytes; MHC class I, IgM, B7, CD19, CD20
b. Cytotoxic T lymphocytes; MHC class I, TCR, CD3
c. Cytotoxic T lymphocytes; MHC class I, TCR, CD3, CD28
d. Helper T lymphocytes; MHC class I, TCR, CD3
e. Helper T lymphocytes; MHC class I, TCR, CD3, CD28
f. Macrophages; MHC class I, MHC class II, CD14

435. Which of the following best represents the "costimulatory signal" pair that occurs between cellular surface proteins associated with the reduced cell type represented in the CD4:CD8 ratio less than 1?

a. B7 (B cell) and CD28 (T cell)
b. B7 (B cell) and CD4 (T cell)
c. CD40L (B cell) and CD40 (T cell)
d. MHC class I (B cell) and CD4 (T cell)
e. MHC class II (B cell) and CD8 (T cell)

436. A young girl has had repeated infections with *Candida albicans* and respiratory viruses since she was 3 months old. As part of the clinical evaluation of her immune status, her responses to routine immunization procedures should be tested. In this evaluation, the use of which of the following vaccines is contraindicated?

a. Bacillus Calmette–Guerin (BCG)
b. Bordetella pertussis vaccine
c. Diphtheria toxoid
d. Inactivated polio
e. Tetanus toxoid

437. A 7-year-old male developed normally until 7 years of age, after which he suddenly starts suffering from progressive personality and intellect deterioration leading to dementia, and finally death within 1 year of symptoms. His history reveals severe measles attack at the age of 1. Laboratory tests indicate elevated measles antibody levels in both the serum and cerebrospinal fluid (CSF) with no antibody to the M protein. A latent measles-like viral infection and, presumably, a defect in cellular immunity are associated with which of the following diseases?

a. Creutzfeldt–Jakob disease (CJD)
b. Epstein–Barr virus (EBV) infection
c. Multiple sclerosis (MS)
d. Progressive multifocal leukoencephalopathy (PML)
e. Subacute sclerosing panencephalitis (SSPE)

438. A 31-year-old patient suffering from recurrent episodic intestinal hemorrhages attributed to a severe form of Crohn disease decides to undergo surgery to resect his terminal ileum. The surgeon orders two units of blood to be preserved for possible use during the surgery. The patient decides to store one unit of his own blood and one unit of his 35-year-old brother's blood with the blood bank. This type of donation is most likely which of the following transplantation terminology (patient's blood:brother's blood)?

a. Allograft:allograft
b. Allograft:autograft
c. Autograft:allograft
d. Autograft:autograft
e. Autograft:isograft (syngeneic graft)

439. A 27-year-old female presents to the emergency room with a temperature of 103°F, severe fatigue, weight loss, and joint pain. During the history and physical examination, the patient reports that she stopped taking her aspirin and corticosteroids to control her condition. A butterfly-type rash over her cheeks, sensitivity to light, and a heart murmur are apparent. The patient also reports a history of a progressively developing arthritis and glomerulonephritis. Laboratory tests further indicate anemia, leukopenia, and thrombocytopenia. This condition is best diagnosed by the presence of which of the following?

a. Anticentromere antibodies
b. Anti-dsDNA antibodies
c. Antimitochondrial antibodies
d. Antineutrophil antibodies
e. Anti-TSH receptor antibodies

440. A 1-year-old male patient presents with marked susceptibility to opportunistic infections with bacteria such as *Escherichia coli* and *Staphylococcus aureus* and fungal *Aspergillus*. Examination findings reveal granulomatous abscesses in the lungs, ataxia, nystagmus, and photophobia. Biochemical analysis reveals the deficiency of the central enzyme in the respiratory burst pathway via an inability to reduce nitroblue tetrazolium (NBT) dye. The deficient enzyme and reaction are represented by which of the following?

a. $NADPH + 2O_2 \xrightarrow{\text{NADPH oxidase}} NADP^+ + 2O_2^- + H^+$
b. $2O_2^- + 2H^+ \xrightarrow{\text{Superoxide dismutase}} H_2O_2 + O_2$
c. $H_2O_2 + Cl^- \xrightarrow{\text{Myeloperoxidase}} H_2O + OCl^-$
d. $\frac{1}{2}O_2 + \text{arginine} \xrightarrow{\text{NO synthase}} NO + \text{citrulline}$
e. $2H^+ + 2e^- + \frac{1}{2}O_2 \xrightarrow{\text{Oxidase}} H_2O$
f. $2H_2O_2 \xrightarrow{\text{Catalase}} 2H_2O + O_2$

441. Which of the following statements best applies to the following diagram?

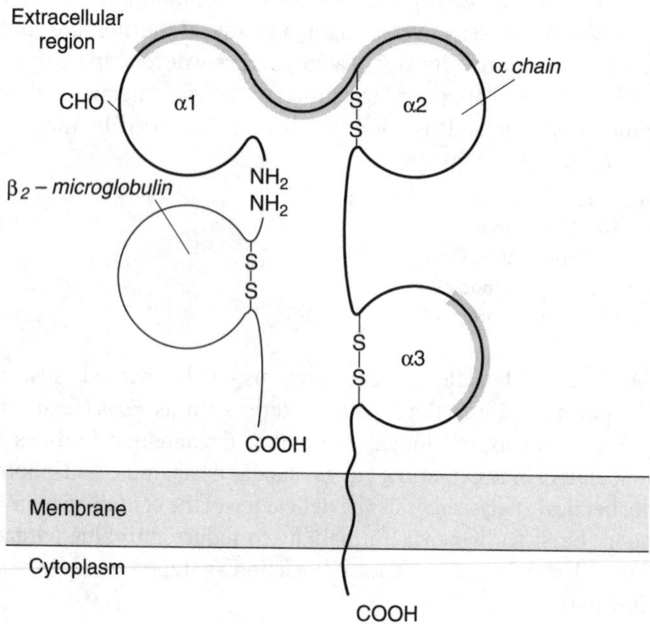

(Modified, with permission, from Parslow TG, et al. Medical Immunology. 10th ed. *New York, NY: McGraw-Hill; 2001:85.)*

a. Depicts the cell-membrane MHC product associated with narcolepsy
b. Essential for the transplacental passage of antibody
c. Found on T and B lymphocytes and all nucleated cells
d. Present on macrophages but not neutrophils
e. Represents the secretory component associated with IgA
f. Required for recognition of processed antigen by TH1 and TH2 lymphocytes

442. A 19-year-old college student develops a rash. She works part-time in a pediatric AIDS clinic. Her blood is drawn and tested for specific antibody to the chicken pox virus (varicella-zoster). Which of the following antibody classes would you expect to find if she is immune to chicken pox?

a. IgG
b. IgA
c. IgM
d. IgD
e. IgE

443. Patients with C5 through C9 complement deficiencies are most likely to be susceptible to which of the following infections?

a. AIDS
b. Giardiasis
c. Histoplasmosis
d. Neisserial infection
e. Pneumococcal infection

444. As part of the management of a 28-year-old male with acute onset of Crohn disease of the small bowel, you decide to treat him with a new cocktail of mouse–human chimeric antibodies to reduce his intestinal inflammation and cachexia. To which of the following sets of proteins are these antibodies directed?

a. IL-1, IL-2, IL-3
b. IL-2, IL-12, TNF-α
c. IL-2, TGF-β, TNF-α'
d. IL-1, IL-6, TNF-α'
e. IL-2, IL-3, IL-12

445. A mother and newborn are exposed to a pathogen while at the hospital for a routine checkup and breastfeeding clinic. This same pathogen had infected the mother about a year previously, and she had successfully recovered from the subsequent illness. Immunity may be innate or acquired. Which of the following best describes acquired immunity with respect to the newborn?

a. Complement cascade
b. Increase in C-reactive protein (CRP)
c. Inflammatory response
d. Maternal transfer of antibody
e. Presence of natural killer (NK) cells

446. A 35-year-old male patient presents with numerous subcutaneous hemorrhages. History and physical examination reveal that he has been taking sedormid (a sedative) for the past week. Laboratory tests indicate normal hemoglobin and white blood cell levels with significant thrombocytopenia (very low platelet count). You suspect that he has developed a drug-induced type II hypersensitivity reaction. This reaction may occur if the drug does which of the following?

a. Activates T cytotoxic cells
b. Acts as a hapten
c. Induces mast cell degranulation, releasing mediators such as histamine, leukotrienes, and prostaglandins
d. Induces oxygen radical production through the respiratory burst pathway
e. Persists in macrophages

447. After learning of a family history of humoral immunity deficiency during an office visit from a patient 6 months pregnant, a radial immunodiffusion assay is ordered on fetal serum. The test reveals no humoral immunity problems and normal results in all respects. According to this test, the normal level of which fetally made immunoglobulin is the highest in the fetus?

a. IgA
b. IgD
c. IgE
d. IgG
e. IgM

448. A 31-year-old male patient complains of fatigue, yeast infection in his mouth, and enlarged lymph nodes under his arms. He says that he was involved in "high-risk" behavior 6 years ago while on a trip to eastern and southern Africa. He also indicates that his "HIV test" was negative. Which of the following options is most appropriate?

a. Initiate treatment for HIV disease
b. Order a test for human T-cell leukemia virus (HTLV)
c. Order an HIV-1 RNA PCR
d. Order an HIV test that would include antibodies to HIV-1 and HIV-2
e. Repeat the test for HIV-1

449. A laboratory analysis report of a specific fraction of a patient's lymphocytes indicates the following: HLA, B, and C+, PHA+, CD3–, CD16+, CD11a/CD18+, CD56+, and in vitro blastogenesis with IL-12. What are the lymphocytes that this set describes?

a. B lymphocytes
b. Cytotoxic T lymphocytes
c. NK cells
d. T helper 1 (TH1) subset
e. T helper 2 (TH2) subset

450. The complement system plays a key role in the host defense process. Which of the following components of this system is the most important in chemotaxis?

a. C1q
b. C3a
c. C3b
d. C4a
e. C5a

451. Soon after birth, a newborn undergoes heart transplantation surgery at a local medical center. Transplantation of tissue and organs is a common procedure whose success depends largely on the "self" versus "nonself" interactions. Survival of allografts is increased by choosing donors with few major histocompatibility complex (MHC) mismatches compared to recipients and by use of immunosuppression in recipients. Which of the following procedures is the most useful measure of immunosuppression in recipients?

a. Administration of corticosteroids to recipient
b. Administration of immunoglobulin to recipient
c. Destruction of donor B cells
d. Destruction of donor T cells
e. Lymphoid irradiation of donor

452. Relative to the primary immunological response, secondary, and later booster responses to a given hapten–protein complex can be associated with which one of the following?

a. Antibodies that are less efficient in preventing specific disease
b. Decreased antibody avidity for the original hapten–protein complex
c. Increased antibody affinity for hapten
d. Lower titers of antibody
e. Maintenance of the same subclass, or idiotype, of antibody produced

453. You are managing a 3-year-old female patient with a fever of unknown origin. Her serum is tested for antibodies against *Haemophilus influenzae*. A precipitation test conducted by the clinical laboratory yields the following results:

Serum (Antibody) Dilutions								
Undiluted serum	1:2	1:4	1:8	1:16	1:32	1:64	1:128	1:256
±	+	+	+	+	+	+	–	–

From these data, which of the following can be concluded?

a. The negative reactions at 1:128 and 1:126 are false negatives
b. The patient has antibodies against *H. influenzae*, the titer is 64, and the dilution 1:64
c. The patient has antibodies against *H. influenzae*, the dilution is 64, and the titer 1:64
d. The patient does not have antibodies against *H. influenzae* since the reaction is negative with undiluted serum
e. The patient should be immunized against *H. influenzae*

454. Of the five immunoglobulin classes, IgA is the main immunoglobulin of secretions from the genital, respiratory, and intestinal tracts. As a result, IgA antibody is the first line of defense against infections at the mucous membrane. It is usually an early specific antibody. Which of the following statements most accurately describes IgA?

a. Complement fixation tests for IgA antibody will be positive if specific IgA antibody is present
b. IgA can be destroyed by bacterial proteases
c. IgA is absent in colostrum
d. IgA is not found in saliva; therefore, an IgA diagnostic test on saliva would have no value
e. IgA is a small molecule with a molecular weight of 30,000 kDa

455. A 60-year-old male presents with severe jaundice to the local walk-in clinic. History and physical examination reveal a 30-year history of alcohol consumption and drug abuse. Blood tests reveal elevated AST and ALT levels and the presence of hepatitis B and, as a result, reduced complement levels. Complement is a series of important host proteins that provide protection from invasion by foreign microorganisms. Which of the following best describes complement?

a. Complement inhibits phagocytosis
b. Complement is activated by IgE antibody classes
c. Complement plays a minor role in the inflammatory response
d. Complement protects the host from pneumococcal infection through C1, C2, and C4
e. Microorganisms agglutinate in the presence of complement but do not lyse

456. Radial immunodiffusion and immunoelectrophoresis is performed on a young patient to evaluate the function of his humoral immune system. Which of the following immunoglobulins has no known function, is found in the serum in low concentrations, and is present on the surface of B lymphocytes (may function as an antigen receptor)?

a. IgG
b. IgA
c. IgM
d. IgD
e. IgE

457. A young patient with severe recurrent pyogenic bacterial infections, but with normal T-cell and B-cell numbers, arrives at the hospital. Testing reveals that this patient's CD4 T-helper cells have a defect in CD40 ligand. As a result, humoral immunity evaluation reveals a significant elevation in the levels of which immunoglobulin that is present as a monomer on B-cell surfaces, as a pentamer in serum, and is initially seen in the primary immune response?

a. IgG
b. IgA
c. IgM
d. IgD
e. IgE

458. A patient with a long history of consuming poorly cooked pork meat presents with generalized myalgia and a low-grade fever. Striated muscle biopsy reveals multiple cysts. Eosinophilia is also present with elevated levels of which of the following immunoglobulins most likely involved in parasitic infections?

a. IgG
b. IgA
c. IgM
d. IgD
e. IgE

459. A patient with cerebellar problems and spider angiomas is diagnosed with a combined T-cell and B-cell deficiency known as ataxia-telangiectasia. In addition to a defect in this patient's DNA repair enzymes, which immunoglobulin is the primary antibody in saliva, tears, and intestinal and genital secretions, and is also deficient in this illness?

a. IgG
b. IgA
c. IgM
d. IgD
e. IgE

460. With four subclasses, which immunoglobulin is the predominant antibody in the secondary immune response and has the greatest concentration of the five immunoglobulin classes in the fetus?

a. IgG
b. IgA
c. IgM
d. IgD
e. IgE

461. A 15-year-old boy is bitten by an *Ixodes* tick while camping with his parents and presents 1 week later with fatigue, fever, headache, and a reddish rash over his trunk and extremities. Positive IgM antibody (1:200) to *Borrelia burgdorferi* is associated with which of the following?

a. Acute Lyme disease
b. Fifth disease
c. Possible hepatitis B infection
d. Possible subacute sclerosing panencephalitis (SSPE)
e. Susceptibility to chicken pox

462. A small child presents with a low-grade fever, coryza, sore throat, a bright red rash on his cheeks, and a less intense erythematous rash on his body. Elevated IgG and IgM antibody titers to parvovirus suggest a diagnosis of which of the following?

a. Acute Lyme disease
b. Fifth disease
c. Possible hepatitis B infection
d. Possible subacute sclerosing panencephalitis (SSPE)
e. Susceptibility to chicken pox

463. Blood from a woman at a local pregnancy clinic is analyzed for antibody titers to known pathogens. A negative varicella antibody titer in this young woman signifies which of the following?

a. Acute Lyme disease
b. Fifth disease
c. Possible hepatitis B infection
d. Possible subacute sclerosing panencephalitis (SSPE)
e. Susceptibility to chicken pox

464. A patient with severe jaundice and liver failure has an increased antibody titer to delta agent. You should suspect which of the following?

a. Acute Lyme disease
b. Fifth disease
c. Possible hepatitis B infection
d. Possible subacute sclerosing panencephalitis (SSPE)
e. Susceptibility to chicken pox

465. A pediatric patient with progressively developing degenerative neurologic disease/disorder has an elevated CSF antibody titer to measles virus. You should suspect which of the following?

a. Acute Lyme disease
b. Fifth disease
c. Possible hepatitis B infection
d. Possible subacute sclerosing panencephalitis (SSPE)
e. Susceptibility to chicken pox

466. A 2-year-old patient presents to the pediatrician for a routine visit. History and physical examination reveals recurrent infections, and enlarged small blood vessels of the skin and conjunctivas. In addition, the physician notices irregular movements most akin to staggering. Suspecting an immune dysfunction, molecular testing reveals a defect in DNA repair enzymes. This autosomal recessive immune deficiency disorder usually is associated with which of the following?

	Humoral Immunity	Cellular Immunity
a.	Normal	Normal
b.	Normal	Deficient
c.	Deficient	Normal
d.	Deficient	Deficient
e.	Elevated	Elevated

467. A 10-month-old male infant with recurrent *H. influenzae* infections presents to the emergency room with otitis media, sinusitis, and in severe respiratory distress. Immunological and genetic testing reveals the absence of B cells and a destructive mutation in the tyrosine kinase gene. This X-linked recessive immune disorder is usually associated with which of the following?

	Humoral Immunity	Cellular Immunity
a.	Normal	Normal
b.	Normal	Deficient
c.	Deficient	Normal
d.	Deficient	Deficient
e.	Elevated	Elevated

468. Amniocentesis conducted during genetic counseling of a pregnant woman reveals a fetal adenosine deaminase deficiency. This autosomal recessive immunodeficiency is usually associated with which of the following?

	Humoral Immunity	Cellular Immunity
a.	Normal	Normal
b.	Normal	Deficient
c.	Deficient	Normal
d.	Deficient	Deficient
e.	Elevated	Elevated

469. A young child with spastic paralysis presents to the emergency room. Blood tests reveal hypocalcemia. This immune disorder is usually associated with which of the following?

	Humoral Immunity	Cellular Immunity
a.	Normal	Normal
b.	Normal	Deficient
c.	Deficient	Normal
d.	Deficient	Deficient
e.	Elevated	Elevated

470. A 10-month-old patient with recurrent pyogenic infections, eczema, and severe bleeding (thrombocytopenia) is diagnosed with Wiskott–Aldrich syndrome. This immune disorder is usually associated with which of the following?

	Humoral Immunity	Cellular Immunity
a.	Normal	Normal
b.	Normal	Deficient
c.	Deficient	Normal
d.	Deficient	Deficient
e.	Elevated	Elevated

471. An autograft of a burn victim is best described by which one of the following?

a. Transplant from one region of a person to another region
b. Transplant from one person to a genetically identical person
c. Transplant from one species to the same species
d. Transplant from one species to another species

472. Transplantation involving tissue from twin brothers possessing identical HLA genes is best described by which one of the following?

a. Allograft: transplant from one species to the same species
b. Autograft: transplant from one region of a person to another region
c. Isograft: transplant from one person to a genetically identical person
d. Xenograft: transplant from one species to another species

473. A 21-year-old patient in severe kidney failure receives a kidney from his 30-year-old brother. This type of transplantation is best described by which of the following?

a. Allograft: transplant from one species to the same species
b. Autograft: transplant from one region of a person to another region
c. Isograft: transplant from one person to a genetically identical person
d. Xenograft: transplant from one species to another species

474. During the infancy days of cardiac transplantation, nonhuman primate hearts were transplanted into humans to save lives. This type of transplantation is best described by which one of the following?

a. Allograft: transplant from one species to the same species
b. Autograft: transplant from one region of a person to another region
c. Isograft: transplant from one person to a genetically identical person
d. Xenograft: transplant from one species to another species

475. Humoral immunity evaluation mainly consists of measuring the amount of IgG, IgM, and IgA in the patient's serum. These three immunoglobulins represent three distinct isotypes. An isotype is characterized by which of the following?

a. Determinant exposed after papain cleavage to an F(ab) fragment
b. Determinant from one clone of cells and probably located close to the antigen-binding site of the immunoglobulin
c. Determinant inherited in a Mendelian fashion and recognized by cross-immunization of individuals in a species
d. Heavy-chain determinant recognized by heterologous antisera
e. Species-specific carbohydrate determinant on the heavy chain

476. An allotype is characterized by which of the following?

a. Determinant exposed after papain cleavage to an F(ab) fragment
b. Determinant from one clone of cells and probably located close to the antigen-binding site of the immunoglobulin
c. Determinant inherited in a Mendelian fashion and recognized by cross-immunization of individuals in a species
d. Heavy-chain determinant recognized by heterologous antisera
e. Species-specific carbohydrate determinant on the heavy chain

477. Antibodies produced from hybridomas are extremely useful clinically for their monoclonal properties. These antibodies have the same idiotype. An idiotype is characterized by which of the following?

a. Determinant exposed after papain cleavage to an F(ab′)2 fragment
b. Determinant from one clone of cells and probably located close to the antigen-binding site of the immunoglobulin
c. Determinant inherited in a Mendelian fashion and recognized by cross-immunization of individuals in a species
d. Heavy-chain determinant recognized by heterologous antisera
e. Species-specific carbohydrate determinant on the heavy chain

478. A 30-year-old male presents to the emergency room with difficulty in breathing and abdominal pain. Upon physical examination, you notice diffuse areas of nondependent, nonpitting swelling without pruritus, with predilection for the face, especially the perioral and periorbital areas. You also notice swelling in the mouth, pharynx, and larynx. Laboratory analysis of blood drawn from this patient indicates a complement problem. Which of the following is most likely?

a. High C4, C2, and C3
b. High C1 and normal level of C1 esterase inhibitor
c. High C1 esterase inhibitor and high C4
d. High C1 esterase inhibitor and low C4
e. Low C1 esterase inhibitor and high C4
f. Low C1 esterase inhibitor and low C4
g. Low C4 and high C2

479. A 45-year-old businesswoman arrives in your office with vague abdominal complaints. She has noticed melenic stool. Upon performing a sigmoidoscopy, you find a 4-cm mass in the upper colon. You should immediately order a blood test for which of the following tumor markers?

a. α-Fetoprotein
b. Antitumor antibody
c. Antitumor light chains
d. Carcinoembryonic antigen (CEA)
e. Human chorionic gonadotropin
f. Prostate-specific antigen

Questions 480 and 481

480. An 18-year-old male heroin addict, who practices the sharing of needles at a "shooting gallery," is positive in the screening test for AIDS. This patient is most likely to be immunodeficient because of which one of the following?

a. A genetic defect in chromosome 14
b. A low T-helper lymphocyte count
c. An atrophied thymus
d. NADPH enzyme deficiency
e. Insufficient B-cell maturation

481. Since a false-positive result is possible in the screening test in the previous vignette, the physician orders a confirmatory test. Which of the following best describes the standard confirmatory test, and what this test checks for, respectively?

a. Complement fixation test; antibodies against the virus
b. Enzyme-linked immunosorbent assay (ELISA); antigens of the virus
c. Radioimmunoassay (RIA); specific antibodies against the virus
d. Western blot; antigens of the virus
e. Western blot; specific antibodies against the virus

482. A pregnant 21-year-old Rh-negative female is about to deliver. The baby's father is determined to be Rh-positive. To reduce the chance for the development of hemolytic disease of the newborn, which of the following procedures should you order?

a. Administration of anti-Rh antibodies to the fetus postdelivery
b. Administration of anti-Rh antibodies to the mother postdelivery
c. Immediate blood transfusion of the suspected father
d. Immediate blood transfusion of the mother with Rh-positive blood
e. Infusion of immune serum globulin into the fetus
f. Intravenous infusion of the Rh antigen into the mother

Questions 483 and 484

483. An 8-month-old male infant with a history of chronic diarrhea, otitis media, and several episodes of pneumonia presents to your clinic with gingivostomatitis (due to herpes simplex virus) and oral candidiasis (thrush). You immediately order an x-ray and a blood workup. X-ray and laboratory blood analysis reveal the absence of a thymic shadow and absence of B lymphocytes, respectively. History taken from the infant's mother reveals a rash evident at birth. Which of the following diseases is most likely present in this infant?

a. Ataxia-telangiectasia
b. Bruton agammaglobulinemia
c. Chediak–Higashi syndrome
d. Chronic granulomatous disease
e. Chronic mucocutaneous candidiasis
f. Hereditary angioedema
g. Severe combined immunodeficiency syndrome (SCID)
h. Thymic aplasia (DiGeorge syndrome)
i. Wiskott–Aldrich syndrome

484. Which of the following is the best therapy for the infant in the previous vignette?

a. Antifungal agents
b. Blood transfusion
c. Bone marrow transplant
d. IgG from pooled random donors
e. Immunization with attenuated vaccines

485. A 5-year-old child arrives at the emergency department minutes after being bitten by a black widow spider. You immediately inject gamma globulin in the form of an antivenom. This type of immunization is referred to as which of the following?

a. Artificial active immunization
b. Artificial passive immunization
c. Natural active immunization
d. Natural passive immunization
e. Adoptive immunization

486. A patient with an increased susceptibility to viral, fungal, and protozoa infection would be expected to have a deficiency in which of the following cell types?

a. B lymphocytes
b. Macrophages
c. NK cells
d. Neutrophils
e. T lymphocytes

487. While walking through a field, a 28-year-old woman is stung by a bee. Within 10 minutes, she has asthmatic-like symptoms. This type of hypersensitivity reaction can be correctly characterized by which of the following sequence of steps?

a. Allergen, chemical mediators, sensitization, allergen, IgE, symptoms
b. Allergen, IgE, sensitization, allergen, chemical mediators, symptoms
c. Allergen, sensitization, IgE, allergen, chemical mediators, symptoms
d. Sensitization, allergen, chemical mediators, allergen, IgE, symptoms
e. Sensitization, IgE, allergen, symptoms, allergen, chemical mediators

488. Findings of IgG antibodies to core antigen, antibodies to e antigen, and antibodies to surface antigen in a hepatitis B patient reflects which of the following?

a. Acute infection (incubation period)
b. Acute infection (acute phase)
c. Postinfection (acute phase)
d. Immunization
e. HBV carrier state

489. Findings of HBsAg-positive and HBeAg-positive test results in a hepatitis B patient reflect which of the following?

a. Acute infection (incubation period)
b. Acute infection (acute phase)
c. Postinfection (acute phase)
d. Immunization
e. HBV carrier state

490. Findings of HBsAg positive, HBeAg positive, and IgM core antibody positive in a hepatitis B patient reflect which of the following?

a. Acute infection (incubation period)
b. Acute infection (acute phase)
c. Postinfection (acute phase)
d. Immunization
e. HBV carrier state

491. Findings of HBsAg positive, no antibodies to HBsAg, and other tests variable in a hepatitis B patient reflect which of the following?

a. Acute infection (incubation period)
b. Acute infection (acute phase)
c. Postinfection (acute phase)
d. Immunization
e. HBV carrier state

492. Findings of antibodies to HBsAg in a hepatitis B patient reflect which of the following?

a. Acute infection (incubation period)
b. Acute infection (acute phase)
c. Postinfection (acute phase)
d. Immunization
e. HBV carrier state

493. A 15-year-old male is rushed to the emergency room with a temperature of 103°F, severe headache, and stiff neck. Upon physical examination, a petechial rash is observed all over his body. Suspecting meningitis, the physician orders a lumbar puncture, revealing gram-negative diplococci (*Neisseria meningitidis*) on Gram stain. The physician wishes to use a more sensitive test to confirm this as the causative agent. Which of the following tests combines features of gel diffusion and immunoelectrophoresis and is applicable only to negatively charged antigens?

a. Coagglutination (COA)
b. Counterimmunoelectrophoresis (CIE)
c. Enzyme-linked immunosorbent assay (ELISA)
d. Latex agglutination (LA)
e. Radioimmunoassay (RIA)

494. A 21-year-old female presents to the emergency room with a high fever, hypotension, and a diffuse, macular, sunburn-like rash that is desquamating. She is also vomiting, has profuse diarrhea, leukocytosis, thrombocytopenia, and elevated BUN and creatinine levels. History from her roommate reveals that these symptoms started soon after the patient began packing her nose to stop chronic nose bleeds. Suspecting *S. aureus*, a nasal swab specimen is obtained and sent to the laboratory. Which of the following rapid tests will be ordered and depends on the presence of protein A on certain strains of *S. aureus*?

a. COA
b. CIE
c. ELISA
d. LA
e. RIA

495. A 50-year-old building contractor arrives in your office complaining of abdominal pain that has increased in severity over the past 3 months. He has noticed melenic stool. Ordering a sigmoidoscopy, a 10-cm mass is visualized in the transverse colon. Surgery is immediately done and the tumor excised. As part of the patient's postsurgical follow through of this resected carcinoma of the colon, blood is obtained and sent to the laboratory to monitor levels of the tumor marker known as CEA. Which of the following tests involves the measurement of very small quantities of CEA through competition of radiolabeled and unlabeled antigen for the same limited amount of antibody?

a. COA
b. CIE
c. ELISA
d. LA
e. RIA

496. A 13-year-old male arrives at his doctor's office with a severe sore throat and very high fever. On physical examination, the physician observes his pharynx to be inflamed with a significant exudate along with tender cervical lymph nodes. Laboratory tests reveal a leukocytosis. Suspecting Group A β-hemolytic *Streptococcus pyogenes*, a throat swab and culture are obtained. Using a rapid diagnostic kit recently obtained, the physician decides to test the specimens himself. This test involves inert particles that are sensitized with either antigen or antibody. Which of the following tests is used extensively to detect microbial antigens rapidly (5 minutes or less)?

a. COA
b. CIE
c. ELISA
d. LA
e. RIA

497. A 7-month-old baby who is failing to thrive is brought into a neighborhood clinic. History reveals that the baby's mother died of AIDS 2 months ago. Blood is obtained and sent to the laboratory to check for HIV infection. The physician orders a test whose detection system is based on enzymatic activity. Which of the following tests is a heterogeneous immunoassay?

a. COA
b. CIE
c. ELISA
d. LA
e. RIA

Questions 498 to 502

A 29-year-old pregnant female gives birth to a stillborn child. History reveals that the woman continued to have close contact with her five cats, by emptying litter boxes and feeding them raw meat, during pregnancy, against her physician's advice. An autopsy is conducted, and multiple cysts are found in the fetal brain, lungs, liver, and eyes. As a confirmatory test, the pathologist orders an enzyme immunoassay to detect the presence of *Toxoplasma gondii*. The diagram below presents the various steps (labeled A-F) of the enzyme immunoassay.

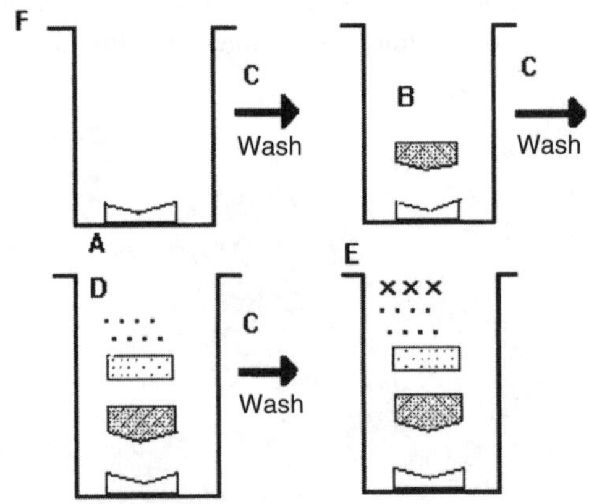

498. Failure of or improper methods for which step in the process is the primary cause of high background color?

a. A
b. B
c. C
d. D
e. E
f. F

499. Where is unlabeled antibody attached if this enzyme immunoassay is intended for detection of antigen?

a. A
b. B
c. C
d. D
e. E
f. F

500. What is the location of the "solid phase"?

a. A
b. B
c. C
d. D
e. E
f. F

501. Addition of reagent at which step will cause color in the positive control well and reactive patient specimens?

a. A
b. B
c. C
d. D
e. E
f. F

502. What is the location of the patient's specimen in the diagram?

a. A
b. B
c. C
d. D
e. E
f. F

503. An 18-year-old male patient with acute lymphocytic leukemia fails all standard chemotherapies. Cells from an HLA-nonidentical donor are used to perform a bone marrow transplant. Prior to transplantation, the patient is given broad-spectrum antibiotics and an immunosuppressive regimen. Within 2 to 4 weeks, lymphocyte and granulocyte numbers begin to rise, confirming bone marrow cell engraftment. However, 1 month later, the patient develops diarrhea, jaundice, and a severe maculopapular rash. Physical examination reveals hepatosplenomegaly. Which of the following is most likely occurring?

a. Acute rejection
b. Chronic rejection
c. Cyclosporine A toxicity
d. Graft versus host disease (GVHD)
e. Hyperacute rejection

504. A 27-year-old male patient (blood group O) arrives at the emergency room with a massive intestinal bleed (hematochezia). Within hours he has lost half of his blood volume, and you decide to transfuse. Due to human error, you transfuse blood group AB into him and within minutes he develops a fever, chills, dyspnea, and a dramatic drop in blood pressure. This reaction is most likely due to which of the following?

a. A cell-mediated response against AB antigens
b. IgG production by the recipient in response to AB antigens
c. Preformed anti-A and anti-B antibodies in the recipient
d. Preformed anti-A and anti-B antibodies of the blood donor
e. Preformed isohemagglutinins of the IgG isotype

505. During a clinic office visit, a 35-year-old male stockbroker shows signs of excessive nervousness and irritability and complains that the office is too hot. History and physical examination reveals the presence of a goiter and exophthalmia. Laboratory analysis of his blood reveals high antibody titers against the thyroid-stimulating hormone (TSH) receptor. Which of the following is the most likely diagnosis?

a. Goodpasture syndrome
b. Graves disease
c. Hashimoto disease
d. Juvenile-onset diabetes mellitus
e. Myasthenia gravis
f. Pernicious anemia
g. Rheumatoid arthritis
h. Systemic lupus erythematosus (SLE)

506. A 9-year-old female with a recent history of weight loss and vision problems arrives at the hospital. Soon after, it is determined that she has low blood glucose, and autoantibodies against β cells are detected in her serum. Which of the following is the most likely diagnosis?

a. Goodpasture syndrome
b. Graves disease
c. Hashimoto disease
d. Juvenile-onset diabetes mellitus
e. Myasthenia gravis
f. Pernicious anemia
g. Rheumatoid arthritis
h. SLE

507. A 35-year-old woman with fever, weight loss, fatigue, and painful joints and muscles presents to her physician's office. The physician notes that she has marked photosensitivity and a rash on the cheeks and over the bridge of her nose. Laboratory tests reveal anemic conditions and the presence of anti-DNA antibodies. Which of the following is the most likely diagnosis?

a. Goodpasture syndrome
b. Graves disease
c. Hashimoto disease
d. Juvenile-onset diabetes mellitus
e. Myasthenia gravis
f. Pernicious anemia
g. Rheumatoid arthritis
h. SLE

Questions 508 to 512

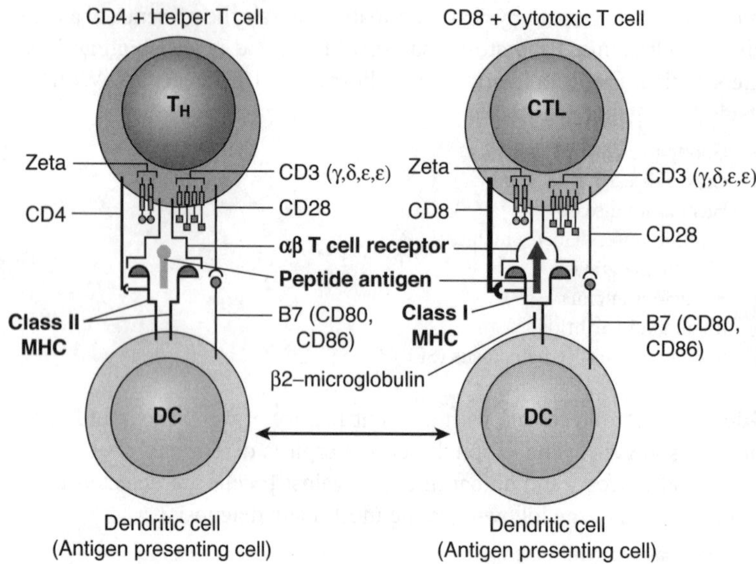

Diagram depicting the process of *T-cell activation by dendritic cells* (professional antigen presenting cells, APC). Shown are a CD4 helper T cell (TH), a CD8 cytotoxic T cell (CTL), and dendritic cells (DC). Major histocompatibility complex (MHC) molecules are also shown. CD4 co-receptor is shown for TH cell activation, and CD8 co-receptor is shown for CTL activation. There are 2 zeta chains and 4 CD3 complex molecules (γ, δ, ε, ε). The rectangles associated with zeta and CD3 are the ITAMs. Costimulation, second signal molecules CD28 and B7 are shown for both TH and CTL activation.

508. Which of the following molecules represent the primary or prototypical members involved in signal 2 mediated activation of naïve T cells?

a. CD28, B7-1 or B7-2
b. CTLA-4, CD28, PD-1
c. CTLA-4, B7-1 or B7-2
d. B7-H1, B7-H3, PD-1

509. The following *best describes* TCR recognition of antigen:

a. Binds to conformational determinants of whole proteins
b. Binds to linear determinants of whole proteins
c. Binds to peptide in the context of MHC
d. Binds to peptide without MHC
e. Binds to large glycoproteins

510. Which of the following *best describes* the TCR complex?

a. αβ TCR covalently linked with CD3 and ζ chains
b. αβ TCR covalently linked with CD2 and CD28
c. αβ TCR noncovalently associated with CD3 and ζ chains
d. αβ TCR noncovalently associated with CD2 and CD28
e. αα TCR noncovalently associated with CD3 and ζ chains

511. The membrane associated T-lymphocyte antigen receptor or TCR is best described asa:

a. Heterodimer consisting of covalently linked α and β chains
b. Homodimer consisting of covalently linked α and β chains
c. Homodimer associated with Igα and Igβ
d. Monomer associated with Igα and Igβ
e. Heavy chain monomer associated with β2m

512. Nearly 95% of mature T cells possess a T-cell receptor (TCR) complex that contains:

a. Igβ and Igα
b. CD28 and TCR γδ
c. A highly variable antigen coreceptor and TCR γδ
d. Four CD3 molecules (γ, δ, ε, ε), each covalently linked to the TCR αβ heterodimer
e. Invariable ζ chain homodimer noncovalently associated with the TCR αβ heterodimer

513. A preschool boy is diagnosed with an immunodeficiency characterized by impaired T-cell activation. The defect is caused by a genetic alteration of a membrane protein whose cytoplasmic tail is involved in signaling associated with TCR recognition of peptide antigen in the context of MHC. Which of the following proteins does NOT fit this description?

a. CD3γ
b. ζ chain
c. TCRβ
d. CD4
e. CD8

514. The germline antigen receptor loci for *both* alpha and beta chains of the TCR are found in:

a. All nucleated cells
b. Double positive T cells only
c. Naïve CD4+ T cells only
d. Naïve CD8+ T cells only
e. Pre-T cells only

515. The processes of negative selection for T lymphocytes eliminates those T cells with TCRs that

a. Do not recognize self-peptide/self-MHC
b. Recognize foreign-peptide/self-MHC complexes with low avidity/affinity
c. Recognize foreign-peptide/self-MHC complexes with high avidity/affinity
d. Recognize self-peptide/self-MHC complexes with low avidity/affinity
e. Recognize self-peptide/self-MHC complexes with high avidity/affinity

516. Cells of the immune system arise in the bone marrow. The cell that finishes its maturation in the thymus is the

a. Follicular B-2 B lymphocyte
b. Marginal zone B lymphocyte
c. NK cell
d. $\alpha\beta$ T lymphocyte
e. Dendritic cell

517. A 1-month-old infant with a bright red rash and purulent conjunctivitis is admitted to the hospital. Examination revealed eosinophilia, low lymphocyte count, and no thymic shadow. Lymphnodes were enlarged and opportunistic infections noted. The diagnosis was a form of SCID termed Omenn syndrome, an autosomal recessive form of SCID. Mutations in which of the following would explain this disease?

a. MHC class I
b. MHC class II
c. CD3 or TCR αβ
d. RAG-1 or RAG-2
e. CD4 or CD8

518. Class-I MHC-restricted CD8+ T cell (CTL) responses to tumors can be demonstrated in patients with various types of tumors, yet most of these tumors do not express costimulatory molecules. Which mechanism most likely explains how naïve CD8+ T cells specific for antigens expressed by these tumors are activated and differentiate into CTLs?

a. Tumor secretion of TGF-β
b. Tumor secretion of IL-12
c. Tumor expression of B7
d. Direct priming of the CTLs
e. Cross priming of the CTLs

519. A 47-year-old woman had a mastectomy because she had breast carcinoma that was previously diagnosed by biopsy. Pathologic examination revealed that several axillary lymph nodes contained metastatic tumors. A test was performed on the tumor cells extracted from the mastectomy specimen, which indicated that the tumor cells overexpressed a certain cellular proto-oncogene. On the basis of this test result, the patient was treated with an FDA-approved monoclonal antibody specific for the protein encoded by that gene. Which of the following was most likely the protein target of the FDA-approved passive antibody therapy?

MONOCLONAL ANTIBODIES APPROVED FOR CANCER TREATMENT

Antibody	Antigen	Antigen Function	Cancer Treated	Year Approved
Rituximab	CD20	B-cell signaling receptor	Non-Hodgkin lymphoma	1997
Trastuzumab	HER2/neu	Growth factor receptor	Breast cancer	1998
Alemtuzumab	CD52	Differentiation antigen	Chronic lymphocytic leukemia	2001
Cetruximab	EGFR	Growth factor receptor	Colorectal cancer Head and neck cancer	2004 2006
Panitumumab	EGFR	Growth factor receptor	Colorectal cancer	2004
Bevacizumab	VEGF	Promotes angiogenesis	Colorectal cancer Non-small cell lung cancer	2004 2006
Ipilimumab	CTLA-4	T-cell inhibition	Metastatic melanoma	2011

EGFR, epidermal growth factor receptor; VEGF, vascular endothelial growth factor.

a. HPV E6, E7
b. Her2/Neu
c. CA-125
d. CD20
e. CEA

520. Which of the following does not describe a documented mechanism of tumor-mediated immune evasion?

a. Down regulation of class I MHC
b. Secretion of TGF-β
c. Secretion of decoy molecules
d. Antigenic variation

521. Which of the following best describes the mechanism(s) of action of CTLA-4?

a. Signal 1 and costimulation
b. Competition and inhibition
c. Activation and proliferation
d. ZAP-70 and ITAMs
e. PD-1 and PD-L1

Immunology

Answers

428 to 431. The answers are 428-a, 429-c, 430-c, and 431-d. (*Kindt, pp 372-396. Parham, pp 365-398.*) Reactions to small amounts of drugs can occur, as illustrated in the skin test using penicilloyl polylysine to reveal a penicillin allergy or type I hypersensitivity reaction. In Question 429, the girl was likely exposed to poison ivy or poison oak (contact dermatitis) which is attributed to a type IV hypersensitivity reaction. An Arthus reaction is a localized type of reaction mediated by aggregates of antibody and antigen and is characteristic of type III hypersensitivity reactions. In Question 430, only hypersensitivity reactions type I and IV are associated with skin tests. Type I is commonly referred to as a challenge in which a specific antigen is injected intradermally into a sensitized individual, creating a "wheal and flare" (erythema and edema) reaction. Type IV hypersensitivity is commonly associated with tuberculin injections to recognize the presence of delayed type hypersensitivity. In Question 431, Rh disease and Goodpasture syndrome are the result of antibodies that have formed against normally present host antigens on red blood cells and the kidney's glomerular basement membrane, respectively. Thus, these two diseases are associated with type II reactions. The table below describes these reactions in detail.

HYPERSENSITIVITY REACTIONS		
Mediator	**Type**	**Reaction**
Antibody (IgE)	I (immediate, anaphylactic)	IgE antibody is induced by allergen and binds to mast cells and basophils. When exposed to the allergen again, the allergen cross-links the bound IgE, which induces degranulation and release of mediators, eg, histamine
Antibody (IgG)	II (cytotoxic)	Antigens on a cell surface combine with antibody; this leads to complement-mediated lysis, eg, transfusion or Rh reactions, or autoimmune hemolytic anemia
Antibody (IgG)	III (immune complex)	Antigen–antibody immune complexes are deposited in tissues, complement is activated, and polymorphonuclear cells are attracted to the site. They release lysosomal enzymes, causing tissue damage
Cell	IV (delayed)	Helper T lymphocytes sensitized by an antigen release lymphokines upon second contact with the same antigen. The lymphokines induce inflammation and activate macrophages, which, in turn, release various mediators

(Reprinted, with permission, from *Levinson W, Jawetz E.* Medical Microbiology. *7th ed. New York, NY: McGraw-Hill; 2002:415.)*

432 and 433. The answers are 432-b and 433-a. (*Kindt, pp 284, 498. Parham, pp 170-171, 341-342.*) Bruton agammaglobulinemia is a congenital defect that becomes apparent at approximately 6 months of age, when maternal IgG is diminished. It occurs in males and is characterized by a defective *btk* gene, very small tonsils, low levels of all five classes of immunoglobulins, and no mature B cells. Thus, the child is unable to produce immunoglobulins and develops a series of bacterial infections characterized by recurrences and progression to more serious infections such as septicemia. The most common organisms responsible for infection are *H. influenzae* and *S. pneumoniae.* Treatment consists of pooled IgG. Cell-mediated immunity is not affected, and the child is able to respond normally to diseases that require this immune response for resolution, such as the measles virus, varicella-zoster virus, and *M tuberculosis*. The other diagnoses do not describe the specific clinical scenario outlined in this case. Also, it is important to note that since the main defect in this child's immunity is in the B-cell line, in that, the child is unable to produce immunoglobulins. The organism that would be most dangerous to the child is *C. trachomatis* because the B-cell line (antibodies) is typically responsible for its elimination from the host.

Note: Immunodeficiency is characterized by unusual and recurrent infections:

- B-cell (antibody) deficiency—bacterial infections
- T-cell deficiency—viral, fungal, and protozoal infections
- Phagocytic cell deficiency—pyogenic infections (bacterial), skin infections, systemic bacterial opportunistic infections
- Complement deficiencies—pyogenic infections (bacterial)

434 and 435. The answers are 434-e and 435-a. (*Kindt, pp 30-40. Parham, pp 220-230, 352-356.*) Cells can be differentiated based on unique cell surface markers (antigens). In this case, a CD4:CD8 ratio of less than 1 indicates a significant reduction in the helper T-lymphocyte population. The surface proteins that best represent this pool are MHC I, TCR, CD3, and CD28. CD4 is also associated with helper T lymphocytes. B lymphocytes have MHC I, IgM, B7 CD19, and CD20. Cytotoxic T lymphocytes have MHC I, TCR, CD3, and CD8, while macrophages have MHC I, MHC II, and CD14. An important fact to remember is that all healthy cells other than mature red cells have class I MHC. The B7 surface protein on the antigen-presenting cell is the costimulatory molecule and must interact with the CD28 on the helper T cell for full activation to occur (see the following figures.)

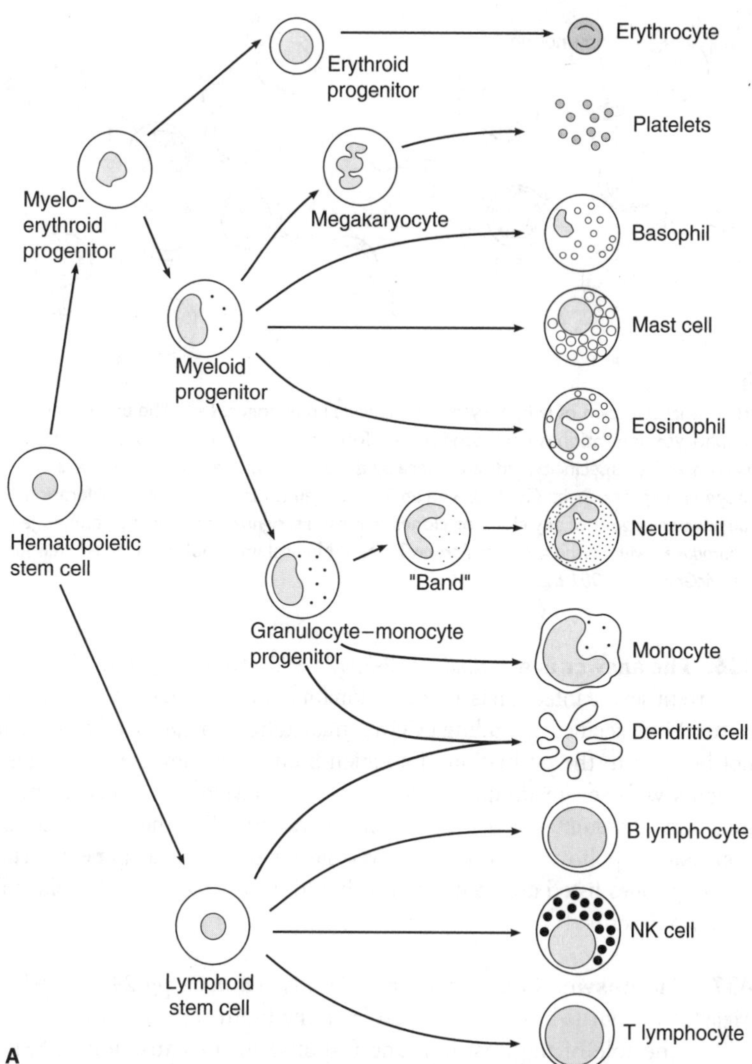

(**A**) Schematic overview of hematopoiesis, emphasizing the erythroid, myeloid, and lymphoid pathways. This highly simplified depiction omits many recognized intermediate cell types in each pathway. All of the cells shown here develop to maturity in the bone marrow, except T lymphocytes, which develop from marrow-derived progenitors that migrate to the thymus. A common lymphoid stem cell serves as the progenitor of T and B lymphocytes and of NK cells. Dendritic cells arise from both the myeloid and lymphoid lineages. *(Reproduced, with permission, from Parslow TG, et al.* Medical Immunology. *10th ed. New York, NY: McGraw-Hill; 2001:3.)*

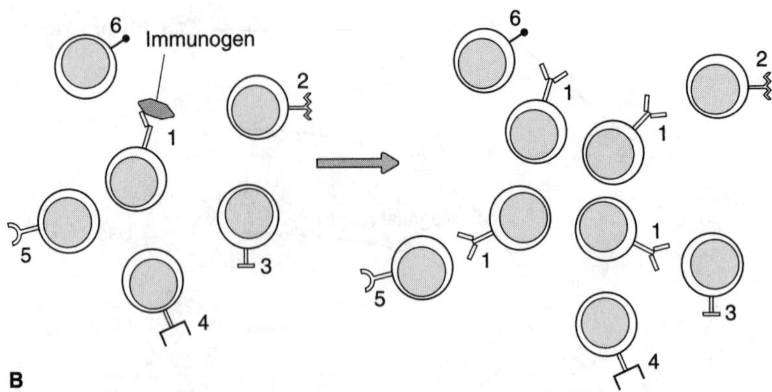

(**B**) Clonal selection of lymphocytes by a specific immunogen. *Left*: The unimmunized lymphocyte population is composed of cells from many different clones, each with its own antigen specificity, indicated here by the distinctive shapes of the surface antigen receptors. *Right*: Contact with an immunogen leads to selective proliferation (positive selection) of any clone or clones that can recognize that specific immunogen. *(Reproduced, with permission, from Parslow TG, et al.* Medical Immunology. *10th ed. New York, NY: McGraw-Hill; 2001:62.)*

436. The answer is a. (*Kindt, pp 2-3, 475-490. Parham, pp 1-7, 437-441.*) Recurrent severe infection is an indication for clinical evaluation of immune status. Live vaccines, including BCG attenuated from *M. tuberculosis*, should not be used in the evaluation of a patient's immune competence because patients with severe immunodeficiencies may develop an overwhelming infection (disseminated disease) from the vaccine. For the same reason, oral (Sabin) polio vaccine is not advisable for use in such persons. The other vaccines listed are acellular and should be safe to use in this clinical scenario described.

437. The answer is e. (*Kindt, pp 475-484. Parham, pp 24, 437-445.*) Measles-like virus has been isolated from the brain cells of patients with SSPE. The role of the host immune response in the causation of SSPE has been supported by several findings including the following: (1) progression of disease despite high levels of humoral antibody; (2) presence of a factor that blocks lymphocyte-mediated immunity to SSPE-measles virus in SSPE-CSF; (3) lysis of brain cells from SSPE patients by SSPE serum or CSF in the presence of complement (a similar mechanism could cause in vivo tissue injury). SSPE is particularly common in those who acquired measles before 2 years of age and is very rare after measles vaccination.

Higher-than-normal levels of serum antibodies (Ab) to measles virus and local synthesis of measles Ab in CSF, as evidenced by the oligoclonal IgG, imply a connection between the virus and MS. However, the other studies have implicated the other viruses. Several studies of cell-mediated hypersensitivity to measles and other viruses in MS have been done, but the results have been conflicting. Definite conclusions regarding defects in cellular immunity in this disease cannot be reached until further research is completed.

CJD is caused by the prion, which is an altered host protein that becomes infectious in nature. It is characterized by myoclonic jerking along with characteristic EEG changes. PML is associated with the JC virus (JCV), while this clinical scenario is not characteristic of EBV infection.

438. The answer is c. (*Kindt, pp 426-440. Parham, pp 455-459.*) Transplantation terminology is being tested in this question. An autograft is a transfer of an individual's own tissue to another site in the body. An isograft (syngeneic graft) is the transfer of tissue between genetically identical individuals, such as monozygotic twins. An allograft is the transfer of tissue between genetically different members of the same species (ie, brother to sister, dizygotic twins, etc), while a xenograft is the transfer of tissue between different species (eg, pig valve to human heart). In this case, one unit is the patient's own blood (an autologous donation) while the second unit is his older brother's blood (most like an allograft donation). If his brother had been an identical twin, then (e) would be the correct answer.

439. The answer is b. (*Kindt, pp 403, 410-412. Parham, pp 403-416.*) This clinical case represents a patient suffering with SLE. The diagnosis of SLE is best supported by detecting the presence of anti-dsDNA and anti-Smith (anti-Sm) antibodies. The presence of anti-dsDNA antibodies are very specific for SLE and represent a poor prognosis for disease. Antinuclear antibodies (ANA) can also be detected using fluorescent antibody tests. The other antibodies listed are related to other autoimmune diseases as follows: anticentromere antibodies in CREST syndrome and occasionally in systemic scleroderma, antimitochondrial antibodies in primary biliary cirrhosis, antineutrophil antibodies in antineutrophil cytoplasmic antibodies

(ANCA)-associated vasculitis (systemic vasculitis), and anti-TSH receptor antibodies in Graves disease (hyperthyroidism).

440. The answer is a. (*Kindt, pp 66, 495t, 501-503. Parham, pp 57, Ch 13.*) The patient in this case has chronic granulomatous disease (CGD), an X-linked (65%) or autosomal recessive (35%) inherited disease. Patients with CGD are not able to generate a respiratory burst after granulocyte and monocyte stimulation. Thus, they are unable to kill microorganisms. Answers a, b, and c are all involved in the respiratory burst; however, the central enzyme is the NADPH oxidase (answer a). Without this enzyme, hydrogen peroxide (answer b), superoxide (answer c), and other microbial reactive oxygen species would not be generated. Answer d depicts the synthetic pathway for nitric oxide, a potent vasodilator. Answers e and f are reactions involving common metabolic enzymes in various bacteria.

441. The answer is c. (*Kindt, pp 193-195. Parham, pp 133-139.*) The figure shown in the question is a schematic representation of the MHC class I molecule, which has a CD8 binding site (α_3) and a peptide-binding site (α_1 and α_2). MHC class I is active on all nucleated cells.

442. The answer is a. (*Kindt, pp 85-89. Parham, pp 95-105.*) The initial response to a new infection is with an IgM class antibody. IgM develops quickly and usually disappears within a few months. The secondary response is IgG and reflects the patient's immune status or, in the case of chicken pox, a vaccination given.

443. The answer is d. (*Kindt, pp 168, 185-186, 502. Parham, pp 343-345.*) Patients with complement deficiencies such as C5 through C9, which form the membrane attack complex (MAC), are predisposed to disseminated meningococcal (neisserial) disease. These patients may also be susceptible to gonococcal (neisserial) infection. There appears to be no disposition to AIDS or to fungal, parasitic, or pneumococcal infections.

444. The answer is d. (*Kindt, pp 346-347. Parham, pp 58-60.*) The acute-phase response is a primitive, nonspecific defense reaction, mediated by the liver, which increases innate immunity and other protective functions in stressful times. It can be triggered by chronic autoimmune disorders such as rheumatoid arthritis and Crohn disease. This response occurs when hepatocytes are exposed to IL-6 and IL-1 or TNF-α. LPS is a potent inducer of these cytokines. They are responsible for fever, somnolence, loss of appetite, and, if the response is prolonged, anemia and cachexia (wasting). A traditional assay known as the *erythrocyte sedimentation rate* (ESR) may be used as an indicator of an acute-phase response. The ESR involves measuring the rate at which the red blood cells fall through plasma, which increases as fibrinogen concentration rises. Currently, Crohn disease may be treated with infusions of a drug known as infliximab, which is a mouse-human chimeric antibody against human TNF-α or adalimumab, a fully humanized monoclonal antibody against human TNF-α. The FDA has approved these monoclonal antibody drugs in the treatment of Crohn disease, rheumatoid and psoriatic arthritis, ankylosing spondylitis, moderate to severe chronic psoriasis, and juvenile idiopathic arthritis.

445. The answer is d. (*Kindt, pp 99-100. Parham, pp 117-118, 267-268.*) Maternal transfer of antibody (secretory IgA in the colostrum of breast milk), however, is passive but still confers specific immunity. It is termed *passive acquired* immunity. Natural immunity is nonspecific. The natural immune functions described are not specific for a certain antigen. For example, certain proteins such as C-reactive protein (CRP) are acute-phase reactants. While elevated CRP is seen in infection, it is not disease specific.

446. The answer is b. (*Kindt, pp 77-78.*) Haptens (incomplete antigens) are not themselves antigenic, but when coupled to a cell or carrier protein become antigenic and induce antibodies that can bind the hapten alone (in the absence of the carrier protein). They are small molecules that are generally less than 1000 kDa. While haptens react with antibodies, they are not immunogenic because they do not activate T cells and cannot bind the MHC. Haptens are significant in disease; penicillin is a hapten and can cause severe life-threatening allergic reaction by destruction of erythrocytes. Catechols in the oils of poison ivy plants are haptens and cause a significant skin inflammatory response. Chloramphenicol is a hapten that can lead to the destruction of leukocytes and cause agranulocytosis. Sedormid is a hapten that can cause thrombocytopenia and purpura (bleeding) through the destruction of platelets.

447. The answer is e. (*Kindt, pp 87, 95-100. Parham, pp 115-118.*) The radial immunodiffusion and immunoelectrophoresis are two tests used to evaluate humoral immunity. Evaluating humoral immunity consists of measuring the levels of IgM, IgG, and IgA in the patient's serum. Whereas total IgG is greater than total IgM in the fetus due to the maternal transfer of IgG and not IgM across the placenta, it is important to remember that IgM is the antibody produced in the greatest amounts by the fetus. The fetus also produces IgG and IgA, but the fetus produces greater amounts of IgM than these other two important antibodies.

448. The answer is d. (*Kindt, pp 508-509, 512. Parham, pp 25-26, 351-361.*) HIV-2 disease is very rare in the United States. However, HIV-2 is present in Africa, the Far East, and some parts of the Caribbean. Many of the screening tests for HIV-1 will not detect antibodies to HIV-2. Either a separate HIV-2 antibody test or a combination HIV-1/2 is necessary. While HTLV disease is also seen in the same geographic areas, the symptoms displayed by this patient are more akin to HIV disease. While an HIV-1 RNA PCR is a useful test for monitoring the results of HIV therapy, it is not approved for diagnosis, nor will it detect HIV-2 nucleic acid.

449. The answer is c. (*Kindt, pp 30, 35-36, 360-363. Parham, pp 16, 65-66.*) NK cells do not express a cell surface TCR/CD3 complex and are CD4–. About half of human NK cells are CD8+. Also, most NK cells express an Fc IgG receptor, known as CD16, and CD56, a neural cell adhesion molecule variant. NK cells are generally CD16+, CD56+, and CD3–, which contrasts them with T cells, which are CD3+, CD16–, and CD56–. In addition, B cells are associated with CD19 and CD20.

450. The answer is e. (*Kindt, pp 175-176, 338-339. Parham, pp 39-42.*) C3a and C5a are potent mediators of inflammation; that is, they have anaphylatoxin activity. This activity is characterized by smooth-muscle contraction and the degranulation of mast cells and basophils leading to the release of histamine and other vasoactive substances, causing increased vascular (capillary) permeability. C5a is the most potent of these anaphylatoxins; however, it also serves another role as a potent chemotactic agent, attracting polymorphonucleated neutrophils and macrophages to the site of inflammation.

451. The answer is a. (*Kindt, pp 33, 426-440. Parham, pp 460-469.*) Allograft rejection is primarily a T-cell response to foreign tissue. Many immunosuppressive measures exist, including cyclosporine, tacrolimus, sirolimus, azathioprine, monoclonal antibodies, radiation, and corticosteroids. Commonly used, the corticosteroids reduce inflammatory response and are generally administered by cytotoxic drugs, such as cyclosporine. Corticosteroids function as immunosuppressive agents by inhibiting cytokine production, such as IL-1 and TNF, and also by lysing certain T-cell types. Lymphoid irradiation is usually done so that the bone marrow is shielded. This removes lymphocytes from lymph nodes and spleen while allowing the patient to have the capacity to regenerate new T and B cells. Likewise, antilymphocyte globulin will destroy the recipient's lymphocytes, especially T cells. Destruction of donor B cells and T cells would not play a role in the immunosuppression of the graft recipient. In graft crises, monoclonal antibody to CD3 is sometimes given. This targets mature T lymphocytes for destruction.

452. The answer is c. (*Kindt, pp 77-78. Parham, pp 115-119.*) With repeated immunization, higher titers of all antibodies are observed, and, as priming is repeated, the immune response recruits B cells of progressively greater affinity. The affinity of antibody for a hapten–protein complex rises, polyclonal cross-reactivity also rises, and the response becomes wider in specificity. As the number of antigenic sites detected per reacting particle increases, the avidity increases. In addition to shifts in the class of immunoglobulin synthesized in response to an antigen (IgM-IgG), shifts also may occur in the idiotype of antibody.

453. The answer is b. (*Kindt, pp 151-153.*) In precipitation reactions, both the antigen and the antibody are soluble. The antibody cross-links antigen molecules, creating an increasing lattice that eventually forms an insoluble precipitate. The antigen must be divalent, and the antigen/antibody proportion is critical in order for detectable precipitate to form. The prozone is the zone of antibody excess. The postzone is the zone of antigen excess. The zone of equivalence is the zone where the proportion of antibody and antigen is optimal for precipitate formation. Titer is the reciprocal of the highest dilution (ratio) of antibody (or antigen) at which there is still a detectable reaction (see figure on the next page).

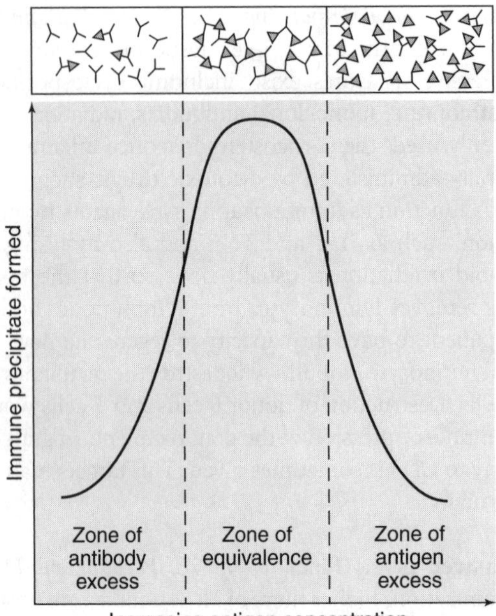

(Modified and reproduced, with permission, from Stites D, Terr A, Parslow T (eds). Basic and Clinical Immunology. *9th ed.* Originally published by Appleton & Lange. *Copyright © 1997 by The McGraw-Hill Companies.)*

454. The answer is b. (*Kindt, pp 96t, 99-100. Parham, pp 117-118.*) Each secretory IgA molecule has a molecular weight of 400,000 and consists of two H2L2 units and one molecule each of J chain and secretory component. Some IgA exists in serum as a monomer H2L2 with a molecular weight of 160,000. Some bacteria, such as *Neisseria*, can destroy IgA-1 by producing protease. It is the major immunoglobulin in milk, saliva, tears, mucus, sweat, gastric fluid, and colostrum. IgA does not fix complement, so one would anticipate that a complement fixation test would not be useful for IgA antibody. It is important to remember that of the five classes of immunoglobulins, only IgG and IgM are complement-fixing/activating antibodies.

455. The answer is d. (*Kindt, pp 9, 55, 168-187. Parham, pp 33-41.*) Both IgG and IgM activate complement by the classic pathway, while IgA activates it by the alternative pathway. IgA, IgD, and IgE cannot activate complement. Complement is a system of several proteins that is activated by either an immune or a nonimmune pathway. Both of these pathways result in the production of many biologically active components that cause cell lysis and death. Thus, it plays a significant role in the inflammatory process. In addition, products of the complement cascade are associated with enhancing opsonization, neutralization of invading pathogens, and clearance of debris by the CR1 on erythrocytes. In this clinical case, the patient is suffering from severe liver failure. This significant reduction in liver function has led to a reduced ability by the patient to produce sufficient complement proteins, and as a result the patient is predisposed to infections caused by pyogenic bacteria. See the below figure.

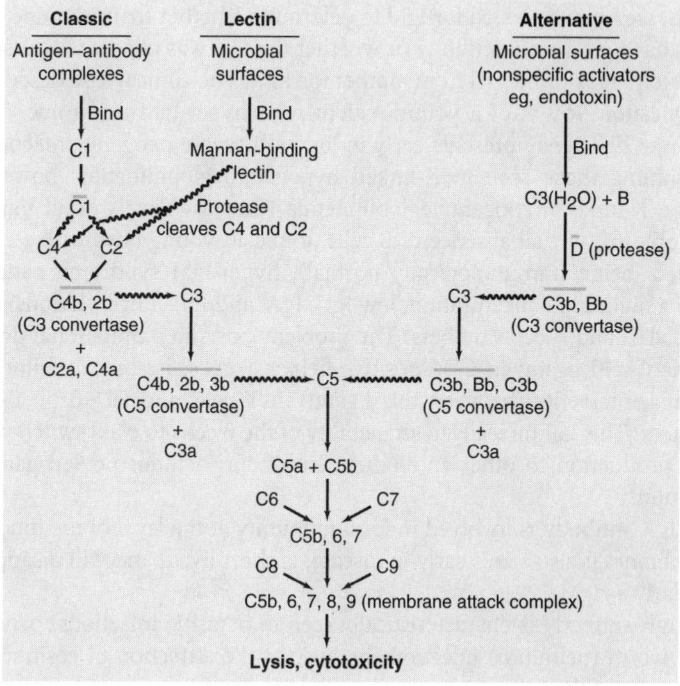

The classic and alternative pathways of the complement system indicate that proteolytic cleavage of the molecule at the tip of the arrow has occurred; a line over a complex indicates that it is enzymatically active. Note that the nomenclature of the cleavage products of C2 is undecided. Some call the large fragment C2a and others call it C2b. The C3 convertase is depicted here as C4b,2b. Note that proteases associated with the mannose-binding lectin cleave C4 as well as C2. *(Reprinted, with permission, from Levinson W, Jawetz E.* Medical Microbiology and Immunology. *7th ed. New York, NY: McGraw-Hill; 2002:401.)*

456 to 460. The answers are 456-d, 457-c, 458-e, 459-b, and 460-a. (*Kindt, pp 95-100, 170-173. Parham, pp 115-120, 264-271.*) IgG antibody provides an "immune history." That is, IgG antibody persists in most people and indicates the antigens to which they have been exposed. IgG is not formed early in infection but is a secondary response arising weeks to months after antigenic challenge. IgG also has a built-in memory. Even people with very low levels of specific IgG will respond to an antigen challenge with an IgG response.

IgM antibody, in contrast, arises early in infection and then disappears within a couple of months. IgM is intravascular and does not cross the placental barrier. For this reason, infants with specific IgG responses to disease must be tested for IgM to determine whether their immune systems have produced antibody or whether the test was positive because of passively transferred IgG from mother to child. The clinical case described in Question 465 is of a young patient with hyper-IgM syndrome. This immune deficiency presents early in life with severe pyogenic infections, resembling those seen in X-linked hypogammaglobulinemia; however, unlike X-linked hypogammaglobulinemia (very low levels of all immunoglobulins, virtual absence of B cells, found in young boys with female carriers being immunologically normal), hyper-IgM syndrome patients have a high IgM concentration, low IgG, IgA, and IgE concentrations, and normal T- and B-cell numbers. The problem exists in a mutational defect in the CD40 ligand in CD4-positive helper T cells, leading to failure of normal interaction between this ligand on T cells and CD40 on B-cell surfaces. This failure leads to an inability of the B cells to class switch from IgM production to other antibodies. Treatment includes pooled gamma globulin.

IgA antibody is involved in local immunity at the level of the mucous membrane. It also arises early in disease, is short lived, and will disappear similarly as IgM.

IgE antibody is characteristically seen in parasitic infections, particularly worm (helminth) infections because of the attraction of eosinophils to the site of the infestation. Certain allergies are due to excessive production of IgE. The patient in this case has irichinosis as a result of consuming undercooked pork and ingesting the parasite *Trichinella spiralis*. IgE specific for worm proteins binds to receptors on eosinophils, promoting the release of worm-destroying enzymes involved in the antibody-dependent cellular cytotoxicity (ADCC) response.

IgD antibody consists of two light chains and two heavy chains. Its role is not known, but it can be found on the surface of lymphocytes, where it may act as a surface receptor.

IgG is susceptible to proteolytic enzymes, which may explain why it is present in such low levels in serum. In addition, the fetus has more total IgG, than IgM, as a result of maternal placental IgG transfer, even though IgM is produced in greater amounts by the fetus.

461 to 465. The answers are 461-a, 462-b, 463-e, 464-c, and 465-d. (*Kindt, pp 455-460, 448-454.*) *Borrelia burgdorferi*, the causative agent of Lyme disease, elicits an acute antibody response. IgM appears within days to a few weeks following tick bite, and IgG appears a few weeks later. IgG persists; IgM does not. Cross-reactions occur with other treponemes.

Fifth disease is a viral exanthem commonly seen in children 8- to 12-year-old. Children are ill for a few days but recover without incident, usually within about 1 week. Unfortunately, if a pregnant female acquires the disease in the first trimester of pregnancy, the fetus is at risk. The causative agent is thought to be a parvovirus (Parvovirus B19). Fifth disease is also known as erythema infectiosum or slapped cheek syndrome. The four other maculopapular or macular rash diseases of childhood are measles, roseola, rubella, and scarlet fever.

Adults with no titer to varicella (VZV) are at risk for acquisition of chicken pox. If they are health care workers, there is additional risk of transmitting VZV to immunodeficient children. Antibodies to VZV are readily detected by both enzyme immunoassay (EIA) and fluorescent antibody (FA) techniques.

Delta agent is a recently discovered antigen associated with HBsAg. Its presence usually correlates with HBsAg chronic carriers who have chronic active hepatitis. EIA and RIA tests are available to detect antibodies to delta agent.

SSPE is thought to be caused by a measles-related virus present in the central nervous system. Most SSPE patients show elevated measles virus antibodies in serum and CSF. In patients with MS, lower CSF antibody titers have been observed, suggesting a possible etiologic role for measles virus in MS.

466 to 470. The answers are 466-d, 467-c, 468-d, 469-b, and 470-d. (*Kindt, pp 185-186, 493-504. Parham, pp 403-418.*) Immunodeficiency disorders can be categorized according to whether the defect primarily involves humoral immunity (bone marrow derived, or B lymphocytes) or cellular immunity (thymus derived, or T lymphocytes) or both. Swiss-type hypogammaglobulinemia, ataxia-telangiectasia, the Wiskott-Aldrich syndrome, and severe combined immunodeficiency disorders all involve defective B-cell and T-cell function. Infantile X-linked agammaglobulinemia is caused chiefly by deficient B-cell activity, whereas thymic hypoplasia is mainly a T-cell immunodeficiency disorder.

In Question 466, this 2-year-old patient has ataxia (staggering)-telangiectasia (spider angiomas), an autosomal recessive immune disorder associated with both a lymphopenia (cellular) and IgA deficiency (humoral). Question 467 describes a patient with X-linked hypogammaglobulinemia or Bruton agammaglobulinemia, which only occurs in boys and is characterized by low levels of all immunoglobulin classes and the absence of almost all B cells. Pre-B cells are present; however, they fail to differentiate into B cells. Cell-mediated immunity is relatively normal. Recurrent bacterial infections occur after about 6 months of age when protective maternal IgG antibody declines. The fetus represented in Question 468 has severe combined immunodeficiency disease (SCID) characterized by defects in early stem cell differentiation. As a result, B cells and T cells are both defective, immunoglobulins are very low, and tonsils and lymph nodes are absent. Thymic aplasia or DiGeorge syndrome marks the young child in Question 469. Failed development of the thymus and the parathyroids lead to hypoparathyroidism, hypocalcemia, and ultimately a spastic paralysis (strong muscle contractions or tetany). Finally, Wiskott–Aldrich syndrome (Question 470), an X-linked defect, is associated with reduced IgM levels and variable cellular-mediated immunity.

471 to 474. The answers are 471-a, 472-c, 473-a, and 474-d. (*Kindt, pp 33, 426-440, 443-444. Parham, pp 465-475.*) Transplantation from one region of a person to another region of that same person is an *autograft* and has the best chance of succeeding. When a transplant is done between monozygotic twins, it is an *isograft* and has a complete MHC compatibility and a good chance of success. *Allografts* are between members of the same species, and *xenografts* are between members of different species. Both of these transplants have a high rate of rejection unless immunosuppression accompanies the transplant.

475 to 477. The answers are 475-d, 476-c, and 477-b. (*Kindt, pp 101-102.*) Isotypes are determined by antigens of the immunoglobulin classes found in all individuals of one species. In addition to heavy-chain isotypes of IgA, IgD, IgE, IgG, and IgM, two light-chain isotypes exist for κ and λ chains.

Allotypes are differentiated by antigenic determinants that vary among individuals within a species and are recognized by cross-immunization of individuals in a species. Allotypes include the Gm marker of IgG and the Inv marker of light chains.

Idiotypes are antigenic determinants that appear only on the F(ab) fragments of antibodies and appear to be localized at the ligand-binding site; thus, anti-idiotype antisera may block reactions with the appropriate hapten. The carbohydrate side chains of immunoglobulins are relatively nonimmunogenic. New determinants may be exposed after papain cleavage of immunoglobulins, but these determinants are not included in the classification of the native molecule.

478. The answer is f. (*Kindt, pp 186. Parham, pp 33-42, 344.*) This patient has a classic case of hereditary angioedema. This disease is characterized by a deficiency of complement control proteins such as C1 esterase inhibitor, leading to overactive complement (reduced C4 levels). Uncontrolled generation of vasoactive peptides (C3a and C5a) causes increased blood vessel permeability, causing hereditary angioedema. Edema, especially of the larynx, obstructs the airways. Abdominal pain may indicate that the patient has angioedema of the gut.

479. The answer is d. (*Fauci, pp 483, 577-578. Kindt, pp 536-537. Parham, p 503.*) The best-characterized human tumor-associated antigens are the oncofetal antigens. CEA is a glycoprotein and member of the immunoglobulin gene superfamily and is elevated in colorectal cancer. α-Fetoprotein (AFP) is analogous to albumin and elevated in hepatocellular carcinoma. Prostate-specific antigen (PSA) is elevated in prostatic cancer. CEA, AFP, and PSA are all glycoproteins. Melena refers to altered (black) blood per rectum, indicative of an upper gastrointestinal bleed. A patient's tumor markers are best used clinically in the monitoring of the efficiency of the antitumor therapy and remission periods posttreatment.

480 and 481. The answers are 480-b and 481-e. (*Kindt, pp 493-495, 500-502. Parham, pp 350-361.*) HIV infection affects mainly the immune system and the brain. The main immunologic feature of HIV infection is progressive depletion of the CD4 subset of T lymphocytes (T-helper cells), causing a reversal in the normal CD4:CD8 ratio, leading to immunodeficiency. Currently, ELISA is the basic screening test to detect anti-HIV antibodies. Repeated reactive ELISA tests should be confirmed using either western blot or immunofluorescence. The western blot detects specific antibodies against the various HIV proteins (antigens). As stated previously, the western blot is positive when two or more of the p14, gp41, gp120, or gp160 bands are present in the gel.

482. The answer is b. (*Kindt, pp 389-391. Parham, pp 309-310.*) Anti-Rh antibodies (IgG are reactive at 98.6°F [37°C]) are the leading cause of hemolytic disease of the newborn (HDN). Currently, Rh immunization can be suppressed in antepartum or postpartum Rh– women if high-titer anti-Rh immunoglobulin (RhIg) is administered within 72 hours after the potentially sensitizing dose of Rh+ cells (ie, the birth of the child). The other choices will do nothing to prevent the development of HDN in future pregnancies.

483 and 484. The answers are 483-g and 484-c. (*Kindt, pp 29-30, 440-442, 494-498. Parham, pp 347-350, 476-477.*) Immune deficiency disorders occur as a result of impaired function in one or more of the major immune system components such as B lymphocytes, T lymphocytes, B and T lymphocytes, phagocytic cells, and complement. Unusual and recurrent infections are the hallmark of immunodeficiency. SCID occurs as a result of an early defect in stem cell differentiation and may be caused as a result of defective IL-2 receptors, adenosine deaminase deficiency, or failure to make MHC class II antigens. This condition is characterized by B- and T-cell deficiency and presents with recurrent infections. The other disorders listed do not have both B- and T-cell deficiency with an absence of a thymus gland. Definitive treatment of SCID consists of stem cell transplantation, with the ideal donor being a sibling with identical human leukocyte antigens (HLA).

485. The answer is b. (*Kindt, pp 95-98, 477-480. Parham, p 272.*) There are three forms of immunity: active, passive, and adoptive. Active immunity involves an individual making his or her own antibodies, either naturally, by infection, or artificially by immunizations. Passive immunity refers to the transfer of preformed antibodies from one individual to another either naturally (transplacental or enteromammary antibodies from mother to fetus) or artificially through gamma globulin injections such as antitoxins, anti-Rh, and antivenoms (black widow spider bites and the like, etc). Finally, adoptive immunity refers to the transfer of lymphoid cells from an actively immunized donor and does not involve antibody transfer.

486. The answer is e. (*Fauci, pp 2054-2058. Kindt, pp 495-500. Parham, pp 346-360.*) Patients with T-cell defects are generally susceptible to viral, fungal, and protozoan infections. This can be especially visible in patients with primary immunodeficiency diseases such as SCID. For further explanation of immunodeficiencies, please refer to the answer explanations for Questions 431 and 432, 474 to 478, 491 and 492.

487. The answer is b. (*Kindt, pp 372-388. Parham, pp 367-385.*) This is an example of a type I hypersensitivity reaction. Type I hypersensitivity is also referred to as anaphylaxis or immediate-type hypersensitivity. Major components include IgE, mast cells/basophils, and pharmacologically active mediators. Exposure to antigen causes IgE production, followed by sensitization of mast cells and basophils. Subsequent encounter with the same allergen (antigen) leads to chemical mediator release (histamine and the like, etc) and also leads to clinical symptoms associated with asthma, allergic rhinitis, and so on. This reaction can occur within minutes and can be extremely severe and life-threatening.

488 to 492. The answers are 488-c, 489-a, 490-b, 491-e, and 492-d. (*Kindt, pp 477-479. Parham, pp 243-439.*) The following table presents the patterns of hepatitis B virus (HBV) serologic markers observed in various stages of infection with HBV. The diagnosis of HBV infection is usually based on three tests: hepatitis B surface antigen (HBsAg), antibodies to surface antigen (HBsAg), and antibodies to core antigen (HBcAg). Tests are available, however, for e antigen and antibodies to e antigen. A variety of testing methods are available and include enzyme immunoassay, RIA, hemagglutination, LA, and immune adherence. The delta agent has recently been described. The delta agent exacerbates infection with HBV, apparently in a synergistic manner. Commercial tests are now available for the delta agent.

	Serologic Markers					
Interpretation	HBsAg	Anti-HBeAg	IgM Anti-HBc	Total Anti-HBc	Anti-HBe	HBs
Acute infection						
Incubation period	+[a]	+[a]	–	–	–	–
Acute phase	+	+	+	+	–	–
Early convalescent phase	+	–	+	+	+	–
Convalescent phase	–	–	+	+	+	–
Late convalescent phase	–	–	–[b]	+	+	+
Long past infection	–	–	–	+[c]	+ or –	+[c]
Chronic infection						
Chronic active hepatitis	+[d]	+ or –	+ or –	+[d]	+ or –	–[d]
Chronic persistent hepatitis	+[e]	+ or –	+ or –	+	+ or –	–
Chronic HBV carrier state	+[e]	+ or –	+ or –	+	+ or –	–
HBsAg immunization	–	–	–	–	–	+

[a]HBsAg and HBeAg are occasionally undetectable in acute HBV infection.

[b]IgM anti-HBc may persist for over a year after acute infection when very sensitive assays are employed.

[c]Total anti-HBc and anti-HBs may be detected together or separately long after acute infection.

[d]HBsAg-negative chronic active hepatitis may occur where total anti-HBc and anti-HBs may be detected together, separately, or not at all.

[e]HBsAg-negative chronic persistent hepatitis and chronic HBV carriers have been observed.

493 to 497. The answers are 493-b, 494-a, 495-e, 496-d, and 497-c. (*Kindt, pp 145-164.*) Of the many methods available for antigen and antibody detection, LA, ELISA, RIA, CIE, and COA are the most widely used. LA employs latex polystyrene particles sensitized by either antibody or antigen. LA is more sensitive than CIE and COA, but slightly less sensitive than either RIA or EIA. LA has been used to detect *H. influenzae*, *N. meningitidis*, and *S. pneumoniae* antigens in CSF. LA has also been used for detection of cryptococcal antigen. Most recently, LA has been widely used for rapid detection of group A streptococcal antigen directly from the pharynx. The test is rapid (5 minutes), sensitive (approximately 90%), and specific (99%).

COA, also an agglutination test, is slightly less sensitive than LA but is less susceptible to changes in the environment (eg, temperature). Most strains of coagulase-positive staphylococci have protein A in their cell wall. Protein A binds the Fc fragment of microbial antigens in body fluids. COA has also been used to rapidly type or group bacterial isolates.

Enzyme immunoassays (EIAs) can be either homogeneous (EMIT) or heterogeneous (ELISA). EMIT has been used primarily for assays of low-molecular-weight drugs. Its primary use in microbiology has been for assays of aminoglycoside antibiotics. EIAs vary as to the solid support used. A variety of supports can be used, such as polystyrene microdilution plates, paddles, plastic beads, and tubes. The number of layers in the antibody–antigen sandwich varies; usually as additional layers are added, detection sensitivity is increased. The two most common enzymes are horseradish peroxidase (HRP) and alkaline phosphatase (AP). β-Galactosidase has also been employed. *O*-phenylenediamine is the most common substrate for HRP and *p*-nitrophenyl phosphate for AP. Because EIAs are usually read in the visible color range, the tests can be read qualitatively by eye or quantitatively by machine.

CIE was originally used for "Australia antigen" (HBsAg) but was soon replaced by RIA. For a decade, CIE was used to detect antigens in body fluids. CIE is not an easy technique. Its success depends on the control of many variables, including solid support, voltage, current, buffer, affinity and avidity of antibodies, charge on the antigen, and time of electrophoresing.

RIA involves the radiolabeling of either antibody or antigen (Ag) using ^{131}Iodine (^{131}I) or ^{125}I (radioisotopes). It measures very small quantities and can be used to detect hormones, CEA, hepatitis B Ag, steroids, prostaglandins, and morphine-related drugs in patient sera.

498 to 502. The answers are 498-c, 499-a, 500-f, 501-e, and 502-b. (*Kindt, pp 155-158.*) The enzyme immunoassay (EIA, ELISA) has become a common method for the detection of either antibody or antigen in a patient specimen. The technique is based on building a "sandwich." For example, the following sandwich is made on what is called the *solid phase.* The solid phase is usually a plastic microtiter plate but can be a plastic paddle or even a nitrocellulose membrane. First, whole *Toxoplasma* organisms or purified antigenic components of *Toxoplasma* are added to the plate and the plate is washed off. Failure of one or more of the washing steps or inadequate washing usually causes high background color in the developed plate.

The *Toxoplasma* antigen–antibody complex must be detected by the addition of a second antibody to which is linked an enzyme such as horseradish peroxidase or alkaline phosphatase. The nature of this second antibody is dependent on whether one wishes to measure IgG or IgM. If the test is for IgG, then the second antibody is antihuman IgG conjugated to an enzyme. Following another wash cycle, the enzyme substrate is added to the plate and color develops in those wells where the sandwich is complete. If the patient's serum does not contain specific antibody, then the sandwich is not completed and there is no development of color. If the EIA is for detection of antigen, then the layers of the sandwich are as follows:

Specific antibody
Patient specimen (contain antigen)
Enzyme-labeled antibody specific for the antigen enzyme substrates

There are many variations of the test using a variety of antibodies, indicators such as fluorescence, and magnetic beads as solid phases. EIA is more sensitive than agglutination methods or complement fixation and slightly less sensitive than RIA.

503. The answer is d. (*Kindt, pp 19, 33, 367-368, 441-442. Parham, pp 456, 478-479.*) GVHD occurs due to attack by the graft against the recipient. There are three requirements for GVHD rejection: (1) histocompatibility differences between the graft (donor) and host (recipient), (2) immunocompetent graft cells, and (3) immunodeficient host cell. Immunocompetent graft cells may be "passenger" lymphocytes or major cells transplanted, and must be present in the graft. Prevention of GVHD is essential, as there is no adequate treatment once it is established.

504. The answer is c. (*Kindt, pp 398-391. Parham, pp 455-458.*) All blood for transfusion should be carefully matched to avoid transfusion reaction. As shown in the tables below, persons with group O blood have no A or B antigens on their erythrocytes and are thus considered to be universal donors. In contrast, persons with group AB blood have neither A nor B antibody and thus are universal recipients.

505 to 507. The answers are 505-b, 506-d, and 507-h. (*Fauci, pp 1960-1967, 2037-2040, 2071-2073. Kindt, pp 403, 408-411, 442-443. Parham, pp 408-413.*) Loss of tolerance by the immune system to certain self-components can lead to the formation of antibodies, causing tissue and organ damage. Such diseases are referred to as *autoimmune diseases.* There are a host of autoimmune diseases characterized by the autoantibodies. The presence of a "butterfly" rash is a classic cutaneous sign of SLE and is characterized by a rash over the bridge of the nose and on the cheeks.

ABO BLOOD GROUPS

Group	Antigen on Red Cell	Antibody in Plasma
A	A	Anti-B
B	B	Anti-A
AB	A and B	No anti-A or anti-B
O	No A or B	Anti-A and anti-B

COMPATIBILITY OF BLOOD TRANSFUSIONS BETWEEN ABO BLOOD GROUPS[a]

	Recipient			
Donor	O	A	B	AB
O	Yes	Yes	Yes	Yes
A (AA or AO)	No	Yes	No	Yes
B (BB or BO)	No	No	Yes	Yes
AB	No	No	No	Yes

[a]"Yes" indicates that a blood transfusion from a donor with that the blood group to a recipient with that blood group is compatible, that is, no hemolysis will occur. "No" indicates that the transfusion is incompatible and that hemolysis of the donor's cells will occur. (Reprinted, with permission, from *Levinson W, Jawetz E. Medical Microbiology and Immunology. 7th ed. New York, NY: McGraw-Hill; 2002:412.*)

508 to 512. The answers are 508-a, 509-c, 510-c, 511-a, and 512-e. (*Kindt, pp 254-260. Parham, pp 211-230.*) Naïve T cells are activated by interaction with dendritic cells in lymphnodes. Activation requires signal 1, which is mediated by CD3, zeta chains and a co-receptor following interaction of the TCR with MHC and peptide. Signal 2 is critical for complete activation of naïve T cells. The CD28 receptor is expressed by naïve T cells and sends activating signal 2 to the T cells after it is engaged by either B7-1 (CD80) or B7-2 (CD86). PD-1 and CTLA-4 are inhibitory receptors expressed by naïve T cells that send signals that block T cell activation, representing a key mechanism of peripheral tolerance, for example, when normal self-peptide antigens are expressed in MHC I or MHC II by dendritic cells. CTLA-4 competes with B7-1 and B7-2 for CD28. B7-H1 and B7-H3 are inhibitory ligands expressed by dendritic cells. PD-1 is bound by B7-H1 (PD-L1). B7-H3 binds a distinct receptor on naïve T cells. T cells, via their surface expressed TCR, only recognize peptide fragments of proteins expressed by dendritic cells in the context of MHC I (CD8+ T cells) or MHC II (CD4+ T cells). The majority of TCRs are comprised of a surface expressed, nonsecreted, covalently linked alpha–beta (α, β) heterodimer. However, a functional TCR complex is made up of an alpha–beta heterodimer, noncovalently associated with the CD3 complex (γ, δ, ε, ε) and 2 zeta (ζ) chains. 95% of all T cells express an α, β heterodimer TCR. Approximately 5% of T cells express an γ, δ heterodimer TCR. This rare subset of T cells is primarily associated with the gut. Igα and Igβ are associated with the B-cell receptor (BCR).

513. The answer is c. (*Kindt, pp 254-259. Parham, pp 222-224.*) Although antigen (MHC-peptide) recognition by T cells is mediated by the TCR it is incapable of signaling. Signaling occurs via the CD3 complex and zeta chains. Signaling is also augmented by the TCR-co-receptors, CD4 and CD8. Therefore, the TCR-β chain (as well as the TCR-α chain) is incapable of signal transduction.

514. The answer is a. (*Kindt, pp 223-232. Parham, pp 125-131.*) Like all genes, TCR genes are found in all cells with a nucleus, all cells except red blood cells.

515. The answer is e. (*Kindt, pp 245-251. Parham, pp 187-205.*) Thymic selection shapes the peripheral T cell repertoire. The goal is to positively select those T cells expressing TCRs that recognize peptides from foreign proteins (eg, microbial pathogens). Negative selection of T cells in the thymus is the primary process for preventing autoimmunity and is a key mechanism of central tolerance. T cells with TCRs that possess too high affinity for normal self-peptides are eliminated by inhibitory signals that results in the T cells death.

516. The answer is d. (*Kindt, pp 245-253. Parham, pp 187-197.*) T cells all mature in the thymus and B cells mature in the bone marrow, hence the origin of their names. It remains unclear where NK cells mature. Dendritic cells mature is peripheral lymph tissues such as the spleen and lymph nodes.

517. The answer is d. (*Kindt, pp 493-504. Parham, pp 125-128, 347-348.*) This is characterized by the lack of a functional TCR and BCR. Defects in recombination activating genes 1 and 2 (RAG-1 and RAG-2) would result in the lack of TCR and BCR gene rearrangement and subsequent protein expression. The outcome is T and B cells absent of antigen receptors making them absent of immune function.

518. The answer is e. (*Kindt, pp 208-217. Parham, pp 137-145.*) Cross-priming or cross-presentation allows endogenously acquired antigens to be presented in the context of MCH I. This was first described for pathogenic microbes but is now a recognized mechanism for activating CD8+ T cells against cancer cell-associated antigens. Tumor cells direct priming would require that the tumor cell expresses ligands for CD28 for the second signal. Tumor cells rarely express B7-1 or B7-2. Tumors are not commonly known to express IL-12 as this would result in TH1 type cell-mediated immunity, which would result in elimination of the tumor cells. Tumors often secrete TGF-β1, a potent immune suppressor.

519. The answer is b. (*Kindt, pp 542-543. Parham, pp 502-505.*) The immune system is capable of recognizing and destroying tumor (cancer) cells. Cancer cells express protein antigens that range in immunogenicity. Some are of viral origin (though rare) and are vary immunogenic others (most) are of self-origin and much less immunogenic. Tumor antigens can be expressed on the tumor cell surface or only intracellularly, thus both humoral (B cells) and cellular (T cells) are important for tumor cells killing. Listed are examples of defined tumor-associated antigens. HPV E6, E7 are associated with cervical cancer. CA-125 is associated with ovarian cancer. CD20 is associated with B-cell lymphomas. CA-125 is associated with colon cancer. Her2/neu is a surfaced expressed growth factor receptor that is commonly overexpressed in breast cancer. Her2/neu overexpressing breast cancers are successfully treated with passive immunotherapy comprised of administration of an monoclonal antibody (mAb) specific for Her2/neu. The mAb is commonly known as herceptin or trastuzumab.

520. The answer is d. (*Kindt, p 538. Parham, pp 498-500.*) Tumor cells have evolved mechanisms to escape and evade immune recognition. These mechanisms include various molecular genetic processes of eliminating MHC I from the tumor cell surface. Mutations inhibit efficient antigen processing and presentation. Tumor cells also block immune cells by secretion of suppressor proteins, most commonly TGF-β1, and other cytokine like "decoy" molecules to confuse the immune system. Antigenic variation is an immune escape mechanism ascribed to pathogenic microbes such as viruses for example.

521. The answer is b. (*Kindt, pp 259, 406. Parham, pp 220-223, 419-420, 501.*) CTLA-4 is an antagonistic/inhibitory receptor normally expressed by T cells that competes with CD28 for binding of B7-1 and B7-2 and thus prevents the second signal and subsequent T-cell activation. This is a key mechanism of peripheral tolerance and plays role in preventing T-cell activation against cancer cells. Administration of antibodies that bind and block CTLA-4 allows CD28 to bind B7-1 and B7-2 and mediate costimulation resulting in the augmentation of antitumor T-cell responses. This passive immunotherapy approach has been approved to treat advanced melanoma skin cancers. Signal 1 is TCR complex and co-receptor mediated. Co-stimulation (signal 2) is via CD28-B7 engagement, follows signal 1, and results in activation and proliferation. PD-1/PD-L1 are a distinct T-cell inhibitory receptor and its ligand. ZAP-70 and ITAMs are involved in intracellular T-cell activation signal transduction.

Bibliography

Andary MT. Guillain–Barré Syndrome. Updated Aug 29, 2012; http://emedicine.medscape.com/article/315632-overview#a0101.

Beckwith CG, Wing EJ, Rodriguez B, Lederman MM. Human immunodeficiency virus infection and acquired immunodeficiency syndrome. In: Andreoli TE, et al, eds. *Andreoli and Carpenter's Cecil Essentials of Medicine*. 8th ed. Philadelphia, PA: Saunders; 2010:1008–1027.

Brooks GF, Carroll KC, Butel JS, et al, eds. *Jawetz's Medical Microbiology.* 24th ed. New York, NY: McGraw-Hill; 2007.

Engleberg NC, DiRita V, Dermody TS, eds. *Schaechter's Mechanism of Microbial Disease.* 4th ed. Philadelphia, PA: Lippincott, Williams & Wilkins; 2007.

Fauci, AS, Braunwald E, Kasper DL, et al, eds. *Harrison's Principles of Internal Medicine.* 17th ed. New York, NY: McGraw-Hill; 2008.

Garcia LS. *Diagnostic Medical Parasitology*. 5th ed. Washington, DC: ASM Press; 2007.

Guidelines for the Use of Antiretroviral Agents in HIV-1-Infected Adults and Adolescents. Developed by the HHS Panel on Antiretroviral Guidelines for Adults and Adolescents—A Working Group of the Office of AIDS Research Advisory Council (OARAC). Last updated March 27, 2012. Available from http://aidsinfo.nih.gov/guidelines.

Katzung BG, Masters SB, Trevor AJ, eds. *Basic and Clinical Pharmacology*. 12th ed. New York, NY: McGraw-Hill; 2012.

Kindt TJ, Goldsby RA, Osborne BA, et al, eds. *Kuby Immunology*. 6th ed. New York, NY: WH Freeman and Co; 2007.

Kumar V, Abbas AK, Aster JC, eds. *Robbins Basic Pathology*. 9th ed. Philadelphia, PA: Saunders Elsevier; 2013.

Levinson W. *Review of Medical Microbiology and Immunology*. 12th ed. New York, NY: McGraw-Hill; 2012.

Li X, Brown N, Chau AS, et al. Changes in susceptibility to posaconazole in clinical isolates of *Candida albicans. J Antimicrob Chemother.* 2004; 53:74–80.

Mokrousov I, Narvskaya O, Otten T, Limeschenko E, Steklova L, Vyshnevskiy B. High prevalence of KatG Ser315Thr substitution among isoniazid-resistant *Mycobacterium tuberculosis* clinical isolates from northwestern Russia, 1996 to 2001. *Antimicrob Agents Chemother*. 2002;46(5): 1417–1424.

Murray PR, Baron EJ, Jorgensen JH, et al. *Medical Microbiology.* 6th ed. St. Louis, MO: Mosby; 2009.

Murray PR, Baron EJ, Pfaller MA, et al, eds. *Manual of Clinical Microbiology.* 8th ed. Washington, DC: ASM Press; 2003.

Murray PR, Rosenthal KS, Pfaller MA. *Medical Microbiology.* 7th ed. Philadelphia, PA: Saunders Elsevier; 2013.

Parham P, ed. *The Immune System.* 3rd ed. New York, NY/London, UK: Garland Science/Taylor and Francis Group, LLC; 2009.

Ryan KJ, Ray CG, eds. *Sherris Medical Microbiology.* 5th ed. New York, NY: McGraw-Hill; 2010.

Schneider E, Whitmore S, Glynn MK, Dominguez K, Mitsch A, McKenna MT [Division of HIV/AIDS Prevention, National Center for HIV/AIDS, Viral Hepatitis, STD, and TB Prevention]. Revised surveillance case definitions for HIV infection among adults, adolescents, and children aged <18 months and for HIV infection and AIDS among children aged 18 months to <13 years—United States, 2008. *MMWR* 2008;57(RR10):1–8. Available from http://www.cdc.gov/mmwr/preview/mmwrhtml/rr5710a1.htm.

Toy EC. *Case Files: Microbiology.* 2nd ed. New York, NY: McGraw-Hill; 2008.

Weiner DL. Reye Syndrome. Updated Jan 22, 2013. http://emedicine.medscape.com/article/803683-overview#a0101.

Index

C

F

H